Drug Hypersensitivity

Editor

PASCAL DEMOLY

IMMUNOLOGY AND ALLERGY CLINICS OF NORTH AMERICA

www.immunology.theclinics.com

Consulting Editor
RAFEUL ALAM

August 2014 • Volume 34 • Number 3

ELSEVIER

1600 John F. Kennedy Boulevard • Suite 1800 • Philadelphia, Pennsylvania, 19103-2899

http://www.theclinics.com

IMMUNOLOGY AND ALLERGY CLINICS OF NORTH AMERICA Volume 34, Number 3

August 2014 ISSN 0889–8561, ISBN-13: 978-0-323-32015-3

Editor: Jessica McCool

Developmental Editor: Stephanie Carter

Immunology and Allergy Clinics of North America (ISSN 0889–8561) is published quarterly by Elsevier Inc., 360 Park Avenue South, New York, NY 10010-1710. Months of issue are February, May, August, and November. Periodicals postage paid at New York, NY and additional mailing offices. Subscription prices are $320.00 per year for US individuals, $454.00 per year for US institutions, $150.00 per year for US students and residents, $395.00 per year for Canadian individuals, $220.00 per year for Canadian students, $577.00 per year for Canadian institutions, $445.00 per year for international individuals, $577.00 per year for international institutions, $220.00 per year for international students. To receive student/resident rate, orders must be accompanied by name of affiliated institution, date of term, and the *signature* of program/residency coordinator on institution letterhead. Orders will be billed at individual rate until proof of status is received. Foreign air speed delivery is included in all *Clinics* subscription prices. All prices are subject to change without notice. **POSTMASTER:** Send address changes to *Immunology and Allergy Clinics of North America,* Elsevier Health Sciences Division, Subscription Customer Service, 3251 Riverport Lane, Maryland Heights, MO 63043. **Customer Service: 1-800-654-2452 (U.S. and Canada); 314-447-8871 (outside U.S. and Canada). Fax: 314-447-8029. E-mail: journalscustomerservice-usa@elsevier.com (for print support); journalsonlinesupport-usa@elsevier.com (for online support).**

Reprints. For copies of 100 or more, of articles in this publication, please contact the Commercial Reprints Department, Elsevier Inc., 360 Park Avenue South, New York, New York 10010-1710. Tel. 212-633-3874, Fax: 212-633-3820, E-mail: reprints@elsevier.com.

Immunology and Allergy Clinics of North America is covered in MEDLINE/PubMed (Index Medicus), Current Contents/Life Sciences, Science Citation Index, ISI/BIOMED, Chemical Abstracts, and EMBASE/Excerpta Medica.

Contributors

CONSULTING EDITOR

RAFEUL ALAM, MD, PhD
Professor and Chief, Division of Allergy and Immunology, National Jewish Health and University of Colorado Denver, Denver, Colorado

EDITOR

PASCAL DEMOLY, MD, PhD
Allergy Unit, Département de Pneumologie et Addictologie, Hôpital Arnaud de Villeneuve, University Hospital of Montpellier, Montpellier; Sorbonne Universités, Paris, France

AUTHORS

MICHAEL AUERBACH, MD
Clinical Professor of Medicine, Georgetown University School of Medicine, Washington, DC; Hematology and Oncology, Private Practice, Baltimore, Maryland

BRIAN A. BALDO, PhD
Retired, Formerly - Head, Molecular Immunology Unit, Kolling Institute of Medical Research, Royal North Shore Hospital of Sydney; Department of Medicine, University of Sydney, Sydney, Australia

ANNICK BARBAUD, MD, PhD
Dermatology and Allergy Department, Brabois Hospital, University Hospital of Nancy, Lorraine University, Vandoeuvre les Nancy, France

ESTHER BARRIONUEVO, MD
Allergy Unit, University Hospital-IBIMA, Malaga, Spain

ANDREAS J. BIRCHER, MD
Allergy Unit, Dermatology Clinic, University Hospital Basel, Basel, Switzerland

MIGUEL BLANCA, MD, PhD
Allergy Unit, University Hospital-IBIMA, Malaga, Spain

CHRIS H. BRIDTS, MLT
Department of Immunology, Allergology, Rheumatology, Faculty of Medicine and Health Science, Antwerp University Hospital, University of Antwerp, Antwerpen, Belgium

KNUT BROCKOW, MD
Department of Dermatology and Allergy Biederstein, Technische Universität München, Munich, Germany

MARIANA C. CASTELLS, MD, PhD
Program Director, Allergy and Clinical Immunology Training; Associate Professor in Medicine; Director, Drug Hypersensitivity and Desensitization Center; Associate Director, Mastocytosis Center, Brigham and Women's Hospital, Harvard Medical School, Boston, Massachusetts

JEAN-CHRISTOPH CAUBET, MD
Department of Pediatrics, University Hospitals of Geneva and Medical School, University of Geneva, Geneva, Switzerland

ANCA M. CHIRIAC, MD
Allergy Unit, Département de Pneumologie et Addictologie, Hôpital Arnaud de Villeneuve, University Hospital of Montpellier, Montpellier; Sorbonne Universités, Paris, France

PASCAL DEMOLY, MD, PhD
Allergy Unit, Département de Pneumologie et Addictologie, Hôpital Arnaud de Villeneuve, University Hospital of Montpellier, Montpellier; Sorbonne Universités, Paris, France

DIDIER G. EBO, MD, PhD
Department of Immunology, Allergology, Rheumatology, Faculty of Medicine and Health Science, Antwerp University Hospital, University of Antwerp, Antwerpen, Belgium

R. AN GOOSSENS, Pharm, PhD
Contact Allergy Unit, Department of Dermatology, University Hospital, Katholieke Universiteit Leuven, Leuven, Belgium

CYNTHIA HADDAD, PharmD
RegiSCAR Network; Reference Center for Blistering Diseases, Hôpital Henri Mondor, Créteil, France

MAREK KOWALSKI, MD, PhD
Department of Immunology Rheumatology and Allergy, Medical University of Lodz, Lodz, Poland

PAUL MICHEL MERTES, MD, PhD
Service d'anesthésie-réanimation chirurgicale, Hôpitaux Universitaires de Strasbourg, Nouvel Hôpital Civil, Strasbourg Cedex, France

BRIGITTE MILPIED-HOMSI, MD
Department of Dermatology, Saint-André Hospital, Bordeaux, France

MAJA MOCKENHAUPT, MD
Professor, RegiSCAR Network; Department of Dermatology, Dokumentationszentrum schwerer Hautreaktionen (dZh), Medical Center–University of Freiburg, Germany

ELLEN M. MORAN, PhD
Institute of Immunology and Infectious Disease, Murdoch University, Murdoch, Western Australia

DEAN J. NAISBITT, PhD
Department of Clinical and Molecular Pharmacology, MRC Centre for Drug Safety Science, University of Liverpool, Liverpool, England

RYAN G. NATTRASS, MR
Department of Clinical and Molecular Pharmacology, MRC Centre for Drug Safety Science, University of Liverpool, Liverpool, England

MONDAY O. OGESE, MR
Department of Clinical and Molecular Pharmacology, MRC Centre for Drug Safety Science, University of Liverpool, Liverpool, England

MAURO PAGANI, MD
Head Physician of General Medicine Ward, Medicine Department, Pieve di Coriano Hospital, Azienda Ospedaliera C.Poma, Mantova, Italy

HAE-SIM PARK, MD, PhD
Department of Allergy and Clinical Immunology, Ajou University School of Medicine, Suwon, Republic of Korea

MAREN PAULMANN, Dipl.Biol
RegiSCAR Network; Department of Dermatology, Dokumentationszentrum schwerer Hautreaktionen (dZh), Medical Center–University of Freiburg, Germany

ELIZABETH J. PHILLIPS, MD
Institute of Immunology and Infectious Disease, Murdoch University, Murdoch, Western Australia; Division of Infectious Diseases, Vanderbilt University Medical Center, Nashville, Tennessee

CLAUDE PONVERT, MD, PhD
Pulmonology & Allergology Service, Department of Pediatrics, Sick Children's Hospital, Paris, France

ANTONINO ROMANO, MD
Professor, Allergy Unit, Complesso Integrato Columbus, Rome; IRCCS Oasi Maria S.S., Troina, Italy

JEAN-CLAUDE ROUJEAU, MD
Professor, Université Paris-Est Créteil, France; RegiSCAR Network

VITO SABATO, MD
Department of Immunology, Allergology, Rheumatology, Faculty of Medicine and Health Science, Antwerp University Hospital, University of Antwerp, Antwerpen, Belgium

MARIO SÁNCHEZ-BORGES, MD
Allergy and Clinical Immunology Department, Centro Médico Docente La Trinidad, Clínica El Avila, Caracas, Venezuela

BERNARD YU-HOR THONG, MBBS, FRCP(Edin)
Department of Rheumatology, Allergy and Immunology, Tan Tock Seng Hospital, Singapore, Singapore

MARIA JOSE TORRES, MD, PhD
Allergy Unit, University Hospital-IBIMA, Malaga, Spain

ASTRID P. UYTTEBROEK, MD
Department of Immunology, Allergology, Rheumatology, Faculty of Medicine and Health Science, Antwerp University Hospital, University of Antwerp, Antwerpen, Belgium

GERALD W. VOLCHECK, MD
Chairman, Division of Allergic Diseases; Associate Professor of Medicine, Mayo Medical School, Mayo Clinic, Rochester, Minnesota

ALESSANDRA VULTAGGIO, MD, PhD
Immunoallergology Unit, Department of Biomedicine, Azienda Ospedaliero-Universitaria Careggi, Florence, Italy

RICHARD WARRINGTON, MB,BS, PhD
Professor, Allergy & Clinical Immunology, Health Sciences Centre, Winnipeg; Departments of Medicine and Immunology, University of Manitoba, Manitoba, Canada

YOUNG-MIN YE, MD
Department of Allergy and Clinical Immunology, Ajou University School of Medicine, Suwon, Republic of Korea

Contents

Anca M. Chiriac and Pascal Demoly

Poorly documented and often self-reported drug hypersensitivity (DH) is a frequent problem in daily clinical practice and has a considerable impact on prescription choices. Little is known about the natural history of true DH. The suspicion of DH starts on clinical grounds. When assessing a patient with a presumed DH reaction in the symptomatic phase, it is mandatory to look for severity signs and, after doing so, to update the risk/benefit balance of exploring the suspected drug(s) on a case-by-case basis. With the help of allergy tests and a careful approach, a firm diagnosis is often possible.

Jean-Claude Roujeau, Cynthia Haddad, Maren Paulmann, and Maja Mockenhaupt

Nonimmediate hypersensitivity to drugs has a huge diversity of clinical presentations affecting exclusively or predominantly a single organ (most often the skin) or multiple organs. The latter is the rule with drug reaction with eosinophilia and systemic symptoms, and with drug-induced vasculitis. The management includes a dozen successive steps. Finally, the patient should be provided clear information on the suspected cause of the reaction, recommendations for follow-up after severe reactions associated with a risk of sequelae, and clear recommendations for future use of medications. Pharmacovigilance networks should be informed.

Antonino Romano and Richard Warrington

Although allergy to β-lactam and non-β-lactam antibiotics is commonly claimed, true allergy to these drugs is often absent. Reactions to antibiotics can be classified according to the interval between the last administration of the drug and the onset of symptoms, but except for immediate reactions occurring within an hour of exposure, which are almost always either IgE-mediated or due to direct stimulation of mast cells, reactions occurring later than 1 hour probably have multiple mechanisms, including being IgE-mediated or involving cell-mediated reactions. The latter are likely caused by drug-specific T lymphocytes. The diagnosis of antibiotic allergy can be difficult.

Maria Jose Torres, Esther Barrionuevo, Marek Kowalski, and Miguel Blanca

Nonsteroidal anti-inflammatory drugs (NSAIDs) are the drugs most commonly involved in hypersensitivity drug reactions. Such reactions can be due to the release of inflammatory mediators in the absence of specific immunologic recognition, or immunoglobulin E (IgE)- or T-cell–selective responses. The former include upper and lower airway symptoms in patients with chronic underlying respiratory disease, the exacerbation of chronic spontaneous urticaria, and the induction of cutaneous symptoms. The latter include selective responses to a single NSAID with good tolerance to strong cyclooxygenase-1 inhibitors, with a putative IgE or T-cell mechanism proposed. These reactions can be acute or delayed.

Intraoperative anaphylaxis and hypersensitivity reactions in the setting of anesthesia contribute significantly to the morbidity and mortality of surgeries and surgical procedures. Because multiple medications and products are given in a short period of time, identifying the specific cause can be difficult. Neuromuscular blocking agents, antibiotics, and latex are the most common causes of anesthesia-related reactions, though other medications or exposures could be involved. Careful review of anesthetic charts and allergy testing can help identify the underlying cause. The identification of the cause and subsequent prevention of reactions are critical to reduce overall mortality and morbidity related to anesthesia.

This article updates current knowledge on hypersensitivity reactions to diagnostic contrast media and dyes. After application of a single iodinated radiocontrast medium (RCM), gadolinium-based contrast medium, fluorescein, or a blue dye, a hypersensitivity reaction is not a common finding; however, because of the high and still increasing frequency of those procedures, patients who have experienced severe reactions are nevertheless frequently encountered in allergy departments. Evidence on allergologic testing and management is best for iodinated RCM, limited for blue dyes, and insufficient for fluorescein. Skin tests can be helpful in the diagnosis of patients with hypersensitivity reactions to these compounds.

Use of cytotoxic agents is associated with potential hypersensitivity reactions which are common with platinum compounds, L-asparaginase, taxanes, procarbazine and epipodophyllotoxins. Mechanisms underlying the reactions may involve IgE, non-allergic or a number of pathogenetically unclear events. Targeted therapies produce less collateral damage but demonstrate their own unique reactions. Cytopenias occur less often and mucocutaneous reactions to EGFR inhibitors, including papulopustular rash, are common. Fifteen currently approved mAbs provoke all four types of hypersensitivities including immune cytopenias, vasculitis, serum sickness and pulmonary events. Some successful desensitization protocols have been developed. Prevention of hypersensitivity reactions is based on skin testing, premedication and/or desensitization.

with heavy uterine bleeding and pregnancy. Free iron is associated with unacceptable high toxicity inducing severe, hemodynamically significant symptoms. Subsequently, formulations that contain the iron as an iron carbohydrate nanoparticle have been designed. With newer formulations, including low-molecular-weight iron dextran, iron sucrose, ferric gluconate, ferumoxytol, iron isomaltoside, and ferric carboxymaltose, serious adverse events are rare.

IMMUNOLOGY AND ALLERGY CLINICS OF NORTH AMERICA

NOW AVAILABLE FOR YOUR iPhone and iPad

Foreword

The Complexity of Drug Hypersensitivity

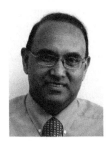

Rafeul Alam, MD, PhD
Consulting Editor

Drug allergy remains one of the most important contributors to iatrogenic morbidity and mortality. Significant progress has been made in understanding the immunopathogenesis of allergy to certain drugs. The identification of specific HLA loci that predispose to drug hypersensitivity has greatly contributed to our knowledge about of drug hypersensitivity. The association of HLA-B5701 with Abacavir[1] and HLA-B1502 with Carbamazepine[2] is now well established. Structural studies have demonstrated the binding of these drugs to the MHC antigen-presenting groove. The screening for these HLA genotypes prevents serious drug allergic reactions. However, our knowledge remains incomplete as only 55% of patients with positive HLA-B5701 treated with Abacavir develop hypersensitivity reaction. Similarly, only 3% to 7% of patients with positive HLA-B1502 treated with Carbamazepine develop Stevens-Johnsons syndrome and toxic epidermal necrolysis.[2] It is likely that a complex of a self-peptide associated with the drug in the MHC groove is the ultimate trigger for T-cell activation. This hypothesis needs identification of the self-peptide and demonstration of the trimolecular complex. Viral reactivation in the context of drug reaction with eosinophilia and systemic symptoms (DRESS)/drug-induced hypersensitivity syndrome is an intriguing subject, which could account for some of the manifestations and complications.

When a patient presents with an allergic skin rash, especially a delayed maculopapular rash, and is on multiple medications, the identification of the causative drug remains a challenge. A number of diagnostic approaches are being pursued. They include skin test, delayed-read intradermal test, patch test, lymphocyte proliferation test, and ELISPOT. Although progress has been slow, standardization and validation of these tests will greatly aid the diagnosis and proper management of drug allergy. An initial approach was to reach a consensus on definition, diagnostic approaches, and management of drug hypersensitivity reactions. An international consensus has

Supported by NIH Grants RO1 AI091614 and N01 HHSN272200700048C.

Immunol Allergy Clin N Am 34 (2014) xiii–xiv
http://dx.doi.org/10.1016/j.iac.2014.04.014 **immunology.theclinics.com**

recently been published, which will greatly facilitate this process.[3] To update us on this important topic, I have invited Dr Pascal Demoly, who is a leader in the field. He has brought together an outstanding group of scientists and clinical investigators, who present the latest in the field.

Rafeul Alam, MD, PhD
Division of Allergy and Immunology
National Jewish Health and
University of Colorado Denver
1400 Jackson Street
Denver, CO 80206, USA

E-mail address:
alamr@njhealth.org

REFERENCES

1. Mallal S, Phillips E, Carosi G, et al. HLA-B*5701 screening for hypersensitivity to abacavir. N Engl J Med 2008;358:568–79.
2. Hung SI, Chung WH, Jee SH, et al. Genetic susceptibility to carbamazepine-induced cutaneous adverse drug reactions. Pharmacogenet Genomics 2006;16: 297–306.
3. Demoly P, Adkinson NF, Brockow K, et al. International Consensus on drug allergy. Allergy 2014;69:420–37.

Preface

Drug Hypersensitivity

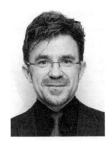

Pascal Demoly, MD, PhD
Editor

Clinicians and researchers working in the field of drug hypersensitivity (DH) are very much aware that they are standing at the limit of repeating iatrogenesis in subjects with histories suggestive, but not always confirmed, of DH. Proper identification of a true DH while upholding the principle of "primum non nocere" is a challenge that weighs heavily in all their considerations. Unnecessary avoidance measures (with their obvious medical consequences) or overlooking alternative diagnoses are at stake. This renders the field of DH diagnosis a very vivid one, whereby universal acceptance of classifications, diagnostic tests, or protocols is difficult to reach.

After an introduction on drug allergy diagnosis and management, this issue of *Immunology and Allergy Clinics of North America* is intended to focus on specific drug classes, rather than specific reactions, for several reasons: first, for the sake of redundancy with the recently published international consensus on drug allergy; and second, it is clear that some medications are often overlooked in DH reviews, although they are of significant importance in clinical practice (vaccines, additives, vehicles) or increasingly used (iron preparations) and therefore deserve our attention. Last, but not least, one of the major pitfalls in the DH area, namely the lack of availability of sufficient numbers of accurately phenotyped patients, is starting to be addressed by emerging single- or multi-center large databases, mostly tackling either frequent (eg, antibiotics, nonsteroidal anti-inflammatory drugs, anaesthetic agents) or emerging (contrast media agents, iron preparations, biologicals) elicitors or severe clinical manifestations. Lessons learned from drugs prescribed to specific populations, in peculiar clinical contexts (eg, chemotherapeutic and biological agents, antiepileptic or antiviral drugs), shed some light on the issue of the natural history of DH (with desensitization and treating through being highly specialized therapeutic approaches and easily accessible pharmacogenetic screening becoming possible for carbamazepine and abacavir) as well as on pathophysiologic concepts (eg, the recently described "altered peptide repertoire model" for abacavir hypersensitivity, possibly shared by other drugs). These two aspects rank next to one another in importance for DH prevention and treatment.

Immunol Allergy Clin N Am 34 (2014) xv–xvi
http://dx.doi.org/10.1016/j.iac.2014.03.001
immunology.theclinics.com
0889-8561/14/$ – see front matter © 2014 Elsevier Inc. All rights reserved.

The articles in this issue of *Immunology and Allergy Clinics of North America* evolve naturally from what we do know and can diagnose, to the active acknowledgment of our limits in this field, which represent the unmet needs of our patients. Articles focus on clinical topics that will help practitioners answer questions at the point of care. Each article follows, as much as possible, a similar structure from epidemiology, pathophysiology, to diagnosis and management. "Author pairs" were carefully selected not only because of their expertise in a specific DH domain but also because they are coming from different teams/continents to catch the worldwide flavor of how to diagnose DH and not just how this author/team manages them. The gaps in our understanding of DH have been identified and will most likely be addressed in the future. *Immunology and Allergy Clinics of North America* will cover them too. We wish you an agreeable reading and most of all hope that this issue will stay on your desk to answer the questions raised during your daily DH activities.

Pascal Demoly, MD, PhD
Allergy Unit, Département de Pneumologie et Addictologie
Hôpital Arnaud de Villeneuve
University Hospital of Montpellier
France and Sorbonne Universités
UPMC Paris 06, UMR-S 1136, IPLESP
Equipe EPAR
75013 Paris, France

E-mail address:
pascal.demoly@inserm.fr

Drug Allergy Diagnosis

Anca M. Chiriac, MD[a], Pascal Demoly, MD, PhD[a,b],*

KEYWORDS

- Drug hypersensitivity reaction • Natural history • Severity signs
- Drug allergy work-up • Imputability

KEY POINTS

- There is no substitute for a proper assessment of the clinical history when a drug hypersensitivity reaction is suspected.
- When assessing a patient with a presumed drug hypersensitivity reaction in the symptomatic phase, it is mandatory to look for severity signs, because they portend a poor prognosis.
- Confirmation of a drug hypersensitivity relies mostly on in vivo tests, and their contraindications must be rigorously observed.
- The available literature does not answer the numerous questions regarding the natural history of drug hypersensitivity. When the diagnosis is confirmed, lifelong avoidance of the drug causing the reaction is recommended.

INTRODUCTION

Drug allergy that is poorly documented and often self-reported is a frequent problem in daily clinical practice and has a considerable impact on prescription choices. When drug reactions resembling allergy occur, they are called drug hypersensitivity (DH) reactions (DHRs) before showing evidence of either drug-specific antibodies or T cells. The term drug allergies should be reserved for immunologically mediated DHRs. The diagnostic work-up of DHRs allows a better classification of the reactions and provides patients with more reliable information and recommendations for future treatments. Several guidelines and consensus documents on general or specific drug class–induced DHRs are available to support the diagnosis. This article is based on the recent International Consensus (iCON) on Drug Allergy,[1] a consensus that was reached by leading allergy organizations worldwide (the European Academy of Allergy

Disclosure Statement: The authors declare no conflict of interest for this work.
a Allergy Unit, Respiratoty and Addictology Department, Hôpital Arnaud de Villeneuve, 371, Avenue du Doyen Gaston Giraud, University Hospital of Montpellier Cedex 5, Montpellier 34295, France; b Sorbonne Universités, UPMC Paris 06, UMR-S 1136, IPLESP, Equipe EPAR, Paris 75013, France
* Corresponding author. Allergy Unit, Département de Pneumologie et Addictologie, Hôpital Arnaud de Villeneuve, 371, Avenue du Doyen Gaston Giraud, University Hospital of Montpellier Cedex 5, Montpellier 34295, France.
E-mail address: pascal.demoly@inserm.fr

and Clinical Immunology [EAACI], the American Academy of Allergy Asthma and Immunology [AAAAI], the American College of Allergy Asthma and Immunology [ACAAI] and the World Allergy Organization [WAO]) to synthesize multiple guidelines into 1 generally approved and accepted consensus document.

CLINICAL MANIFESTATIONS

DHRs are classified artificially into 2 types, according to the delay of onset of the reaction after the last administration of the drug: (1) immediate reaction, occurring less than 1 hour after the last drug intake, usually in the form of isolated urticaria, angioedema, rhinitis, conjunctivitis, bronchospasm, gastrointestinal symptoms (nausea, vomiting, diarrhea), or anaphylaxis with or without cardiovascular collapse (anaphylactic shock); and (2) nonimmediate reaction, with variable cutaneous symptoms occurring after more than 1 hour and up to several days after the last drug intake, such as late-occurring urticaria, maculopapular eruptions, fixed drug eruptions, vasculitis, blistering diseases (such as toxic epidermal necrolysis [TEN], Stevens-Johnson syndrome [SJS], and generalized bullous fixed drug eruptions), drug reaction with eosinophilia and systemic symptoms (DRESS), acute generalized exanthematous pustulosis (AGEP), and symmetric drug-related intertriginous and flexural exanthemas. Internal organs can be affected either alone or with cutaneous symptoms including hepatitis, renal failure, pneumonitis, anemia, neutropenia, and thrombocytopenia. The first category is mostly mediated through specific immunoglobulin E (IgE), whereas the second is specific T cell mediated. For specific descriptions, the readers are referred to previous issues of *The Clinics of North America*.[2,3]

SEVERITY SIGNS OF DHRS

When assessing a patient with a presumed DHR in the symptomatic phase, it is mandatory to look for severity signs and, after doing so, to update the risk/benefit balance of exploring the suspected drug(s) on a case-by-case basis.

Severity (danger) signs may include both clinical symptoms and biological/laboratory parameters, according to the type of reaction.[1] Some are well-established criteria and have been assigned individual weights in scoring systems for classifying the severity of delayed reactions.[4]

Severity signs are either obvious to the naked eye (clinical), or invisible (mainly biological) (**Table 1**). The latter must be looked for thoroughly, to reveal internal organ damage.

In immediate reactions, the clinical picture is self-explanatory. Symptoms develop rapidly and cutaneous and mucosal involvement may quickly escalate toward life-threatening airway, breathing, or circulatory problems. Measurements of histamine or tryptase have no value for the therapeutic management in the acute setting, but may a posteriori support the diagnosis of allergic anaphylaxis, especially in cases of drug allergy in perioperative settings.[5]

Nonimmediate reactions are more heterogeneous and there may be overlap between different patterns. When confronted with a suspicion of a delayed DHR, both general and organ-specific severity/danger signs must be systematically looked for (see **Table 1**). Daily reevaluation is mandatory to identify progression or signs of recovery.

Regardless of the type of reaction, the presence of severity signs warrants the immediate withdrawal of the suspected drug(s), appropriate supportive treatment of the patient, and special care later during the exploration phase. However, in the absence of these signs and if the drug is mandatory, treating through might be an option.

Table 1
Severity/danger signs in DHR

	Visible Severity Signs	Invisible Severity Parameters
Immediate reactions	Sudden onset of multisystem symptoms (respiratory, skin, and mucosal) Reduced blood pressure Dyspnea Dysphonia Sialorrhea	High levels of serum tryptase[a]
Nonimmediate reactions	General Lymphadenopathy Fever >38.5°C Organ specific Painful skin Skin extension >50% Atypical target lesions Erosions of mucosa Skin blisters, bullae Centrofacial edema Purpuric infiltrated papules, cutaneous necrosis	Changes in blood count[b] Cytopenia Eosinophilia Alteration of liver function tests[b] Alteration of kidney function[b]

[a] No clinical utility in the acute setting.
[b] If a severe delayed DHR is suspected, all patients should have complete blood count and liver and kidney function tests.
  Adapted from Bircher AJ. Symptoms and danger signs in acute drug hypersensitivity. Toxicology 2005;209(2):204; with permission.

NATURAL HISTORY OF DHRS

The natural history of DHR is difficult to assess, for several reasons, and can only be analyzed by a firm initial diagnosis and later reexposures. The current knowledge in this area is scant but needs to be understood when diagnosing a DHR.

First, unlike respiratory or food allergy, for which the ubiquitous nature of certain allergens makes it difficult to adhere to strict avoidance of the culprit allergen (which can easily be encountered at eliciting doses in everyday life), in DHR, once the diagnosis has been established, lifelong avoidance of the causative drug is recommended and generally observed, both by the patient and by health care professionals in therapeutic settings. Medicolegal consequences are involved. However, an unpredictable subliminal contact is thought to occur because certain drugs, namely antibiotics, are present in small and hidden amounts in foods. It is not known to what extent this ongoing contact may influence the natural history of DH to antibiotics in the absence of therapeutic exposure.

Second, DH is a heterogeneous clinical entity (in terms of clinical manifestations and eliciting drugs) and although the frame is virtually the same (clinical history, drug allergy work-up, avoidance), it is difficult, if not impossible, to put all drugs in the same category and extrapolate the existent data on some antibiotics or nonsteroidal antiinflammatory drugs (NSAIDs) to, for instance, drugs like biological agents.

In addition, instances in which the drug is given despite a previous DH provide some insight into how patients may evolve and sometimes outgrow their DH.

Data regarding the natural history of DHRs arises from articles addressing this question in a direct or indirect way.

Follow-up of Patients with a Confirmed DH: Skin Test Conversion

When nonirritant concentrations are used for skin testing (eg, β-lactams), the positive predictive value of skin tests in the presence of a history compatible with a DH has been reported to be 100% for immediate reactions and more than 92% for delayed reactions.[6]

However, little is known about the clinical consequences of the negativization of a previous positive immunologic response, either assessed by means of skin or biological tests. The IgE antibody response is not permanent over time, and prospective studies of skin test and/or specific IgE reactivity showed that decreased antibody levels may occur months to years after the occurrence of a DH. This finding was mainly reported for penicillin allergy,[7] with patients having a selective response to the amino-penicillin side chain switching from positive to negative skin responses sooner than in patients with reactivity to several penicillin determinants. After 5 years, none of the selective responders had positive skin tests. Submitting these patients to reexposure would not be acceptable in the absence of highly specific therapeutic indications because it is suspected that the lack of skin reactivity does not warrant the systemic tolerance of the drug. Vultaggio and colleagues[8] reported the case of a patient in whom retreatment after negativization of serum-specific IgE to rituximab led to the development of a new and more severe reaction associated with higher levels of serum IgE antibodies and positive skin tests. The same team[9] observed a rapid decrease of specific IgE antibodies to infliximab with none of the patients showing skin test positivity or specific serum IgE within 1 year after the first analysis. However, IgE sensitization may also persist for years, as shown for neuromuscular blocking agents.[10] T-cell memory seems to be even stronger for delayed DHRs.[11]

Follow-up of Patients After Drug Desensitization

Once it is achieved, tolerance through desensitization is maintained by continuous administration of the drug. The process is reversible and, when the drug is discontinued, tolerance is lost over hours or days.[12] When the drug is mandatory, as is often the case for chemotherapeutic or biological agents, and in the absence of contraindications, it is common practice that patients undergo desensitization at each cure. Although experts recommend it, it is not clear whether repeat desensitization is required for each drug infusion in all patients. It is known that a subset of patients continues to have reactions during successive desensitizations, suggesting persistent DH. However, some investigators[13] reported patients in whom skin test results convert from positive to negative after repeated desensitization and the drug is subsequently tolerated through standard infusion with no reaction. It is unclear whether this tolerance is compatible with a natural loss of sensitivity and instead the investigators put forward the hypothesis of the maintenance of the desensitized state caused by the long half-life of monoclonal therapeutics.

Influence of the Underlying Disease

Aspirin-exacerbated cutaneous disease is an entity per se within the large spectrum of ASA/NSAID hypersensitivity. Up to one-third of the patients with chronic spontaneous urticaria (CSU) experience exacerbation of their skin symptoms on ingestion of ASA/NSAIDs. In contrast, up to 37% of NSAID-hypersensitive patients may develop CSU in the future.[14] The degree of sensitivity to NSAIDs may show temporary fluctuations related to the activity of their underlying CSU and sensitivity may even disappear in some patients.[15,16]

Influence of Age

Proven DHR seems to be less common in children compared with adults. However, the validity of a negative drug allergy work-up performed in adults who have had a reaction suggesting DH in childhood can be questioned because of the time elapsed since the occurrence of the reaction. In a study involving 3275 patients, Rubio and colleagues[17] reported that, when the first reaction occurred during childhood, the prevalence rate of positive tests was similar whether the test was during childhood (10.6%) or adulthood (10.6%); thus, it could be argued that DH in childhood does not resolve with time.

The Multiple Drug Hypersensitivity Syndrome

The immune response in drug allergy is highly specific and often restricted to a drug or drug class. However, under certain circumstances, sensitizations for different drugs occur simultaneously, accounting for the multiple DH (MDH) syndrome.[18] Recent studies place severe cutaneous adverse reactions (SCARs), and particularly DRESS, at high risk of inducing multiple drug sensitizations. Antimicrobials or antiepileptics are often involved and are considered the primary eliciting drugs, but neosensitizations also involve drugs given as concomitant therapy for several weeks before the onset of the SCAR.[11] Thus, MDH with simultaneous sensitizations could be regarded as a model of how an acquired DH facilitates a new DH. In these patients, drug sensitization (as proved by either positive skin tests or lymphocyte transformation test) is persistent and detectable for many years after the allergic reaction.[11,19,20]

EVALUATION OF THE CLINICAL HISTORY

The suspicion of DHR arises on a constellation of data that make up the clinical history. Two main situations occur in everyday practice: the patient is seen during the symptomatic phase, or the patient is referred to the allergy consultation after recovery. When patients are seen during the symptomatic phase, physical examination is mandatory to provide invaluable information (ie, the presence/absence of danger signs) and to help ensure that a severe reaction is not overlooked. Otherwise, diagnosis is more difficult and, in this case, photographs taken at the time of the reaction are helpful. In addition, there are inpatients and outpatients. For hospitalized patients, data can more easily be tracked from medical records. For outpatients, it is especially important to enquire about over-the counter medications and health supplements, because patients often do not report these as medications.

The approach to assessing a suspicion of DHR could be conceived as a pyramid.

The first step (ie, the basis) is as exhaustive as possible. It encompasses symptoms, physical examination, and a complete drug administration history, including starting and stopping points of each medication. Then, several things help narrow down the list of potential causes of a DHR. Among them, the timing is of paramount importance, with its multifaceted distribution: the temporal relationship between the administration of each drug and the onset of symptoms, the effect of stopping the treatment, and the time to recovery. Several chronologies have been described,[1] and they refer typically to naive patients (ie, those experiencing the DHR for the first time). However, if the causative drug is readministered by mistake, the delay can be considerably shorter.

Although any drug can cause a DHR, the nature of the drugs involved and the knowledge of the classes most likely to be associated with the type of reaction may help in establishing extrinsic imputability. Special attention should be paid to dose changes, because for certain drugs and clinical presentations, dose changes are known to accelerate the onset of symptoms. Procedures involving administration of contrast media or dyes should be tracked, because these agents are potential elicitors. Moreover, iodinated radiocontrast media (RCM) have been reported to elicit very delayed DHRs (ie, several days after a single administration) and this kind of peculiarity should be kept in mind when considering imputability related to timing.[21]

A history of previous uneventful exposure and/or prior DHR is equally important. For instance, patterns of reaction have been established for certain drugs, such as the occurrence of DHRs to platinum salts or biological agents.[13,22]

Besides the differential diagnosis (eg, food allergy, infection), the circumstances surrounding the onset of the reaction should be recorded. Cofactors like physical effort or exposure to light should not be overlooked.

In addition, interpreting the data in the medical/genetic background of the patient produces additional information. Specific questioning for a medical condition, such as chronic urticaria/chronic rhinosinusitis (which can be aggravated by the intake of certain drugs; eg aspirin and non–cyclooxygenase-2–selective NSAIDs), or autoimmune or infectious disease (eg, patients infected with human immunodeficiency virus) facilitates the interpretation. Moreover, recent findings have shown a strong genetic association between human leukocyte antigen alleles and susceptibility to specific immune-mediated DHRs.[23,24]

Data should ideally be recorded in a uniform format and, in order to harmonize the DHR diagnostic procedures, members of EAACI-DAIG/ENDA have developed a questionnaire[25] that is available in many different languages.

In complex situations, a flow diagram including clinical manifestations and biological parameters should be drawn, for a more comprehensive overall view of the available data.

There is no substitute for a proper assessment of the clinical history. However, in most cases clinical history alone is not reliable, for various reasons (concomitant medication, imprecise information, heterogeneity of the clinical manifestations).[26]

PHARMACOVIGILANCE ALGORITHMS

Causality assessment methods performed by pharmacovigilance authorities are based principally on the clinical history (which may be insufficient or inaccurate) and are not designed to make definite decisions but rather to classify adverse drug reactions from the likelihood of a causal relationship between the drug and the reaction, as well as to detect new alerts. Moreover, they do not specifically address DHR. Therefore their sensitivity to ascertain DHRs is low, and allergy testing is often necessary.[26] An algorithm tailored to SJS/TEN, with parameters chosen from clinicians' knowledge of experts and available scoring systems, has been proposed by the RegiSCAR Study Group.[27]

SKIN TESTS

Skin tests (STs) are of utmost importance for the diagnosis of DHRs. Their use and interpretation is sometimes hampered by lack of data regarding nonirritant concentrations and vehicles. To address this pitfall, the EAACI-DAIG/ENDA experts recently reviewed the available literature in order to recommend appropriate concentrations for systemically administered drugs.[28] The conclusions are summarized in **Table 2**.

The sensitivity of STs seems to be moderate to high for immediate DHRs to β-lactam antibiotics, perioperative drugs, heparins, and platinum salts but low for many other drugs. For most drugs, the sensitivity of STs is higher in immediate DH compared with nonimmediate DH.[28] A recent multicenter study to determine the

Table 2
Nonirritating skin test concentrations for some systemically administered drugs

Drug or Drug Class	SPT	IDT	Patch
Anticoagulants			
Heparins[a]	Undiluted	1/10 diluted	Undiluted
Heparinoids[b]	Undiluted	1/10 diluted	Undiluted
Platinum Salts			
Carboplatin	10 mg/mL	1 mg/mL	NA
Oxaliplatin	1 mg/mL	0.1 mg/mL	NA
Cisplatin	1 mg/mL	0.1 mg/mL	NA
NSAIDs			
Pyrazolones[c]	Powder	0.1 mg/mL	10%
Coxibs[d]	Powder	—	10%
Other NSAIDs[e]	Powder	0.1 mg/mL	10%
Biologics			
Adalimumab	50 mg/mL	50 mg/mL	Undiluted
Etanercept	25 mg/mL	5 mg/mL	NA
Infliximab	10 mg/mL	10 mg/mL	NA
Omalizumab	1.25 µg/mL	1.25 µg/mL	NA
Others			
Local anesthetics	Undiluted	1/10 diluted	Undiluted
Iodinated RCM	Undiluted	1/10 diluted	Undiluted
Gadolinium chelates	Undiluted	1/10 diluted	NA
Patent blue	Undiluted	1/10 diluted	NA
Methylene blue	—	1/100 diluted	—
Fluorescein	Undiluted	1/10 diluted	Undiluted
PPI[f]	Undiluted	40 mg/mL	10%
Anticonvulsants[g]	NA	NA	10%
Chlorhexidine digluconate	5 mg/mL	0.002 mg/mL	1%

Abbreviations: IDT, intradermal test; NA, not applicable or no test concentration recommended; PPI, proton pomp inhibitors; SPT, skin prick test.

[a] Heparins: heparin sodium, nadroparin, dalteparin, and enoxaparin; testing contraindicated in heparin-induced thrombopenia.

[b] Heparinoids: danaparoid and fondaparinux.

[c] Pyrazolones: metamizol, paracetamol, propyphenazone, aminopyrine, phenazone, and phenylbutazone.

[d] Coxibs: celecoxib, etoricoxib, and valdecoxib.

[e] Other NSAIDs: for example, aspirin, ibuprofen, naproxen, indomethacin, diclofenac, fenoprofen, meloxicam, mefenamic acid, and nimesulide.

[f] For lansoprazole and rabeprazole, no intravenous solution is available: SPT with powder; IDT not possible.

[g] In case of history of severe reaction, test first with 1%.

From Brockow K, Garvey LH, Aberer W, et al. Skin test concentrations for systemically administered drugs - an ENDA/EAACI Drug Allergy Interest Group position paper. Allergy 2013; 68(6):705; with permission.

value and safety of drug patch tests for the 3 main classes of SCARs found a sensitivity of 64% among cases with DRESS, 58% for AGEP, and 24% for SJS/TEN. For nonimmediate reactions, delayed-reading intradermal tests have a higher sensitivity than patch tests.[29]

Preliminary results regarding the satisfactory negative predictive value (NPV) of STs in immediate DHR to iodinated RCM, gadolinium contrast agents, or myorelaxants[30–32] await confirmation in larger series.

Although there is general agreement among Allergology Societies and Academies on the importance of ST in drug allergy work-up, it is still a matter of debate for some drugs. The US Practice Parameters[33] suggest that immediate DHRs to iodinated RCM are all nonallergic (described as anaphylactoid) and therefore STs are not included in the management of patients who have experienced a previous DHR to iodinated RCM. The European experience[34] challenges this position.

Testing patients without a prior history of DHR is not supported by available studies and therefore is not recommended, in particular in preoperative settings.[5]

BIOLOGICAL TESTS

There is no universal biological test either to diagnose or to predict DHRs. With some exceptions, the currently available biological methods to diagnose drug allergy lack sensitivity, although they are normally considered to be specific.[1] A negative test does not exclude the imputability of the drug, whereas a positive result shows a sensitivity to the drug but does not reliably confirm its causality. For specific descriptions, readers are referred to previously published guidelines and reviews.[1,35]

PROVOCATION TESTS

The drug provocation test (DPT) comes at the end of a stepwise approach in the drug allergy work-up. It is the procedure with the highest sensitivity among all the other available diagnostic tools, but its use as the gold standard to establish (rather than just to exclude) the diagnosis of DHR is not unanimously accepted, mostly because of the reactions it may trigger, ranging from mild to severe.

Although protocols are not standardized among centers, and the precise challenge procedure varies from one team to another, there is general consensus with regard to 2 prerequisites: contraindications must be strictly observed before deciding whether or not to perform a DPT, and immediate treatment must be available, allowing complete and rapid recovery.

Several recent studies discussed the concerns that had already been raised about DPT protocols and methodology. There is some controversy among different groups about whether 1 full therapeutic dose of a tested drug is sufficient to elicit reactions in nonimmediate responders. Hence, full therapeutic courses have been suggested to increase the sensitivity of DPTs.[36] However, such an indication must be regarded cautiously, in terms of diagnostic improvement, cost, and medical implications, and is yet to be debated. In contrast, groups[37,38] performing DPTs in the pediatric population suggest that a 1-dose DPT in children with a history of delayed-onset benign reaction to β-lactams (assessed by a careful primary evaluation in the acute phase by an experienced allergist) can be considered sufficient and safe, even in the absence of an ST.[37] Although tempting, this approach needs validation in larger studies.

Patients do not like to be reexposed to drugs that they consider harmful. However, recent data collected from 3 centers in Europe revealed that most patients accepted DPTs for diagnostic purpose irrespective of the test results, and 95% of them thought that DPT was useful and that they would recommend it to others.[39]

A negative DPT does not prove tolerance to the drug in the future, but rather that there is no DH at the time of the challenge and to the doses challenged. Nevertheless, a high NPV of β-lactam DPT of 94% to 98% was found in large studies involving both children and adults,[40,41] and most of the reactions reported by patients were both mild and nonimmediate. The NPV of DPT with NSAIDs similarly seems to be high (more than 96%) whatever the NSAID (the one negatively tested or an alternative), and none of the false-negative patients described a life-threatening reaction.[42]

SUMMARY

The diagnosis of DHR remains largely clinical. Reasoning is almost identical for all drugs and all clinical presentations. With the help of some allergy tests that are available for some of the drug classes and a careful approach, a firm diagnosis is often possible no matter which drug is involved. However, a lot still needs to be done for severe cutaneous reactions for which DPTs are contraindicated and in biological diagnosis.[43]

Clinicians and researchers working in DH are aware that there is a risk of iatrogenesis in subjects with histories that suggest but are not always confirmed as DH. Proper identification of a DH upholds the principle of primum non nocere, and this principle is a challenge that weighs heavily in all their considerations. The attitude of not evaluating a suspicion of DH carries the risk of using unnecessary avoidance measures (with the obvious medical consequences) or overlooking alternative diagnoses. All this renders the field of DH diagnosis a very vivid one, because universal acceptance of classifications, diagnostic tests, or protocols is difficult to achieve.

REFERENCES

1. Demoly P, Adkinson NF, Brockow K, et al. International consensus on drug allergy. Allergy 2014;69:420–37.
2. Limsuwan T, Demoly P. Acute symptoms of drug hypersensitivity (urticaria, angioedema, anaphylaxis, anaphylactic shock). Med Clin North Am 2010;94(4): 691–710.
3. Scherer K, Bircher AJ. Danger signs in drug hypersensitivity. Med Clin North Am 2010;94(4):681–9.
4. Kardaun SH, Sidoroff A, Valeyrie-Allanore L, et al. Variability in the clinical pattern of cutaneous side-effects of drugs with systemic symptoms: does a DRESS syndrome really exist? Br J Dermatol 2007;156(3):609–11.
5. Mertes PM, Malinovsky JM, Jouffroy L, et al. Reducing the risk of anaphylaxis during anesthesia: 2011 updated guidelines for clinical practice. J Investig Allergol Clin Immunol 2011;21(6):442–53.
6. Chiriac AM, Demoly P. Positive predictive value of skin testing with β-lactams. Abstract P17:45–6. Programme of the 5th Drug Hypersensitivity Meeting, Munich 2012. Available at: http://www.eaaci.org/images/files/Abstract_Books/2012/DHM2012.pdf. Accessed April 27, 2014.
7. Blanca M, Torres MJ, Garcia JJ, et al. Natural evolution of skin test sensitivity in patients allergic to beta-lactam antibiotics. J Allergy Clin Immunol 1999;103(5 Pt 1):918–24.
8. Vultaggio A, Matucci A, Nencini F, et al. Drug-specific Th2 cells and IgE antibodies in a patient with anaphylaxis to rituximab. Int Arch Allergy Immunol 2012;159(3):321–6.
9. Matucci A, Pratesi S, Petroni G, et al. Allergological in vitro and in vivo evaluation of patients with hypersensitivity reactions to infliximab. Clin Exp Allergy 2013; 43(6):659–64.
10. Guttormsen AB, Johansson SG, Oman H, et al. No consumption of IgE antibody in serum during allergic drug anaphylaxis. Allergy 2007;62(11):1326–30.

11. Barbaud A, Collet E, Milpied B, et al. A multicentre study to determine the value and safety of drug patch tests for the three main classes of severe cutaneous adverse drug reactions. Br J Dermatol 2013;168(3):555–62.

12. Cernadas JR, Brockow K, Romano A, et al. General considerations on rapid desensitization for drug hypersensitivity - a consensus statement. Allergy 2010; 65(11):1357–66.

13. Brennan PJ, Rodriguez Bouza T, Hsu FI, et al. Hypersensitivity reactions to mAbs: 105 desensitizations in 23 patients, from evaluation to treatment. J Allergy Clin Immunol 2009;124(6):1259–66.

14. Asero R. Intolerance to nonsteroidal anti-inflammatory drugs might precede by years the onset of chronic urticaria. J Allergy Clin Immunol 2003;111(5):1095–8.

15. Kowalski ML, Makowska JS, Blanca M, et al. Hypersensitivity to nonsteroidal anti-inflammatory drugs (NSAIDs) - classification, diagnosis and management: review of the EAACI/ENDA(#) and GA2LEN/HANNA*. Allergy 2011;66(7):818–29.

16. Setkowicz M, Mastalerz L, Podolec-Rubis M, et al. Clinical course and urinary eicosanoids in patients with aspirin-induced urticaria followed up for 4 years. J Allergy Clin Immunol 2009;123(1):174–8.

17. Rubio M, Bousquet PJ, Gomes E, et al. Results of drug hypersensitivity evaluations in a large group of children and adults. Clin Exp Allergy 2012;42(1):123–30.

18. Chiriac AM, Demoly P. Multiple drug hypersensitivity syndrome. Curr Opin Allergy Clin Immunol 2013;13(4):323–9.

19. Gex-Collet C, Helbling A, Pichler WJ. Multiple drug hypersensitivity–proof of multiple drug hypersensitivity by patch and lymphocyte transformation tests. J Investig Allergol Clin Immunol 2005;15(4):293–6.

20. Gaig P, Garcia-Ortega P, Baltasar M, et al. Drug neosensitization during anticonvulsant hypersensitivity syndrome. J Investig Allergol Clin Immunol 2006;16(5): 321–6.

21. Kanny G, Pichler W, Morisset M, et al. T cell-mediated reactions to iodinated contrast media: evaluation by skin and lymphocyte activation tests. J Allergy Clin Immunol 2005;115(1):179–85.

22. Castells MC, Tennant NM, Sloane DE, et al. Hypersensitivity reactions to chemotherapy: outcomes and safety of rapid desensitization in 413 cases. J Allergy Clin Immunol 2008;122(3):574–80.

23. Mallal S, Phillips E, Carosi G, et al. HLA-B*5701 screening for hypersensitivity to abacavir. N Engl J Med 2008;358(6):568–79.

24. Chen P, Lin JJ, Lu CS, et al. Carbamazepine-induced toxic effects and HLA-B*1502 screening in Taiwan. N Engl J Med 2011;364(12):1126–33.

25. Demoly P, Kropf R, Bircher A, et al. Drug hypersensitivity: questionnaire. EAACI interest group on drug hypersensitivity. Allergy 1999;54(9):999–1003.

26. Benahmed S, Picot MC, Dumas F, et al. Accuracy of a pharmacovigilance algorithm in diagnosing drug hypersensitivity reactions. Arch Intern Med 2005; 165(13):1500–5.

27. Sassolas B, Haddad C, Mockenhaupt M, et al. ALDEN, an algorithm for assessment of drug causality in Stevens-Johnson Syndrome and toxic epidermal necrolysis: comparison with case-control analysis. Clin Pharmacol Ther 2010;88(1):60–8.

28. Brockow K, Garvey LH, Aberer W, et al. Skin test concentrations for systemically administered drugs - an ENDA/EAACI Drug Allergy Interest Group position paper. Allergy 2013;68(6):702–12.

29. Torres MJ, Gomez F, Dona I, et al. Diagnostic evaluation of patients with nonimmediate cutaneous hypersensitivity reactions to iodinated contrast media. Allergy 2012;67(7):929–35.

30. Caimmi S, Benyahia B, Suau D, et al. Clinical value of negative skin tests to iodinated contrast media. Clin Exp Allergy 2010;40(5):805–10.
31. Chiriac AM, Audurier Y, Bousquet PJ, et al. Clinical value of negative skin tests to gadolinium contrast agents. Allergy 2011;66(11):1504–6.
32. Ramirez LF, Pereira A, Chiriac AM, et al. Negative predictive value of skin tests to neuromuscular blocking agents. Allergy 2012;67(3):439–41.
33. Joint Task Force on Practice Parameters, American Academy of Allergy, Asthma and Immunology, American College of Allergy, Asthma and Immunology, et al. Drug allergy: an updated practice parameter. Ann Allergy Asthma Immunol 2010;105:259–73.
34. Brockow K, Romano A, Aberer W, et al. Skin testing in patients with hypersensitivity reactions to iodinated contrast media - a European multicenter study. Allergy 2009;64(2):234–41.
35. Ebo DG, Leysen J, Mayorga C, et al. The in vitro diagnosis of drug allergy: status and perspectives. Allergy 2011;66(10):1275–86.
36. Hjortlund J, Mortz CG, Skov PS, et al. One-week oral challenge with penicillin in diagnosis of penicillin allergy. Acta Derm Venereol 2012;92(3):307–12.
37. Caubet JC, Kaiser L, Lemaitre B, et al. The role of penicillin in benign skin rashes in childhood: a prospective study based on drug rechallenge. J Allergy Clin Immunol 2011;127(1):218–22.
38. Ponvert C, Perrin Y, Bados-Albiero A, et al. Allergy to betalactam antibiotics in children: results of a 20-year study based on clinical history, skin and challenge tests. Pediatr Allergy Immunol 2011;22(4):411–8.
39. Gomes ER, Kvedariene V, Demoly P, et al. Patients' satisfaction with diagnostic drug provocation tests and perception of its usefulness. Int Arch Allergy Immunol 2011;156(3):333–8.
40. Ponvert C. Diagnosis of allergic and non-allergic hypersensitivity reactions to commonly used drugs and biological substances in children: diagnostic algorithm. Arch Pediatr 2011;18(4):486–92 [in French].
41. Demoly P, Romano A, Botelho C, et al. Determining the negative predictive value of provocation tests with beta-lactams. Allergy 2010;65(3):327–32.
42. Defrance C, Bousquet PJ, Demoly P. Evaluating the negative predictive value of provocation tests with nonsteroidal anti-inflammatory drugs. Allergy 2011;66(11):1410–4.
43. Papadopoulos NG, Agache I, Bavbek S, et al. Research needs in allergy: an EAACI position paper, in collaboration with EFA. Clin Transl Allergy 2012;2(1):21.

Management of Nonimmediate Hypersensitivity Reactions to Drugs

Jean-Claude Roujeau, MD[a,b,*], Cynthia Haddad, PharmD[b,c],
Maren Paulmann, Dipl.Biol[b,d], Maja Mockenhaupt, MD[b,d]

KEYWORDS

- Drug-allergic liver injury (DALI) • Drug-induced nephritis (DIN)
- Drug-induced vasculitis
- Drug reaction with eosinophilia and systemic symptoms (DRESS)
- Stevens-Johnson syndrome (SJS) • Toxic epidermal necrolysis (TEN)

KEY POINTS

- Early diagnosis, early identification, and early withdrawal of suspect drug or drugs are essential.
- Severe reactions need an immediate referral to specialized centers.
- Patients should be provided with clear recommendations for follow-up, when needed, and for future use of medicines.

Disclosure: J.C. Roujeau and M. Mockenhaupt had/have financial links with several pharmaceutical companies that are detailed elsewhere. They consider that such links, related to causality of medications in severe cutaneous adverse reactions, do not affect the present topic.
J.C. Roujeau: For the past 5 years, *Punctual expertise of cases of SCAR* for: AB-Science, Negma, Johnson & Johnson, Hoffman La Roche, Boehringer-Ingelheim; *Safety boards*: Vertex (2008–2011), OM-Pharma (2008–2012), Servier (2009–2011), Janssen (2010–2012), Boehringer-Ingelheim (2010–2013), Menarini (2012), Pfizer (2013); *Expert witness* in 5 cases of litigation in the United States concerning McNeil Consumers/Johnson & Johnson; *Research:* member of the RegiSCAR International study group funded in France by GSK, Novartis, Boehringer Ingelheim, OM-Pharma, Science & Technologie, Astellas Pharma.
M. Mockenhaupt: For *Expert panels and advisory boards*: Vertex (2008–2011), Merck/MSD (since 2009), Boehringer-Ingelheim (since 2013), Pfizer (since 2013); *Expert witness* in 5 cases of litigation in the United States concerning McNeil Consumers/Johnson & Johnson; *Research:* coordinator of the RegiSCAR International study group funded in Germany by Berlin Chemie/Germany; Cephalon/USA; Grünenthal/Germany; GSK/UK; MSD Sharpe & Dohme/Germany; Negma/France; Novartis/Spain and USA; Pfizer/USA.

[a] Université Paris-Est Créteil, France; [b] RegiSCAR Network; [c] Reference Center for Blistering Diseases, Hôpital Henri Mondor, Créteil, France; [d] Department of Dermatology, Dokumentationszentrum schwerer Hautreaktionen (dZh), Medical Center–University of Freiburg, Hauptstr 7, Freiburg 79104, Germany
* Corresponding author. 19 Avenue d'Alembert, Antony 92160, France.
E-mail address: jean-claude.roujeau@wanadoo.fr

Immunol Allergy Clin N Am 34 (2014) 473–487
http://dx.doi.org/10.1016/j.iac.2014.04.012
0889-8561/14/$ – see front matter © 2014 Elsevier Inc. All rights reserved.
immunology.theclinics.com

INTRODUCTION

The denomination "nonimmediate hypersensitivity" explicitly refers to idiosyncratic, type B, reactions mediated by a drug-specific immune response belonging to types II, III, and IV of the classification proposed by Coombs and Gell.[1]

Type II reactions, antibody-mediated reactions, are considered responsible for a variety of drug-induced blood dyscrasias (eg, thrombocytopenia).[2] Type III reactions, involving depositions of immune complexes, are definitely the cause of serum-sickness, a reaction that is quite rare nowadays. For "serum-sickness-like syndromes" and drug-induced vasculitis, often quoted as other examples of type III hypersensitivity, the pathomechanisms are actually more complex, with T cells playing a role and drug-specific antibodies being rarely detected. Most nonimmediate reactions to drugs are actually type IV, delayed, T-cell-mediated reactions.

The present review focuses on these "type IV," T-cell-mediated reactions that are not only by far the most frequent but also diverse enough to justify the subclassification proposed by Pichler[3] in subtypes IVa to IVd. Nonimmediate drug hypersensitivity may affect a single organ, most often the skin, or present as a complex multisystem disease (eg, DRESS, abacavir hypersensitivity, systemic vasculitis).

Table 1 presents the incidence of the reactions discussed in the present review.[4–13]

Management includes the following steps: accurate diagnosis of the type of the reaction, evaluation of severity, identification of the most suspect drug or drugs, decision on drug discontinuation, treatment, confirmation of drug causality, reporting to regulatory agencies, and counseling patients on future use of medications.

CLINICAL DIAGNOSIS
Skin

As demonstrated by a large prospective study, 90% of reactions affecting the skin manifest as benign "maculopapular eruptions."[4] Such eruptions most often occur 4 to 20 days after the first intake of the inducing drug with a peak around 7 days. They are difficult to distinguish from viral eruptions, which are more common in childhood. A skin biopsy would be useless, because histologic changes are very mild and nonspecific.

Many other phenotypes may occur, including delayed urticaria, eczematous eruptions, lichenoid reactions, fixed drug eruptions (round, well-demarcated patches of erythema usually leaving pigmented areas). Whatever the clinical presentation, pruritus is almost constantly observed.

Table 1
Incidence of reactions included in this review

	Phenotype	Population	Exposed to "High-Risk Drugs"
Single organ			
Skin	Maculopapular eruption	2%–4%[a,4]	5%–10%
	AGEP	<10/million/y	Unknown
	SJS/TEN	2/million/y[5]	1/100,000 to 1/1,000[6]
Liver	Drug-induced liver injury	10–20/million/y[7,b]	1/100,000 to 1/10,000[8]
Kidney	Acute interstitial nephritis	NA	1/100,000 to 1/5,000[9]
Multisystem	DRESS	9/million/y[10,c]	1/10,000 to 1/1,000[11]
	Vasculitis	NA	Up to 3/100[12]

[a] Overestimated since obtained among hospitalized patients (higher rate of exposure to medications than general population).
[b] Overestimated since including "toxic" and "allergic" cases.
[c] Probably overestimated since obtained from West Indies in a population likely at increased risk.

Severe cutaneous adverse reactions (SCARs) are defined as life-threatening effects that most often lead to hospitalization. They are very rare but may initially resemble a trivial eruption (see evaluation of severity later in discussion). They include the following:

- Epidermal necrolysis (from less severe Stevens-Johnson syndrome [SJS] to toxic epidermal necrolysis [TEN]) characterized by high fever, skin pain, erosions of mucous membranes, targetlike lesions, blisters, positive Nikolsky sign, and large erosions resulting from detachment of dead epidermis (**Fig. 1**).[14]
- Acute generalized exanthematous pustulosis (AGEP) with fever and rapid progression of large patches of burning erythema covered by dozens of small pustules.[15]
- Drug reaction with eosinophilia and systemic symptoms (DRESS), also sometimes called drug-induced hypersensitivity syndrome (DIHS).[16]

If not useful in mild eruptions, a skin biopsy is mandatory for all cases of severe reactions. It will allow a retrospective validation of the diagnosis and in some cases may help to exclude nondrug causes of a reaction pattern.

Taking photographs of the lesions is also of tremendous importance, because it may help in making an earlier diagnosis, if transmitted to an expert center, and also allowing for better retrospective evaluation.

Liver

Drug-induced liver diseases are often reported under the denomination of DILI (drug-induced liver injury),[7] with the limitation of not only immune-mediated reactions but also toxic injuries (such as "type A" acetaminophen-related liver failure). Calling the former DALI (for drug-allergic liver injury[8]) would be more appropriate. Usually, definition and classification are based on liver test alterations. Cases are classified

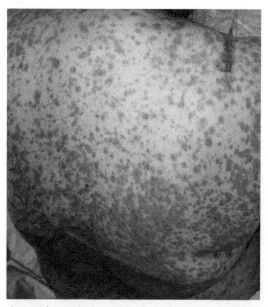

Fig. 1. SJS/TEN overlap with atypical targets and macules as well as large areas of skin detachment.

depending on dominant biologic alterations as "hepatocellular" (ALT greater than twice the upper limit of normal range), "cholestatic" (AP greater than twice the upper limit of normal or ALT/AP ratio <2), or "mixed."[7]

Kidney

Immune-mediated reactions affecting the kidney most often present as acute interstitial nephritis. It is generally considered that 70% of cases of acute interstitial nephritis are caused by drugs.[17] Hence, the denomination of "drug-induced interstitial nephritis" (DIN) was coined.[9] Clinical signs appear 2 to 3 weeks, or even later, after initiation of the inducing medication. Patients with DIN typically present with nonspecific symptoms of acute renal failure, including oliguria, malaise, anorexia, nausea, and vomiting. Alteration of renal function may also be totally asymptomatic, but detected because of other symptoms of hypersensitivity (fever, rash, arthralgia, etc). The latter symptoms, even if mild and transient, should not be missed because they are good markers for suggesting that the mechanism is more likely hypersensitivity than toxicity. A definitive diagnosis of DIN can be established only by kidney biopsy. Eosinophiluria is frequently used as a surrogate marker, but its sensitivity is probably low.[18]

Multisystem

DRESS

DRESS (formerly known as "hypersensitivity syndrome" and also called DIHS in Japan) is a multisystem drug reaction beginning typically 3 to 6 weeks after the use of a new drug and characterized by the varying association of fever, skin eruption of variable severity (**Fig. 2**), enlarged lymph nodes, and visceral lesions (liver, kidney, and lung being the most frequent, whereas gut, pancreas, and the peripheral and central nervous systems are rarely involved). Blood counts show leukocytosis with marked eosinophilia, lymphocytosis, activated "atypical" lymphocytes, and strong elevation of inflammation markers. A frequent characteristic of DRESS is the reactivation of latent viral infections (human herpesvirus 6 [HHV6], Epstein-Barr virus (EBV), cytomegalovirus [CMV]) that can be detected by elevation of serology at 2-week intervals and/or viremia (evidenced by quantitative polymerase chain reaction on serum or plasma). The course of DRESS is often prolonged with partial remissions and relapses, which are often associated with viral activation and also occasionally with the introduction of a new medication. A scoring system was proposed for retrospective validation of suspected cases of DRESS.[19]

   Abacavir hypersensitivity, occasionally reported as DRESS, is actually different by a shorter time latency between the beginning of drug use and the reaction onset,

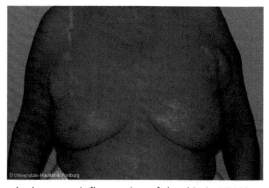

Fig. 2. Infiltrated and edematous inflammation of the skin in DRESS.

infrequent eosinophilia, lymphadenopathy, visceral involvement, and shock in the case of rechallenge.[20,21]

On the other hand, DALI and DIN have a rather long latency. DALI often displays eosinophilia, rash, and fever[7]; lymphadenopathy and atypical lymphocytes are also reported.[8] DIN is associated with rash (42%), fever (46%), and eosinophilia (40%).[9] Further evaluation of the degree of overlap between DRESS, DALI, and DIN is obviously needed.

Drug-induced vasculitis

This reaction usually manifests with skin purpura, arthralgia, and myalgia with possible involvement of kidney and lung combined with features of a lupuslike condition, especially in patients on long-term treatment with antithyroid drugs. Patients affected by drug-induced vasculitis are very often positive for myeloperoxidase–antineutrophil cytoplasma antibodies (MPO-ANCAs). They may also have antinuclear antibodies (ANAs), antihistone antibodies, high levels of immunoglobulin M anticardiolipin antibodies, and low C4 values. This pattern of autoantibodies contrasts with the usual absence of ANAs, antihistone and anticardiolipin antibodies, and normal C4 levels in patients with idiopathic systemic vasculitis.[22]

EVALUATION OF SEVERITY
Skin

The severity of a skin reaction is evaluated on the following:

1. Type of lesions: pustules (suspicion of AGEP or DRESS), vesicles, blisters, erosions (suspicion of epidermal necrolysis), infiltration, facial edema, scaling (suspicion of AGEP or DRESS), purpura (suspicion of vasculitis or DRESS).
2. Associated symptoms and signs: high fever (suspicion of SCAR), intense skin pain (suspicion of epidermal necrolysis), and presence of erosions affecting the mucous membranes (suspicion of SCAR). On this point, it is important to distinguish between peri-orificial skin and true mucous membranes (eg, lips vs mouth, eyelids vs conjunctiva). Only erosive mucous membrane lesions indicate a severe reaction.
3. Extent: evaluated as the proportion of body surface area (BSA) involved. This criterion is prone to errors by excess, resulting from confusion between "dissemination" and surface. An eruption made of small nonconfluent "spots" disseminated to most parts of the body, as seen in measles, is very unlikely to affect more than 10% of the total BSA.[23] The name of exfoliative dermatitis is used when redness and scaling are confluent on more than 90% of the BSA. Exfoliative dermatitis can be caused by several skin diseases, including a drug reaction that most often fulfills the criteria for DRESS. Whatever its cause, exfoliative dermatitis is associated with high morbidity and requires specialized treatment.
4. Rapid progression is a characteristic of SCAR. In case of doubt, severity should be re-evaluated within a few hours.

Any skin lesion is associated with alteration of the "skin barrier," leading to exaggerated water and electrolyte losses and to facilitated systemic penetrations of bacteria colonizing the skin. Such alterations are extreme when erosions (epidermal necrolysis) or scaling (DRESS) affect a high percentage of the BSAs. Sepsis is a frequent cause of death in severe skin reactions, especially SJS/TEN.[24]

Liver

As for hepatitis of any cause, the severity of drug-induced liver disease is most often appreciated on the existence of jaundice and strong elevation of ALT (>10 times ULN) or of AP (>2 times ULN).[8] Any of these alterations requires rapid advice from a liver specialist because of the risk of progression to liver failure (usually defined as international normalized ratio $\geq$1.5, ascites, or encephalopathy) with possible need for emergency transplantation.[25]

Kidney

The absence of a decrease of creatinine level 1 week after discontinuation of the responsible drug suggests severe nephritis and often leads to using systemic corticosteroids with or without prior renal biopsy.[17,18]

Multisystem

Severity of multisystem reactions is logically proportional to that of the most severely involved organ or organs, but multisystem reactions may also be complicated by nonspecific syndromes resulting from inflammation and organ failure, such as systemic inflammatory response syndrome, disseminated intravascular coagulation, or hemophagocytic syndrome.[26]

IS REFERRAL TO SPECIALIZED WARDS NEEDED?

Referral to a specialized center should be considered based on severity at admission and on quickness of progression of signs and symptoms. Acute failure of any organ including the skin needs specialized measures for surveillance and/or management.[26]

As an example, an algorithm evaluating the need for referral to an expert center of cases of SJS or TEN has been proposed. It is based on the main prognosis factors, as evaluated by a disease-specific score (SCORTEN) reliably predicting the risk of death.[27] Recommendations issued by the French health authorities state that SCORTEN of 2 or more indicates the need for immediate transfer to an expert center.[28]

Box 1 presents SCORTEN values.

IDENTIFICATION OF SUSPECT DRUGS

To identify the most likely causing drug is not always easy in the frequent situation of patients exposed to several drugs, not even with the help of diagnostic tests after the patient's recovery. Results of tests, discussed elsewhere, are obviously not available

---

Box 1
SCORTEN

One point for each of the following 7 items:

A score greater than or equal to 2 indicates a risk of death greater than or equal to 10% and the need for referral to a specialized center[28]

1. Age greater than or equal to 40 years

2. Current malignancy

3. Detached/detachable epidermis on greater than 10% of BSA

4. Heart rate greater than 120

5. Serum urea greater than 10 mmol/L

6. Serum glucose greater than 14 mmol/L

7. Serum bicarbonate less than 20 mmol/L

Adapted from Guégan S, Bastuji-Garin S, Poszepczynska-Guigné E, et al. Performance of the SCORTEN during the first five days of hospitalization to predict the prognosis of epidermal necrolysis. J Invest Dermatol 2006;126(2):273; with permission.

to physicians who have to face the early management of a patient with drug hypersensitivity. At this stage there are 4 main criteria helping to consider a drug as a likely suspect. These criteria were integrated in many algorithms, especially a recent one that proved useful for SJS/TEN.[29]

Delay Between Initiation of the Medication and Onset of the Reaction

Studies addressing the time relationship of the risk were done for SJS/TEN and have shown that the odds ratios for "high-risk" drugs were no more significant with long-term treatments (more than 8 weeks).[30] That cannot be extrapolated to all types of drug reactions, but it is patent that most types of reaction have a suggestive "time-window" or delay that is helpful in the evaluation of causality.

Table 2 presents the suggestive time-window by type of reaction.

Is the Medication Still Present in the Patient's Body?

The pertinence of this question is based on the demonstration that most types of nonimmediate hypersensitivity reactions (HSR) are directed by drug-specific T cells. In vitro, these cells react only in the presence of the drug (or a metabolite) at concentrations in the range of the serum level of efficacy. Much lower concentrations do not elicit any response from drug-specific T-cell clones.[31] This strongly suggests that a drug stopped before the onset of reaction for more than 5 times the duration of "elimination half-life" (10 times in the case of alteration in the kinetics of drug elimination) is very unlikely the culprit.[29]

Did the Patient Use the Same Drug in the Past?

The authors' experience with SCAR has been that "associated" drugs were nearly always administered for the first time, with very rare exceptions of recurrent cases with a precipitated onset. The authors, therefore, consider not only that a prior reaction to the same medication increases the probability that it is responsible, but also that prior usage without a problem decreases the probability.

What Is the Notoriety of the Drug for Inducing This Type of Reaction?

Whatever the phenotype of the reaction, a limited number of medications are responsible for most cases (**Table 3**).

Table 3 presents drugs most often responsible for a certain type of reaction.

If initiated within a suggestive "time-window," such drugs are definitely first-rank suspects to be withdrawn in priority.

Table 2
Suggestive "time-windows" (days between beginning of drug use and onset of the reaction) by type of reaction

Nature of Reaction	Suggestive Delay (from First Intake of Medication to Onset of Reaction)
Maculopapular eruption	4–12 d[4]
AGEP	Hours to 2 d (antibiotics), 4–12 d (other drugs)[15]
SJS/TEN	4–28 d[29]
DALI	5–90 d (peak >4 wk)[8]
DIN	2–3 wk or later[9]
DRESS	2–5 wk[16]
Vasculitis	Months with propylthiouracil[22]

Table 3
Drugs most often responsible by type of reaction

MPE[4]	AGEP[a,15]	SJS/TEN[a,30]	DALI[8]	DIN[9,32]	DRESS[b,16]	Vasculitis[22]
Aminopenicillins	Aminopenicillins	Allopurinol	Allopurinol	Penicillins	Carbamazepine	Propylthiouracile
Cephalosporins	Pristinamycine	Lamotrigine	Sulfamethoxazole[c]	Cephalosporins	Allopurinol	Other antithyroid
Other antibiotics	Diltiazem	Sulfamethoxazole[c]	Amoxi/clavulanate	NSAIDs	Lamotrigine	AntiTNF-α
AEDs	(Hydoxy)chloroquine	Phenytoin	Macrolides	Proton pump inhibitors	Salazopyrine	Cefotaxim
	Quinolones	Carbamazepine	AEDs		Phenytoin	Minocycline
	Sulfamethoxazole[a]	Nevirapine	Vitamin K antagonists		Vancomycin	Hydralazine
	Terbinafine	Phenobarbital				
		Oxicam NSAIDs				

Abbreviations: AED, antiepileptic drugs; MPE, Maculopapular eruptions; NSAIDs, nonsteroidal anti-inflammatory drugs; TNF, tumor necrosis factor.
[a] Listed drugs account for 50% of cases.
[b] Listed drugs account for 60% of cases.
[c] And other anti-infectious sulfonamides.

DECISION ON WITHDRAWAL
The Rule

The rule is to withdraw as soon as possible any suspected drug. This attitude was supported in SJS/TEN by a study showing that an early withdrawal of the "culprit drug" was associated with a significantly lower mortality, provided the drug had a rather short elimination half-life.[33]

On the other hand, the authors recommend that drugs that are both *nonsuspected AND important* for future treatment should rather be continued. In the authors' experience, most patients are indeed reluctant to take again any of the medications that were stopped because of the hypersensitivity reaction, even when further tests identify a single one as the most likely culprit. Conversely, they consider easily as "innocent" medications that were not withdrawn during the course of the disease.

A Few Exceptions

It is important to keep in mind that in the context of a mild to moderate drug eruption, not accompanied by systemic symptoms, and attributed to an important medication (eg, for treating HIV infection), patients were sometimes "treated through" the rash.[34] That was usually not followed by progression of the reaction, and resolution of the "rash" occurred in about the same time as expected if the drug had been withdrawn.

A decision of "treating through" depends obviously on a thorough evaluation of the balance between the severity of the adverse reaction, the severity of disease to be treated, and the existence of alternative medications. The decision to treating through needs information of the patient and very close surveillance, preferably in hospital.

TREATMENT
Skin Reactions

Maculopapular eruptions

There is no treatment of proven efficacy for common drug eruptions. Mild to moderate eruptions vanish in a few days without any treatment. Oral antihistamines and topical emollients are often prescribed. There is no evidence that they shorten the evolution, but they may help to alleviate pruritus (as demonstrated for many other skin diseases where pruritus is an important symptom). In the case of severe pruritus, topical corticosteroids of mild or moderate potency are probably useful.

Severe reactions—SCAR

AGEP Most patients with AGEP are hospitalized because the combination of widespread pustules, fever, and high neutrophil count often raises the suspicion of severe sepsis. Investigations for infection are negative; there is no need for antibacterial treatment, and the eruption disappears within 7 to 15 days with or without treatment using oral antihistamines.[15]

SJS/TEN Because these conditions are the most severe forms of drug hypersensitivity with 30% mortality,[35] most physicians are obligated to give "some specific treatment" even though available evidence is that none has demonstrated any benefit and none is free of potentially severe side effects.

Systemic corticosteroids (high oral dosage or intravenous "pulse") and intravenous human immunoglobulins (IVIg) are the immune-modulating treatments most often prescribed. For IVIg, the rationale was based on expected inhibition of Fas-Ligand, a cytokine considered responsible for the widespread death of cells in the epidermis. This rationale has been refuted by recent studies demonstrating that Fas-Ligand had no role or a very minor role in the mechanisms of TEN.[36] Furthermore, one large cohort study[35] and 2 meta-analyses[37,38] observed no benefit from IVIg on mortality. The same cohort[35] and one meta-analysis[37] also evaluated systemic corticosteroids and found no benefit.

Waiting for further results of ongoing studies testing a possible benefit of cyclosporine[39] or etanercept, physicians should focus their efforts on providing the best supportive care as the only treatment that can save the patient's life in such severe diseases. That is best done in specialized hospital settings (intensive care unit or burn units in cases with large amounts of skin detachment, dermatology units in cases not requiring intensive care) with skilled nurses and a multidisciplinary team of physicians capable of managing the multiple complications of "acute skin failure," especially severe sepsis.[24] It is not within of the scope of this review to detail the complex symptomatic measures that resemble in many parts (but not all) what is needed for the management of severe burns.

Liver

Systemic corticosteroids are often used in drug-induced hepatitis, especially with evident markers of hypersensitivity (rash, eosinophilia), but their benefits are still not proven.[8] Management is centered on the prompt withdrawal of the suspected drug. That usually results in a 50% decrease in serum ALT within 8 days of discontinuation in the hepatocellular type. Improvement may require a longer period in the cholestatic type.

In cases with acute liver failure, a randomized controlled trial (RCT) has suggested a significant increase in spontaneous survival of a subgroup of patients (ie, without liver transplantation) with intravenous N-acetylcysteine.[40] However, this trial suffered from some methodological bias and was not confirmed by a further randomized trial that instead suggested worsening with N-acetylcysteine.[41] Based on these RCTs, routine use of N-acetylcysteine cannot be recommended for the treatment of DALI.[42]

Kidney

There is no consensus on the treatment of DIN. On one hand, most cases improve after drug withdrawal without any "specific" treatment. On the other hand, 2 retrospective analyses found that treatments with corticosteroids were followed by more frequent recovery of normal renal function. In the first study, the benefit was restricted to cases with treatment initiated less than 2 weeks after diagnosis.[43] In the second study, a benefit from steroids was observed whatever the delay in initiating treatment.[44] Taking the results of both studies into account, data support the recommendation of (1) withdrawing suspected drugs and (2) initiating steroid treatment if creatinine level is not substantially decreased after 1 week. The typical corticosteroid regimen is "pulse" methylprednisolone (250–500 mg intravenous injection) for 2 to 4 days followed by oral prednisolone 1 mg/kg/d tapered over 8 to 12 weeks.

DRESS

Prompt withdrawal of the offending drug is the mainstay of treatment. The authors also suggest avoiding the introduction of new medications during the course of DRESS because of the risk of a flare-up that may be considered "multiple drug allergy."[45] Patients with severe cutaneous manifestations are usually hospitalized for treatment. Those with exfoliative dermatitis require fluid and electrolyte replacement as well as nutritional support. Additional measures include a warm and humid environment and gentle skin care with warm baths/wet dressings and emollients.

An expert consensus in France proposed that in the absence of clinical, laboratory, or imaging evidence of renal or pulmonary involvement and with only modest elevation of liver enzymes, patients with DRESS can be treated symptomatically.[46]

Relief of pruritus and skin inflammation is obtained with high-potency topical corticosteroids applied 2 to 3 times per day for 1 to 2 weeks. That is enough for obtaining complete recovery in patients without severe organ involvement. For more severe cases, there is consensus among experts on the use of systemic corticosteroids, particularly in patients with renal and/or pulmonary involvement. The optimal dose and duration of corticosteroid therapy are not known. After a usual initial dose of 1 to 2 mg/kg/d of prednisone or equivalent maintained up to the beginning of remission, the daily dose is tapered progressively. Waiting for a better evaluation of treating DRESS with systemic corticosteroids, the authors recommend using them only for the most severe cases.

There are no studies evaluating the treatment of DRESS with antiviral agents active against HHV6 or CMV (eg, ganciclovir, foscarnet, or cidofovir). Given the substantial toxicity of antiviral agents and the natural course of spontaneous resolution, antiviral agents are rarely used in the treatment of DRESS. However, they may be warranted for cases in which virus reactivation is both demonstrated and strongly suspected of contributing to severe complications (eg, severe erosive colitis).[47]

Systemic Vasculitis

In the absence of involvement of kidney or lung, discontinuation of the causal agent is usually enough. A course of systemic corticosteroids is justified in the case of organ involvement. Prednisone or equivalent is used at a daily dose of 1 mg/kg for 4 to 8 weeks. In cases with severe nephritis, the treatment may begin with intravenous "pulse." Corticosteroid therapy is then tapered off over 6 to 12 months. Periodic checking of MPO-ANCA levels may help to accelerate or stop decreasing steroid dosage. In contrast to idiopathic systemic vasculitis, the addition of immune-suppressive agents is rarely necessary.[22]

CONFIRMATION OF CAUSALITY

Before embarking a patient in long and expensive investigations, the authors suggest to clearly define the objectives. What level of evidence is needed and for what aim?

Is it for better understanding the immune mechanisms of an adverse drug reaction? That is a research objective to be explored following the rules of good clinical practice.

Is it for helping the patient and the general practitioner in future use of medicines? In more than 50% of cases, a single medication or a couple of medications is highly suspected on clinical judgment. In such cases, prescribing an alternative treatment without any further investigation is costless and effective.

What will be the interpretation of a negative in vivo or in vitro test? No allergy expert will conclude that the reaction was not allergy.

The authors' experience with SJS/TEN is that the skin biopsies *always* exhibit a pattern of cytotoxic T cells invading the epidermis. When extracted and tested, these T cells revealed drug-specific cytotoxicity. Clinically, one or occasionally 2 medications are strongly suspected in 65% to 70% of cases of SJS/TEN.[29] Patch tests with these drugs are positive in 20% to 25%[48] and lymphocyte transformation test (LTT) in no more than 30% of patients. Rather than concluding that the reaction was not immune-mediated in the case of negative results, the authors consider more plausible that the sensitivity of tests available nowadays is too low to be useful to assess causality. The authors do not doubt that new tests will be developed that will prove more helpful.

REPORTING

After the marketing of a new drug, pharmaceutical companies and regulatory agencies have to reassess its benefit/risk balance in real life, because (1) the most severe reactions are too rare to be detected in premarketing clinical trials and (2) patients with comorbidities that may increase the risk are often not enrolled in clinical trials.

It is, therefore, an essential duty of all physicians interested in drug hypersensitivity to report cases to pharmacovigilance systems.

FOLLOW-UP

There is growing evidence that many nonimmediate HSR may induce some sequelae, which may be long-lasting. Sequelae occur very frequently after SJS/TEN, impairing daily life in most patients. Not only may the eyes be severely affected but also other mucosal sites, skin, appendages, bronchial tract, and others. A follow-up examination is recommended 3 months and 1 year after discharge for the evaluation of sequelae and referral to organ specialists for optimal management.

Many recent case reports have also insisted on the possible development of autoimmune diseases following DRESS. In a retrospective study of 43 patients with DRESS followed up for at least 1 year, 4 patients developed autoimmune diseases (Grave disease, diabetes mellitus type 1, and autoimmune hemolytic anemia) and 2 patients developed chronic renal failure.[49]

FUTURE USE OF MEDICATIONS

Patients who experienced a hypersensitivity reaction to a medication must be educated about future avoidance of that specific medication. In the case of prior severe reaction, re-exposure to the culprit drug may be fatal. Relevant information should be inscribed on an "allergy passport" that patients must carry with them at all times. Patients should be able to report the precise type of hypersensitivity they suffered and the generic name for the causative medication, but this might be a challenge in elderly patients needing assistance.

Whatever the mechanisms (true "cross-reactivity", common genetic susceptibility, or other), the risk of "multiple drug hypersensitivity" exists and should be addressed.[48] Patients with hypersensitivity to one of the following anticonvulsants, such as phenytoin, carbamazepine, phenobarbital, or lamotrigine, should be informed that they have also a risk of similar reaction to the others in the list for themselves certainly and possibly their family members. However, numerous patients have been seen with SJS/TEN after one of these drugs that were treated with another one subsequently without any problems.

The risk of recurrence with structurally distinct agents (within the same therapeutic class of drugs) is unknown but low enough for being acceptable. As an example, the authors recommend patients with past severe reaction to cotrimoxazole avoid other anti-infectious sulfonamides but authorize the use of thiazide diuretics or sulfonylurea-derived antidiabetics.

REFERENCES

1. Mayorga C, Sanz ML, Gamboa P, et al. In vitro methods for diagnosing nonimmediate hypersensitivity reactions to drugs. J Investig Allergol Clin Immunol 2013;23:213–25.
2. Al-Nouri ZL, George JN. Drug-induced thrombocytopenia: an updated systematic review, 2012. Drug Saf 2012;35:693–4.

3. Pichler WJ. Delayed drug hypersensitivity reactions. Ann Intern Med 2003;139: 683–93.
4. Hunziker T, Kunzi UP, Braunschweig S, et al. Comprehensive hospital drug monitoring (CHDM): adverse skin reactions, a 20-year survey. Allergy 1997;52:388–93.
5. Rzany B, Mockenhaupt M, Baur S, et al. Epidemiology of erythema exsudativum multiforme majus, Stevens-Johnson syndrome, and toxic epidermal necrolysis in Germany (1990-1992): structure and results of a population-based registry. J Clin Epidemiol 1996;49(7):769–73.
6. Miller KD, Lobel HO, Satriale RF, et al. Serious cutaneous reactions among American travelers using pyrimethamine-sulfadoxine (Fansidar) for malaria prophylaxis. Am J Trop Med Hyg 1986;35(3):451–8.
7. Fontana RJ, Seeff LB, Andrade RJ, et al. Standardization of nomenclature and causality assessment in drug-induced liver injury: summary of a clinical research workshop. Hepatology 2010;52(2):730–4.
8. Cerny A, Bertoli R. Drug allergic liver injury. In: Pichler WJ, editor. Drug hypersensitivity. Basel (Switzerland): Karger; 2007. p. 278–94.
9. Keller M, Spanou Z, Pichler WJ. Drug-induced interstitial nephritis. In: Pichler WJ, editor. Drug hypersensitivity. Basel (Switzerland): Karger; 2007. p. 295–305.
10. Muller P, Dubreil P, Mahé A, et al. Drug hypersensitivity syndrome in a West-Indian population. Eur J Dermatol 2003;13(5):478–81.
11. Tennis P, Stern RS. Risk of serious cutaneous disorders after initiation of use of phenytoin, carbamazepine, or sodium valproate: a record linkage study. Neurology 1997;49(2):542–6.
12. Lionaki S, Hogan SL, Falk RJ, et al. Vasculitis and anti-thyroid medication. Nephrol Dial Transplant 2008;23(5):1766–8.
13. Mockenhaupt M. Epidemiology of cutaneous adverse drug reactions. Chem Immunol Allergy 2012;97(1):1–17.
14. Mockenhaupt M. Severe drug-induced skin reactions: clinical pattern, diagnostics and therapy. J Dtsch Dermatol Ges 2009;7(2):142–60.
15. Sidoroff A. Acute generalized exanthematous pustulosis. Chem Immunol Allergy 2012;97:139–48.
16. Kardaun SH, Sekula P, Valeyrie-Allanore L, et al, The RegiSCAR study group. Drug reaction with eosinophilia and systemic symptoms (DRESS): an original multisystem adverse drug reaction. Results from the prospective RegiSCAR study. Br J Dermatol 2013;169(5):1071–80.
17. Praga M, González E. Acute interstitial nephritis. Kidney Int 2010;77(11):956–61.
18. Xu B, Murray M. Flucloxacillin induced acute renal failure. Aust Fam Physician 2008;37(12):1009–11.
19. Kardaun SH, Sidoroff A, Valeyrie-Allanore L, et al. Variability in the clinical pattern of cutaneous side-effects of drugs with systemic symptoms: does a DRESS syndrome really exist? Br J Dermatol 2007;156:609–11.
20. Phillips E, Mallal S. Drug hypersensitivity in HIV. Curr Opin Allergy Clin Immunol 2007;7(4):324–30.
21. Peyrière H, Dereure O, Breton H, et al. Variability in the clinical pattern of cutaneous side-effects of drugs with systemic symptoms: does a DRESS syndrome really exist? Br J Dermatol 2006;155(2):422–8.
22. Radic M, Martinovic Kaliterna D, Radic J. Drug-induced vasculitis: a clinical and pathological review. Neth J Med 2012;70(1):12–7.
23. Bastuji-Garin S, Rzany B, Stern RS, et al. Clinical classification of cases of toxic epidermal necrolysis, Stevens-Johnson syndrome, and erythema multiforme. Arch Dermatol 1993;129(1):92–6.

24. de Prost N, Ingen-Housz-Oro S, Duong T, et al. Bacteremia in Stevens-Johnson syndrome and toxic epidermal necrolysis: epidemiology, risk factors, and predictive value of skin cultures. Medicine (Baltimore) 2010;89(1):28–36.

25. Bernal W, Auzinger G, Dhawan A, et al. Acute liver failure. Lancet 2010;376: 190–2.

26. Wei CH, Chung-Yee Hui R, Chang CJ, et al. Identifying prognostic factors for drug rash with eosinophilia and systemic symptoms (DRESS). Eur J Dermatol 2011;21(6):930–7.

27. Guégan S, Bastuji-Garin S, Poszepczynska-Guigné E, et al. Performance of the SCORTEN during the first five days of hospitalization to predict the prognosis of epidermal necrolysis. J Invest Dermatol 2006;126(2):272–6.

28. Haute Autorité de Santé. Nécrolyse épidermique (syndromes de Stevens-Johnson et de Lyell), protocole national de diagnostic et de soins. 2010. Available at: www.has-sante.fr. Accessed on January 17, 2014.

29. Sassolas B, Haddad C, Mockenhaupt M, et al. ALDEN, an algorithm for assessment of drug causality in Stevens-Johnson syndrome and toxic epidermal necrolysis: comparison with case-control analysis. Clin Pharmacol Ther 2010;88(1):60–8.

30. Mockenhaupt M, Viboud C, Dunant A, et al. Stevens-Johnson syndrome and toxic epidermal necrolysis: assessment of medication risks with emphasis on recently marketed drugs. The EuroSCAR-study. J Invest Dermatol 2008;128(1):35–44.

31. Mauri-Hellweg D, Bettens F, Mauri D, et al. Activation of drug-specific CD4+ and CD8+ T cells in individuals allergic to sulfonamides, phenytoin, and carbamazepine. J Immunol 1995;155(1):462–72.

32. Klepser DG, Collier DS, Cochran GL. Proton pump inhibitors and acute kidney injury: a nested case–control study. BMC Nephrol 2013;14(1):150.

33. Garcia-Doval I, LeCleach L, Bocquet H, et al. Toxic epidermal necrolysis and Stevens-Johnson syndrome: does early withdrawal of causative drugs decrease the risk of death? Arch Dermatol 2000;136(3):323–7.

34. Chaponda M, Pirmohamed M. Hypersensitivity reactions to HIV therapy. Br J Clin Pharmacol 2011;71(5):659–71.

35. Sekula P, Dunant A, Mockenhaupt M, et al, RegiSCAR study group. Comprehensive survival analysis of a cohort of patients with Stevens-Johnson syndrome and toxic epidermal necrolysis. J Invest Dermatol 2013;133(5):1197–204.

36. Chung WH, Hung SI, Yang JY, et al. Granulysin is a key mediator for disseminated keratinocyte death in Stevens-Johnson syndrome and toxic epidermal necrolysis. Nat Med 2008;14(12):1343–50.

37. Roujeau JC, Bastuji-Garin S. Systematic review of treatments for Stevens-Johnson syndrome and toxic epidermal necrolysis using the SCORTEN score as a tool for evaluating mortality. Ther Adv Drug Saf 2011;2(3):87–94.

38. Huang YC, Li YC, Chen TJ. The efficacy of intravenous immunoglobulin for the treatment of toxic epidermal necrolysis: a systematic review and meta-analysis. Br J Dermatol 2012;167(2):424–32.

39. Valeyrie-Allanore L, Wolkenstein P, Brochard L, et al. Open trial of ciclosporin treatment for Stevens-Johnson syndrome and toxic epidermal necrolysis. Br J Dermatol 2010;163(4):847–53.

40. Lee WM, Hynan LS, Rossaro L, et al, Acute Liver Failure Study Group. Intravenous N-acetylcysteine improves transplant-free survival in early stage non-acetaminophen acute liver failure. Gastroenterology 2009;137(3):856–64.

41. Squires RH, Dhawan A, Alonso E, et al. Intravenous N-acetylcysteine in pediatric patients with nonacetaminophen acute liver failure: a placebo-controlled clinical trial. Hepatology 2013;57(4):1542–9.

42. Sales I, Dzierba AL, Smithburger PL, et al. Use of acetylcysteine for non-acetaminophen-induced acute liver failure. Ann Hepatol 2013;12(1):6–10.

43. González E, Gutiérrez E, Galeano C, et al. Early steroid treatment improves the recovery of renal function in patients with drug-induced acute interstitial nephritis. Kidney Int 2008;73(8):940–6.

44. Raza MN, Hadid M, Keen CE, et al. Acute tubulointerstitial nephritis, treatment with steroid and impact on renal outcomes. Nephrology (Carlton) 2012;17(8): 748–53.

45. Mardivirin L, Valeyrie-Allanore L, Branlant-Redon E, et al. Amoxicillin-induced flare in patients with DRESS (Drug Reaction with Eosinophilia and Systemic Symptoms): report of seven cases and demonstration of a direct effect of amoxicillin on human herpesvirus 6 replication in vitro. Eur J Dermatol 2010;20(1): 68–73.

46. Descamps V, Ben Saïd B, Sassolas B, et al, groupe Toxidermies de la Société française de dermatologie. Management of drug reaction with eosinophilia and systemic symptoms (DRESS). Ann Dermatol Venereol 2010;137(11):703–8 [in French].

47. Dieterich DT, Kotler DP, Busch DF, et al. Ganciclovir treatment of cytomegalovirus colitis in AIDS: a randomized, double-blind, placebo-controlled multicenter study. J Infect Dis 1993;167(2):278–82.

48. Barbaud A, Collet E, Milpied B, et al, Toxidermies group of the French Society of Dermatology. A multicentre study to determine the value and safety of drug patch tests for the three main classes of severe cutaneous adverse drug reactions. Br J Dermatol 2013;168:555–62.

49. Chen YC, Chang CY, Cho YT, et al. Long-term sequelae of drug reaction with eosinophilia and systemic symptoms: a retrospective cohort study from Taiwan. J Am Acad Dermatol 2013;68:459–65.

Antibiotic Allergy

Antonino Romano, MD[a], Richard Warrington, MB,BS, PhD[b],*

KEYWORDS

- Drug • Hypersensitivity • Allergy • Antibiotics • Immediate • Nonimmediate
- β-lactam • Non-β-lactam

KEY POINTS

- Antibiotic allergy is overdiagnosed, often resulting in the administration of less appropriate and more expensive antibiotics, with increasing costs and development of resistance through the use of more broad-spectrum drugs.
- The appropriate diagnosis and management of patients with reported antibiotic allergy are essential to good medical care and it requires the appropriate use of diagnostic tests, when these are available.
- Unfortunately, appropriate diagnosis and management are often difficult to achieve because of the lack of appropriate reagents, sometimes because of the shortsightedness of regulatory authorities. In other instances, there has been insufficient research carried out to define appropriate diagnostic techniques, except in situations such as β-lactam allergy.
- Differences exist in different parts of the world in regard to the appropriate means to investigate drug allergy, but to a large extent, these may be the result of a lack of access and standardization rather than true differences in the frequency and type of drug-induced hypersensitivity.

INTRODUCTION

Antibiotics may be classified as β-lactams or non-β-lactams. β-Lactam antibiotics contain a 4-membered β-lactam ring and consist of 2 major classes, the penicillins (penams) and cephalosporins (cephems), and the carbapenems, monobactams, oxacephems, and clavams. Non-β-lactam antibiotics, such as macrolides, sulfonamides, quinolines, and aminoglyclosides, are very different chemically and also immunogenically.

PATHOGENESIS OF ANTIBIOTIC ALLERGY

Because most antibiotics are low-molecular-weight chemicals (ie, too small to stimulate an immune response), it has been assumed that the drug or its metabolite first binds

The authors have nothing to disclose.
[a] Department of Internal Medicine and Geriatrics, UCSC-Allergy Unit, Complesso Integrato Columbus, Via G. Moscati 31, Rome 00168, Italy; [b] Allergy & Clinical Immunology, Health Sciences Centre, Winnipeg, Departments of Medicine and Immunology, University of Manitoba, GC319, 820 Sherbrook Street, Winnipeg, Manitoba R3A 1R9, Canada
* Corresponding author.
E-mail address: rwarrington@hsc.mb.ca

Immunol Allergy Clin N Am 34 (2014) 489–506
http://dx.doi.org/10.1016/j.iac.2014.03.003
0889-8561/14/$ – see front matter © 2014 Elsevier Inc. All rights reserved.
immunology.theclinics.com

covalently to a macromolecule such as a circulating serum protein to form a multivalent conjugate, that is processed and presented to T lymphocytes.[1] Probably the clearest example of this occurs with penicillin, which is able to bind to lysine residues on proteins such as serum albumin.[2,3] This binding occurs because the β-lactam ring opens spontaneously and forms a stable covalent conjugate. Haptenation may also occur through the carboxyl and thiol groups to form minor antigenic determinants.[1,4,5] A similar although slower and less efficient process occurs with cephalosporins.[1,6] In the case of sulfamethoxazole, the drug becomes reactive through cytochrome p450 modification to a nitroso-intermediate that modifies thiol groups on proteins.[7–9]

The novel drug-conjugate undergoes antigen processing to form a small but novel Major Histocompatibility Complex (MHC) ligand, loaded on to MHC molecules, where it interacts with antigen-specific T cells.[9,10]

However, not all antibiotics stimulate immune responses in this way. The pharmacologic interaction or p-i hypothesis suggests that chemically inert drugs may bind noncovalently to antigen-interacting structures such as the T-cell receptor or MHC and cause direct stimulation of an immune response.[1,5,11] This situation occurs with sulfamethoxazole.[12] The drug interaction with the receptor is highly specific and may, in some cases, exhibit specificity for certain HLA alleles or receptors, possibly explaining the genetic associations of certain forms of drug hypersensitivity.[13,14]

GENERAL PRINCIPLES

Allergy to antibiotics appears to be very common, according to patient reports, possibly with a prevalence as high as 5% to 10%.[15–18] However, many individuals labeled as drug allergic are not truly allergic any longer or perhaps never were. Hypersensitivity reactions to antibiotics are adverse responses that resemble allergic responses and are categorized as type B according to Rawlins and Thompson classification.[19,20] Strictly speaking, only when a definite immunologic mechanism is demonstrated should a reaction to an antibiotic be considered allergic; however, such mechanisms have not been identified for many drugs, and the assumption is usually made that similarities in presentation indicate an allergic basis. Attempts have been made to fit these reactions into the Gell and Coombs classification of type I (immunoglobulin E [IgE]-mediated), type II (cytotoxic, IgG-mediated, or IgM-mediated), type III (immune complex–mediated by IgG antibodies), and type IV (mediated by drug-specific T cells), which is subdivided into type IVa, IVb, IVc, and IVd.[5]

CLINICAL PRESENTATION

By clinical criteria, antibiotic-induced hypersensitivity reactions can be classified simply as immediate or delayed. Immediate reactions occur quickly, usually within 1 hour after the last intake of the drug and are often mediated by IgE antibodies already present in the patient.[21] They may comprise urticaria, angioedema, bronchospasm, gastrointestinal symptoms, rhinitis, and conjunctivitis and, most seriously, anaphylaxis and anaphylactic shock. Nonimmediate reactions occur later than 1 hour and may also consist of urticaria and angioedema, the common morbilliform eruptions, fixed drug eruptions, and severe delayed reactions such as exfoliative dermatitis, acute generalized exanthematous pustulosis (AGEP), Stevens-Johnson syndrome (SJS), and toxic epidermal necrolysis (TEN) and drug reaction with eosinophilia and systemic symptoms (DRESS). Antibiotics may also cause immune-mediated interstitial nephritis, hepatitis, pneumonitis, and vasculitis.[22,23]

European guidelines currently classify drug reactions into immediate, occurring in less than 1 hour, and delayed, occurring after 1 hour after the last drug intake. It has been frequently implied that these timeframes also indicate likely pathogenesis, with the rapid reactions being IgE-mediated and the delayed reactions being the result of T-cell-driven responses.[21,23,24] Although there is evidence from some studies that this may sometimes be the situation, with regard to nonimmediate reactions occurring after 1 hour, the opinion in North America and of some European experts is that such reactions, occurring even as long as 24 hours after the last drug intake, may still be IgE-mediated, depending on the individual situation.[25-28]

Although maculopapular or morbilliform eruptions can result from rapid responses by previously sensitized T cells, diagnostic testing has shown that skin test reactivity in such cases is often delayed for several hours.[29] It would be difficult to explain the occurrence of hives and angioedema on the basis of a T-cell response occurring after only 1 to 2 hours. Nevertheless, it can be argued that the above classification gives some help in determining the types of skin tests that should be used.

ASSESSMENT OF ANTIBIOTIC ALLERGY

To assess drug allergy in a patient, it is necessary, but not always possible, to obtain a detailed clinical history, including the nature of the reaction, the time between the occurrence of symptoms and the first as well as the last intake of the drug, and concomitant medications.[30] It is also helpful to know why the antibiotic was prescribed, because reactions to many antibiotics are more frequent in the presence of unproven bacterial (and often viral) infections. Some illnesses such as HIV and other virus infections may increase the probability that an allergic reaction will occur.[31-33] Confirmation of the diagnosis is attempted by skin tests, in vitro tests, and drug provocation tests (DPTs).[34-39] The tests themselves are selected because of the known history, the nature of the reactions, and their presumed time of onset, whether immediate or delayed. Although immediate reactions may be assessed by skin tests, in vitro specific IgE assays, or basophil activation flow cytometry, for many antibiotics such tests are either not validated, have a high false-negative rate, or are simply not available.[40-42] Nonimmediate or delayed reactions are even more difficult to assess, by either delayed-reading intradermal skin testing, patch testing, or specialized laboratory investigations such as lymphocyte transformation studies or cytokine release assays.[43-48] Although delayed-reading skin tests have been validated for β-lactam antibiotics, there is less evidence for their utility for other classes of antibiotics. In vitro tests, when available, are less useful in patients with remote histories of antibiotic allergy and can be subject to false-negative/positive results, such as in the ImmunoCAP assay for penicillin, where antibodies were directed against phenylethylamine, rather than penicillin itself.[49] Confirmation or exclusion of the diagnosis of drug allergy often depends on DPT, usually when diagnostic testing is negative, when the previous reaction was not life-threatening or severe, and when there is a reasonable need to readminister the suspected drug.[36,50,51]

β-LACTAM ANTIBIOTICS

Penicillins and cephalosporins are the antibiotics most frequently causing antibiotic-related allergic reactions, because of their ability to form conjugates with serum proteins and their widespread massive use. Penicillin allergy is the most commonly reported drug allergy, with a prevalence rate of 5% to 10% in adults and children.[15-17,52,53]

Benzylpenicillin has progressively been replaced by amoxicillin and to a lesser extent by other penicillins in causing allergic reactions and, in European experience, this is often associated with side-chain-specific allergy.[54,55] There is increasing evidence supporting the role of side chains as the relevant part of the structure of the allergenic determinant. The evaluation of immediate anaphylactic β-lactam allergy combines skin tests and IgE-specific assays (when a penicillin is suspected the culprit) with a panel of common reagents, including classic penicillin reagents, such as penicilloyl-polylysine (PPL), minor determinant mixture (MDM), and amoxicillin, as well other relevant β-lactams.

In both the European Academy of Allergy and Clinical Immunology (EAACI)/ European Network for Drug Allergy (ENDA) and the American Academy of Allergy, Asthma, and Clinical Immunology (AAAAI) Practice Parameters, skin testing is the best method for diagnosing immediate hypersensitivity reactions to β-lactams.[34,36] In patients with a recent history of anaphylactic reaction, it seems reasonable to use serum-specific IgE assays when available, to avoid the risk of reactions to skin testing (**Fig. 1**). The ImmunoCAP technique is the most validated technique for penicillins.

DIFFERENCES IN PRACTICE ACROSS THE WORLD

In Europe, the highest concentration accepted for epicutaneous prick and intradermal testing are 5×10^{-5} M for PPL, 2×10^{-2} M for MDM, 25,000 IU/mL for benzyl penicillin (BP), 25 mg/mL for amoxicillin and other penicillins, and 2 mg/mL for cephalosporins. Both PPL and MDM are available in some but not all countries in Europe (DAP; Diater, Madrid, Spain), whereas in North America, only PPL (PRE-PEN; AllerQuest LLC, West Hartford, CT, USA) is available commercially. In some centers, PPL and MDM may be prepared locally, but standardization is a problem. It has been estimated that skin testing with only PPL and BP, and not using the penilloate and penicilloate, may miss 10% to 20% of penicillin-allergic subjects, but studies from North America have found that DPTs after skin testing only with PPL and BP produce a similar rate

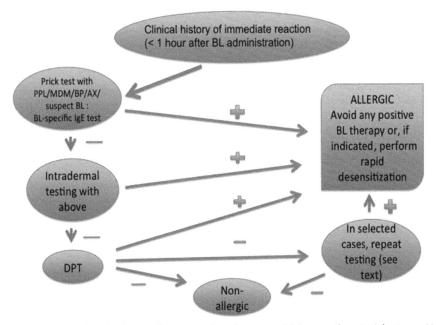

Fig. 1. Algorithm for the diagnosis of immediate hypersensitivity reactions to β-lactams. AX, amoxicillin; BL, β-lactams; BP, benzyl penicillin; DPT, drug provocation test; IgE, immunoglobulin E; MDM, minor determinant mixture; PPL, penicilloyl-polylisine.

of reactions to that seen in patients testing negative to both PPL and BP or MDM reagent.[39,56–60] Lin and colleagues[58] assessed 243 patients with self-reported penicillin allergy, of whom 20.6% reacted to BP derivatives, 9% only to penilloate and penicilloate, and 5.8% to amoxicillin. Even more striking were the findings of Macy,[39] in 242 patients with self-reported penicillin allergy. Only 2 reacted to benzylpenicilloyl polylysine, and on challenge with penicillin or amoxicillin, only 1.66% reacted.[39] The experience of one of the authors, over the last 3 years in Canada, supports these findings. In 350 patients skin test–negative to PPL, BP, and ampicillin, only a single patient suffered a delayed but mild rash after challenges with penicillin V or amoxicillin (Warrington RJ, personal communication, 2013).

It seems clear that over the past 20 years, the incidence of proven allergy to penicillin itself in patients reporting penicillin allergy has fallen steadily from a high of perhaps 20% to 5% or even less.[16] However, European experience suggests an increasing role for side-chain-specific determinants in penicillin allergy, particularly for amoxicillin.[61] In Europe, amoxicillin and ampicillin for intravenous use are used for skin testing, at concentrations of up to 25 mg/mL.[62,63] In North America, although ampicillin is available, the trihydrate of amoxicillin has been used, which limits the concentration that can be prepared for testing to about 4 mg/mL.[38,64] Nevertheless, this is still approximately equivalent to the concentration used for minor determinants and the above DPT studies suggest that allergic patients are not missed by using the lower concentration.[65]

An article by Torres and colleagues,[62] in which 330 patients with a history of immediate hypersensitivity reactions to penicillins were assessed, reported that 78.3% of the initial reactions were caused by either amoxicillin or ampicillin. Sixty-one percent showed positive skin tests to at least one reagent. There were 11.5% who were skin test–negative and ImmunocCAP positive, whereas 14.8% were skin test and ImmunoCAP–negative but reacted to DPT (in 55% cases to amoxicillin). Therefore, 12.1% had a negative drug-allergy workup. A study by Montanez and colleagues[66] of 276 patients with a history of immediate reactions to the association of amoxicillin/clavulanic acid found 19.9% positive to skin tests, 62% of these reacting to amoxicillin and tolerating benzylpenicillin challenge, whereas 29% reacted to clavulanic acid alone and tolerated benzylpencillin and amoxicillin. One hundred ninety patients were negative to all testing. In contrast, Macy and Ngor[39] found a rate of positive skin tests to PPL and BP in only 0.8% of 500 subjects, with only 4 (0.8%) subjects with negative skin tests reacting acutely to challenge. The difference seems to relate to the studied population, with immediate reactions occurring in all positive subjects in the studies by Torres and colleagues,[62] but only in 10.4% in the study of Macy and Ngor.[39]

With regard to cephalosporins, injectable forms are used for testing, usually at approximately 2 mg/mL, or even higher. Solutions can be made from oral capsules or pills.[67–70] However, the latter method is not as straightforward as the use of injectable forms of the drugs and requires careful standardization. Most often, specificity of IgE antibodies to cephalosporins is directed to the side-chain determinants, rather than the β-lactam ring, except in first-generation cephalosporins.[67,71] Studies conducted in both adults and children with histories of immediate reactions to these antibiotics have found the rate of positive skin tests to vary from 30.7% to 72.1%, using 2 mg/mL solutions. However, the negative predictive value of such testing remains uncertain, but may be approximately 82%.[67,71,72]

IgE-mediated hypersensitivity to β-lactams may decrease with time. It is therefore advised in European guidelines that patients who have suffered immediate reactions to β-lactams and are negative on the first evaluation, including provocation test, should be retested later.[73–77] In one of these studies, resensitization in the region of 27%, based on skin testing, was shown, but this was not confirmed when the skin test–positive patients were challenged. In this study, positive challenges were present in only a very small percentage of skin test–positive patients and not significantly more than was seen in skin test–negative patients.[77] These data are also supported by Solensky and colleagues,[78] who found that skin test–negative patients with a history of prior penicillin allergy were not resensitized after 3 full courses of therapy with penicillins. US Practice Parameters state that resensitization after treatment with oral penicillin is rare, and therefore, penicillin skin testing does not need to be routinely repeated in patients who have tolerated one or more courses of treatment with β-lactams.[79] It remains possible that resensitization may be more frequent after parenteral therapy but these data are not available.

It is important to raise the issue of what is considered to be a positive skin test for antibiotic allergy, because differences exist between Europe and North America. This difference is particularly an issue when there is little information available regarding DPT testing in skin test–positive patients. A positive response to skin testing with β-lactam reagents in Europe is considered to be a reaction that is 3 mm or more greater than the saline control, or an increase of 3 mm or more in the intradermal test, whereas in North America, with regard to Pre-Pen, a positive response is defined as a 5-mm or greater increase in either the prick test or the intradermal test. What is known of the reaction rates in skin test–positive subjects? The most recent data come from the study by Goldberg and Confino-Cohen, who used the criteria of a 3-mm increase in skin test reaction for prick tests and 5-mm increase for intradermal tests.[77] Seven of 67 skin test–positive patients reacted to penicillin or amoxicillin challenge (10.4%), whereas 4 of 94 skin test–negative subjects reacted, with positive and negative predictive values of 10.4% and 95.7%, respectively. At a second evaluation 2 to 5 months later, the positive predictive value of the repeated skin tests as assessed by DPT was 2.9%, and the negative predictive value was 97.6%. It is important to note that the patients in this study had non-life-threatening reactions to β-lactams more than 3 years before the allergy workup, and therefore, the results cannot be extrapolated to those individuals with more recent and more serious immediate hypersensitivity reactions.

When it comes to skin testing itself, European guidelines suggest that this can be spread out over several days, because of the risk of reactions occurring from the skin testing itself.[80] Although occasionally a patient may react to skin testing with an anaphylactic reaction, usually but not always this is after intradermal testing, and this would seem to be inordinately rare. It would seem unlikely to result if the testing were carried out using only standardized penicillin reagents and the β-lactam antibiotic to which the patient initially reacted. A review of the data on which this suggestion to delay testing is based indicates that 61% of the subjects who reacted to skin testing reacted to what would be considered to be standard skin test reagents used on the first day of testing.[81] What was striking was that reactions occurred in patients who had had immediate or anaphylactic reactions and who were tested within 5 months of that reaction, whereas in the non-reacting group, the delay to testing was approximately 18 months. Therefore, it is reasonable in patients with a recent history of an immediate reaction to start at lower concentrations and to limit the number of tests to major and minor determinants and the implicated β-lactam.

DPTs or graded challenges are recommended in appropriate cases, according to international guidelines. The AAAAI Practice Parameters recommend that DPT be carried out in patients who, after diagnostic testing or clinical evaluation, are considered unlikely to be allergic to the challenge drug.[36] Therefore, after negative skin and in vitro tests, the patient is given a full dose of the β-lactam in North America. The

EAACI/ENDA guidelines consider the DPT to be the gold standard to establish a definitive diagnosis in patients with convincing histories of drug hypersensitivity but negative diagnostic tests.[50] In such cases, challenge is begun with one-hundredth (or lower if the reaction was of rapid onset and/or severe) of the therapeutic dose, and if negative, one-tenth of the therapeutic dose is given half an hour to 1 hour later, followed by the full dose after a further half an hour to 1 hour. Challenges are obviously prohibited in cases of severe and serious reactions, such as SJS, TEN, AGEP, and DRESS.

Key issues outstanding between European and North American practice are as follows:

1. Availability and need for MDMs
2. Requirement for retesting after skin tests and challenge
3. Challenge protocols after negative testing
4. Importance of side-chain-specific allergy to penicillins

IMMEDIATE β-LACTAM ALLERGY IN CHILDREN

Although immediate β-lactam allergy in children is rare, it may occur and is evaluated by the diagnostic protocols used in adults. Atanaskovic-Markovic and coworkers assessed 1170 children who had histories of immediate reactions to penicillins and/ or cephalosporins by skin tests, specific IgE in vitro testing, and challenge.[82] Positive tests were found in 58.3%; of these, 94.4% were positive to penicillins and 35.3% to cephalosporins (ie, there was some cross-reactivity). Only approximately 40% were positive to amoxicillin or ampicillin. Tests were more likely to be positive when carried out within 6 months of the reaction. A later study by Ponvert and colleagues[83] of 1431 children found positive reactions in 30.9%, most by skin testing. Positive reactions were more likely when the reaction was immediate rather than delayed. The rate of systemic reactions from skin testing is low, only 1% to 3%, and the negative predictive value of challenge testing is high.

NONIMMEDIATE REACTIONS

Nonimmediate reactions to drugs can be extremely heterogeneous and similar to the symptoms of an infectious disease. In addition, the presence of a concomitant viral and possibly also a bacterial infection may favor the development of an apparent allergic reaction.[34]

To investigate a nonimmediate allergic drug reaction, unless the reaction is consistent with a life-threatening reaction, such as SJS, TEN, AGEP, or DRESS, when patch testing with appropriate concentrations of the drug is usually advised, intradermal skin tests and patch tests with the same reagents used to investigate immediate reactions are performed. Reactions to these tests may occur after several hours or days, so patients should be warned appropriately (**Fig. 2**).

Patch tests are administered in those who have suffered severe reactions listed above, and only if it is essential. Usually a concentration of 5% in petrolatum is used. Intradermal testing can be used in AGEP/DRESS, in case of negative results to patch tests and starting with lower concentrations. Intradermal testing is preferred in those with mild morbilliform reactions.

In a study by Romano and colleagues,[61] 36.2% of 433 adults with histories of delayed reactions to penicillins had positive skin tests, 96.9% of which were positive by patch or delayed-reading intradermal testing. Two hundred thirty-nine patients who were negative on skin testing had challenges and only 2.9% reacted.

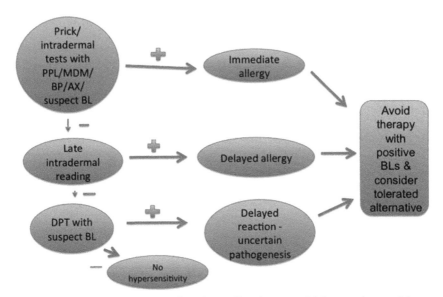

Fig. 2. Algorithm for the diagnosis of nonimmediate hypersensitivity reactions to β-lactams. AX, amoxicillin; BL, β-lactams; BP, benzyl penicillin; DPT, drug provocation test; MDM, minor determinant mixture; PPL, penicilloyl-polylisine.

The same group also assessed 105 adults with delayed reactions to cephalosporins. It was found that 6.6% were positive on skin testing, and of the 86 who were skin test–negative and were challenged, none reacted.[84]

Barbaud and colleagues[43] carried out patch tests to different drugs, including antibiotics, on 134 patients with AGEP, DRESS, and SJS/TEN within 1 year of the reaction. Positive tests were found in 64% of DRESS, 58% of AGEP, and 24% of SJS/TEN, with only one relapse of AGEP.

There are some concerns about whether a single therapeutic-dose drug challenge is sufficient to confirm or exclude a delayed reaction to penicillins. Borch and Bindslev-Jensen[85] found that of 22 patients with negative delayed-reading skin tests and single-dose challenge, 11 reacted during a 10-day therapeutic course. Nevertheless, in a multicenter study of patients with immediate or delayed reactions to β-lactams, the negative predictive value of a 1-day drug challenge was 94.1% (11 false negatives of 118 patients).[86]

Hjortlund and colleagues[87] studied 342 patients of whom 36 were considered to have had immediate reactions, 235 had nonimmediate reactions, and 71 could not be classified. All were assessed by immediate and delayed-reading skin testing, patch testing, and specific serum IgE assays. Of the 291 patients who tested negative, 10 reacted to a single-dose challenge and 23 to a 7-day challenge. There was no correlation between the history of the reaction and the time to reaction on challenge.

HYPERSENSITIVITY REACTIONS TO MONOBACTAMS, CARBAPENEMS

Allergic reactions to these antibiotics also containing the β-lactam ring are relatively uncommon, but are assessed in a similar manner to that used in the diagnosis of penicillin and cephalosporin allergy. Skin testing with aztreonam at 2 mg/mL has been of value in immediate allergy.[88–90] In a case of anaphylaxis to imipenem/cilastatin, this was diagnosed by skin testing at 1 mg/mL and by a positive serum-specific IgE assay.[91]

THE ADMINISTRATION OF ALTERNATIVE β-LACTAMS TO β-LACTAM-ALLERGIC PATIENTS

Cross-reactions may occur between β-lactams, particularly if the specific reaction is directed to the β-lactam ring or identical side-chain determinants.[92] However, in recent years, allergy to the common β-lactam ring seems to have become much less frequent than previously noted. Reactions may still occasionally occur in penicillin-allergic subjects given first-generation cephalosporins, but this is unusual and is rarely seen with second-generation or third-generation cephalosporins.[93–95] A meta-analysis by Pichichero and Casey[96] found an increased incidence of reactions to first-generation cephalosporins in penicillin-allergic subjects (OR = 4.8, CI = 3.7–6.2), but this analysis included studies from the 1970s, when the purity of cephalosporins was in question.[96] Macy and Burchette[79] found that of 42 penicillin skin test–positive patients receiving 129 courses of cephalosporins, 5.4% had reactions, compared with 3.2% in 80 skin test–negative controls who received 221 courses of cephalosporin therapy.[79]

Patients who have been shown to be allergic to amoxicillin should avoid cephalosporins with identical R-group side-chains, which include cefadroxil, cefprozil, and cefatrizine, while ampicillin-allergic subjects should avoid the cephalosporins, cephalexin, cefaclor, cephradine, cephaloglycin, and the carbacephem loracarbef.[82,97] It has also been noted that there is cross-reactivity between the cephalosporins with identical or similar side-chains, such as cefuroxime, cefotaxime, ceftriaxone, and ceftazidime.[67,71]

The best approach in someone with proven β-lactam allergy is to skin test with the drug that it is proposed to use, and if negative, give a graded challenge.[98]

NON-β-LACTAM ANTIBIOTICS
Quinolones

The quinolones are classified in generations: first (cinoxacin and nalidixic acid), second (ofloxacin, norfloxacin, ciprofloxacin, and enoxacin), third (levofloxacin), and fourth (gemifloxacin and moxifloxacin). With increasing use, hypersensitivity reactions have become more frequent.[99]

The main immediate reactions are urticaria, angioedema, and anaphylaxis, particularly in patients with cystic fibrosis.[99,100] Specific IgEs have been demonstrated to be present in more than 50% of patients by radioimmunoassay or basophil activation tests.[101,102] Nonimmediate reactions have also been described, including maculopapular rashes, fixed drug eruptions, AGEP, and SJS/TEN. Gemifloxacin seems to be the more frequent culprit and the incidence of such rashes is reported as 1% to 7%, especially in younger female patients.[103,104] T-cell-mediated responses have been demonstrated by patch testing or lymphocyte transformation testing.[99,105]

Skin testing with presumably nonirritant concentrations of quinolones has been carried out, but this has not been clearly shown to be reliable, because both false positive and false negative results may be obtained based on subsequent drug challenge (**Fig. 3**). In 64 subjects with immediate reactions to these drugs, 3 of 6 patients with positive skin tests tolerated challenges, whereas 3 of 45 subjects with negative skin tests reacted to challenge.[106] A recent study of 218 patients with histories of hypersensitivity reactions to fluoroquinolones using Basophil Activation Test (BAT) and DPTs found that 32.1% (69) had evidence for hypersensitivity, the majority for immediate and only 3 for nonimmediate. Risk factors for true hypersensitivity were an immediate reaction, a reaction to moxifloxacin, and past confirmed reactions to β-lactams.[100]

Cross-reactivity is unpredictable, appearing to be common between first-generation and second-generation quinolones (cinoxacin, nalidixic acid and ofloxacin,

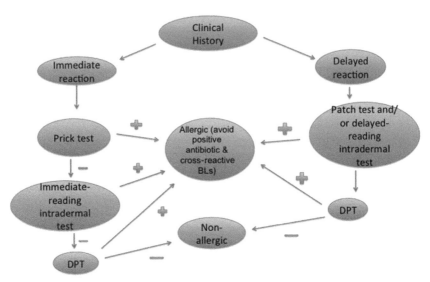

Fig. 3. Algorithm for the diagnosis of hypersensitivity reactions to non-β-lactam antibiotics. DPT, drug provocation test.

norfloxacin, ciprofloxacin, enoxacin), but less common with third (levofloxacin) and fourth generations (gemifloxacin, moxifloxacin).[99,101]

Macrolides

The macrolide antibiotics are classified according to the number of carbon atoms in the lactone ring: 14-membered (erythromycin, troleandromycin, roxithromycin, dirithromycin, and clarithromycin), 15-membered (azithromycin), and 16-membered (spiramycin, rokitamycin, josamycin, and midecamycin).

Hypersensitivity to these antibiotics is relatively uncommon (0.4%–3% of treatments), but immediate and nonimmediate reactions have been reported, including fixed drug eruptions and TEN.[107–110] There is little evidence with regard to the reliability of skin testing, with only single cases reported as positive.[107,111–113] Nonirritating concentrations are 0.05 mg/mL for erythromycin and 0.01 mg/mL for azithromycin. Positive skin tests have been described by patch testing at 10% in petrolatum or dimethylsulfoxide in fixed drug eruptions and contact reactions, but the sensitivity of skin tests is low.[107,109,114] Seitz and colleagues[115] found that only 1 of 125 patients with immediate or delayed reactions to macrolides had a positive skin test and challenges in 47 subjects with immediate reactions were negative, whereas 4 of 66 patients with delayed reactions were positive. In contrast, Mori and colleagues[110] reported that intradermal skin test sensitivity was 75% and specificity was 90% in 64 children with clarithromycin sensitivity.

Cross-reactivity among the 14-membered macrolides has been reported in single cases but it seems likely that there macrolide allergy is not a class hypersensitivity.[108,111,114]

Sulfonamides

Sulfonamide antibiotics are characterized by a sulfonamide (SO_2-NH_2) moiety attached to a benzene ring, carrying an unsubstituted amine at the N4 position.[116,117] Hypersensitivity reactions to sulfonamide antibiotics are common, occurring in 2% to 4% of healthy individuals and even more common in patients with AIDS, affecting as many as 50% to 60%.[118] Although immediate reactions are relatively uncommon, delayed reactions, such as maculopapular rashes, fixed drug eruptions, SJS/TEN, and DRESS, are more frequently reported.[117–119]

Intradermal tests may be useful in immediate and delayed reactions, when used at a concentration of 0.80 mg/mL.[120] Studies have shown IgE antibodies in some patients with immediate reactions.[121] However, Shapiro and colleagues[122] found positive skin tests in 4 of 28 patients tested and positive in vitro tests in 2 of 10. Recently, Kavadas and colleagues[123] reported on 6 of 11 patients with a history of immediate reactions to cotrimoxazole who had positive intradermal skin tests to the drug, but only one was challenged and reacted. Patch testing has been performed but the sensitivity is low, except when applied at the site of fixed drug eruptions.[124] Cross-reactivity between antibiotic sulfonamides has been reported,[116] but does not include nonantibiotic sulfonamides.[117]

Aminoglycosides

Aminoglycosides are subdivided into the streptidine group (streptomycin) and the deoxystreptamine group (kanamycin, amikacin, gentamicin, tobramycin, and neomycin). Immediate and nonimmediate reactions may occur. Immediate reactions may be diagnosed by skin testing, and streptomycin has been used at concentrations ranging from 0.1 ng/mL to 20 mg/mL.[125–127] Anaphylaxis from skin testing has been reported.[126]

Cases of anaphylaxis to other aminoglycosides have been occasionally reported, diagnosed by skin prick tests.[128–131] Hypersensitivity reactions to aminoglycosides occur frequently from contact. Such reactions may be immediate, like those with bacitracin and neomycin, or delayed. In the latter, patch tests are carried out with 20% concentration in petrolatum for neomycin, gentamicin, and tobramycin, but only at 1% for streptomycin.[132] There is significant cross-reactivity within the deoxystreptamine group.[133]

Clindamycin

This antibiotic may cause reactions, usually delayed maculopapular exanthemas. Notman and colleagues[134] have demonstrated the limited usefulness of skin testing in such cases, with only 2 of 31 patients showing positive delayed-reading skin tests, whereas 10 of the 31 reacted to challenge.

Patch testing for clindamycin allergy may have some value, with 30% positive tests at 10% in petrolatum.[135] However, in a study by Seitz and colleagues[135] of 26 patch test–negative subjects, 6 reacted.

Rifamycins

Anaphylactic reactions have occurred with both rifampicin and rifamycin, with positive intradermal skin tests at 0.006 mg/mL for rifampicin and 50 μg/mL to 5 mg/mL for rifamycin.[136–140]

Glycopeptides

Vancomycin most commonly causes "red man syndrome," associated with too rapid intravenous administration of the drug, and characterized by flushing, warmth, pruritus, and hypotension. Rarely, allergic reactions are reported, and a positive intradermal skin test with 0.1 μg/mL has been reported.[141] Nonimmediate reactions, including severe reactions such as SJS, TEN, and DRESS, can occur. Positive patch tests have been reported in delayed eruption.[43,142]

SUMMARY

Antibiotic allergy is overdiagnosed, often resulting in the administration of less appropriate and more expensive antibiotics, with increasing costs and development of resistance through the use of more broad-spectrum drugs. The appropriate diagnosis and management of patients with reported antibiotic allergy is essential to good medical care and it requires the appropriate use of diagnostic tests, when these are available. Unfortunately, this is often difficult to achieve because of the lack of appropriate reagents, often because of the shortsightedness of regulatory authorities. In other instances, there has been insufficient research carried out to define appropriate diagnostic techniques, except in situations such as β-lactam allergy. Differences exist in different parts of the world in regard to the appropriate means to investigate drug allergy, but to a large extent, these may be the result of a lack of access and standardization rather than true differences in the frequency and type of drug-induced hypersensitivity.

REFERENCES

1. Pichler W, Naisbitt D, Park B. Immune pathomechanism of drug hypersensitivity reactions. J Allergy Clin Immunol 2011;127:S74–81.
2. Jenkins R, Yaseen F, Monshi M, et al. beta-Lactam antibiotics form distinct haptenic structures on albumin and activate drug-specific T-lymphocyte responses in multiallergic patients with cystic fibrosis. Chem Res Toxicol 2013; 26:963–75.
3. Meng X, Jenkins R, Berry N, et al. Direct evidence for the formation of diastereoisomeric benzylpenicilloyl haptens from benzylpenicillin and benzylpenicillenic acid in patients. J Pharmacol Exp Ther 2011;338:841–9.
4. Levine B. Immunologic mechanisms of penicillin allergy. A haptenic model system for the study of allergic diseases of man. N Engl J Med 1966;275:1115–25.
5. Pichler WJ. Immune mechanism of drug hypersensitivity. Immunol Allergy Clin North Am 2004;24:373–97, v–vi.
6. Perez-Inestrosa E, Suau R, Montanez M, et al. Cephalosporin chemical reactivity and its immunological implications. Curr Opin Allergy Clin Immunol 2005;5: 323–30.
7. Elsheikh A, Castrejon L, Lavergne S, et al. Enhanced antigenicity leads to altered immunogenicity in sulfamethoxazole-hypersensitive patients with cystic fibrosis. J Allergy Clin Immunol 2011;127:1543–51.e3.
8. Elsheikh A, Lavergne S, Castrejon J, et al. Drug antigenicity, immunogenicity, and costimulatory signaling: evidence for formation of a functional antigen through immune cell metabolism. J Immunol 2010;185:6448–60.
9. El-Ghaiesh S, Monshi M, Whitaker P, et al. Characterization of the antigen specificity of T-cell clones from piperacillin-hypersensitive patients with cystic fibrosis. J Pharmacol Exp Ther 2012;341:597–610.
10. Zaheer-ul-Haq, Khan W. Molecular and structural determinants of adamantyl susceptibility to HLA-DRs allelic variants: an in silico approach to understand the mechanism of MLEs. J Comput Aided Mol Des 2011;25:81–101.
11. Pichler W. Pharmacological interaction of drugs with antigen-specific immune receptors: the p-i concept. Curr Opin Allergy Clin Immunol 2002;2:301–5.
12. Posadas S, Pichler W. Delayed drug hypersensitivity reactions—new concepts. Clin Exp Allergy 2007;37:989–99.
13. Illing P, Vivian J, Dudek N, et al. Immune self-reactivity triggered by drug-modified HLA-peptide repertoire. Nature 2012;486:554–8.

14. Adam J, Eriksson K, Schnyder B, et al. Avidity determines T-cell reactivity in abacavir hypersensitivity. Eur J Immunol 2012;42(7):1706–16.
15. Solensky R. Allergy to beta-lactam antibiotics. J Allergy Clin Immunol 2012;130: 1442-2.e5.
16. Macy E, Schatz M, Lin C, et al. The falling rate of positive penicillin skin tests from 1995 to 2007. Perm J 2009;13:12–8.
17. Gomes E, Demoly P. Epidemiology of hypersensitivity drug reactions. Curr Opin Allergy Clin Immunol 2005;5:309–16.
18. Smyth R, Gargon E, Kirkham J, et al. Adverse drug reactions in children–a systematic review. PLoS One 2012;7:e24061.
19. Rawlins MD, Thompson JW. Pathogenesis of adverse drug reactions. In: Davis DM, editor. Textbook of Adverse Drug Reactions. New York: Oxford University Press; 1977. p. 832–6.
20. Johansson S, Bieber T, Dahl R, et al. Revised nomenclature for allergy for global use: report of the Nomenclature Review Committee of the World Allergy Organization, October 2003. J Allergy Clin Immunol 2004;113:832–6.
21. Romano A, Torres M, Castells M, et al. Diagnosis and management of drug hypersensitivity reactions. J Allergy Clin Immunol 2011;127:S67–73.
22. Pichler W. Delayed drug hypersensitivity reactions. Ann Intern Med 2003;139: 683–93.
23. Romano A, Blanca M, Torres M, et al. Diagnosis of nonimmediate reactions to beta-lactam antibiotics. Allergy 2004;59:1153–60.
24. Demoly P, Bousquet J. Drug allergy diagnosis work up. Allergy 2002;57(Suppl 72): 37–40.
25. Gomez E, Blanca-Lopez N, Salas M, et al. Induction of accelerated reactions to amoxicillin by T-cell effector mechanisms. Ann Allergy Asthma Immunol 2013; 110:267–73.
26. Bircher A, Scherer K. Delayed cutaneous manifestations of drug hypersensitivity. Med Clin North Am 2010;94:711–25, x.
27. Bircher A, Scherer Hofmeier K. Drug hypersensitivity reactions: inconsistency in the use of the classification of immediate and nonimmediate reactions. J Allergy Clin Immunol 2012;129:263–4 [author reply: 255–6].
28. Chang C, Mahmood M, Teuber S, et al. Overview of penicillin allergy. Clin Rev Allergy Immunol 2012;43:84–97.
29. Warrington R, Silviu-Dan F, Magro C. Accelerated cell-mediated immune reactions in penicillin allergy. J Allergy Clin Immunol 1993;92:626–8.
30. Adkinson NJ. Risk factors for drug allergy. J Allergy Clin Immunol 1984;74: 567–72.
31. Pirmohamed M, Park BK. HIV and drug allergy. Curr Opin Allergy Clin Immunol 2001;1:311–6.
32. Jappe U. Amoxicillin-induced exanthema in patients with infectious mononucleosis: allergy or transient immunostimulation? Allergy 2007;62:1474–5.
33. Renn CN, Straff W, Dorfmuller A, et al. Amoxicillin-induced exanthema in young adults with infectious mononucleosis: demonstration of drug-specific lymphocyte reactivity. Br J Dermatol 2002;147:1166–70.
34. Blanca M, Romano A, Torres M, et al. Update on the evaluation of hypersensitivity reactions to betalactams. Allergy 2009;64:183–93.
35. Brockow K, Romano A, Blanca M, et al. General considerations for skin test procedures in the diagnosis of drug hypersensitivity. Allergy 2002;57:45–51.
36. Solensky R, Khan DA. Drug allergy: an updated practice parameter. Ann Allergy Asthma Immunol 2010;105:259–73.

37. Macy E, Richter P, Falkoff R, et al. Skin testing with penicilloate and penilloate prepared by an improved method: amoxicillin oral challenge in patients with negative skin test responses to penicillin reagents. J Allergy Clin Immunol 1997;100:586–91.
38. Macy E. The clinical evaluation of penicillin allergy: what is necessary, sufficient and safe given the materials currently available? Clin Exp Allergy 2011;41: 1498–501.
39. Macy E, Ngor E. Safely diagnosing clinically significant penicillin allergy using only penicilloyl-poly-lysine, penicillin, and oral amoxicillin. J Allergy Clin Immunol 2013;1(3):258–63.
40. Elzagallaai AA, Koren G, Bend JR, et al. In vitro testing for hypersensitivity-mediated adverse drug reactions: challenges and future directions. Clin Pharmacol Ther 2011;90:455–60.
41. Torres M, Padial A, Mayorga C, et al. The diagnostic interpretation of basophil activation test in immediate allergic reactions to betalactams. Clin Exp Allergy 2004;34:1768–75.
42. Macy E, Goldberg B, Poon K. Use of commercial anti-penicillin IgE fluorometric enzyme immunoassays to diagnose penicillin allergy. Ann Allergy Asthma Immunol 2010;105:136–41.
43. Barbaud A, Collet E, Milpied B, et al. A multicentre study to determine the value and safety of drug patch tests for the three main classes of severe cutaneous adverse drug reactions. Br J Dermatol 2013;168:555–62.
44. Pichler W, Tilch J. The lymphocyte transformation test in the diagnosis of drug hypersensitivity. Allergy 2004;59:809–20.
45. Warrington RJ, Tse KS. Lymphocyte transformation studies in drug hypersensitivity. Can Med Assoc J 1979;120:1089–94.
46. Warrington R, Sauder P, McPhillips S. Lymphocyte transformation studies in suspected hypersensitivity to trimethoprim-sulphamethoxazole. Clin Allergy 1983; 13:235–40.
47. Tanvarasethee B, Buranapraditkun S, Klaewsongkram J. The potential of using enzyme-linked immunospot to diagnose cephalosporin-induced maculopapular exanthems. Acta Derm Venereol 2013;93:66–9.
48. Rozieres A, Hennino A, Rodet K, et al. Detection and quantification of drug-specific T cells in penicillin allergy. Allergy 2009;64:534–42.
49. Johansson SG, Adedoyin J, van Hage M, et al. False-positive penicillin immunoassay: an unnoticed common problem. J Allergy Clin Immunol 2013;132:235–7.
50. Aberer W, Bircher A, Romano A, et al. Drug provocation testing in the diagnosis of drug hypersensitivity reactions: general considerations. Allergy 2003;58: 854–63.
51. Messaad D, Sahla H, Benahmed S, et al. Drug provocation tests in patients with a history suggesting an immediate drug hypersensitivity reaction. Ann Intern Med 2004;140:1001–6.
52. Macy E. Penicillin allergy might not be very common in subjects with cephalosporin allergy. J Allergy Clin Immunol 2011;127:1638 [author reply: 1638–9].
53. Warrington RJ, Simons FE, Ho HW, et al. Diagnosis of penicillin allergy by skin testing: the Manitoba experience. Can Med Assoc J 1978;118:787–91.
54. Blanca M, Mayorga C, Torres M, et al. Side-chain-specific reactions to betalactams: 14 years later. Clin Exp Allergy 2002;32:192–7.
55. Torres M, Blanca M. The complex clinical picture of beta-lactam hypersensitivity: penicillins, cephalosporins, monobactams, carbapenems, and clavams. Med Clin North Am 2010;94:805–20, xii.

56. Solley G, Gleich G, Van Dellen R. Penicillin allergy: clinical experience with a battery of skin-test reagents. J Allergy Clin Immunol 1982;69:238–44.
57. Gadde J, Spence M, Wheeler B, et al. Clinical experience with penicillin skin testing in a large inner-city STD clinic. JAMA 1993;270:2456–63.
58. Lin E, Saxon A, Riedl M. Penicillin allergy: value of including amoxicillin as a determinant in penicillin skin testing. Int Arch Allergy Immunol 2010;152:313–8.
59. Bousquet P, Co-Minh H, Arnoux B, et al. Importance of mixture of minor determinants and benzylpenicilloyl poly-L-lysine skin testing in the diagnosis of beta-lactam allergy. J Allergy Clin Immunol 2005;115:1314–6.
60. Torres MJ, Blanca M. The contribution of major and minor determinants from benzylpenicillin to the diagnosis of immediate allergy to beta-lactams. J Allergy Clin Immunol 2006;117:220–1 [author reply: 221].
61. Romano A, Gaeta F, Valluzzi R, et al. The very limited usefulness of skin testing with penicilloyl-polylysine and the minor determinant mixture in evaluating non-immediate reactions to penicillins. Allergy 2010;65:1104–7.
62. Torres M, Mayorga C, Leyva L, et al. Controlled administration of penicillin to patients with a positive history but negative skin and specific serum IgE tests. Clin Exp Allergy 2002;32:270–6.
63. Torres MJ, Romano A, Mayorga C, et al. Diagnostic evaluation of a large group of patients with immediate allergy to penicillins: the role of skin testing. Allergy 2001;56:850–6.
64. Montanez M, Torres M, Perez-Inestrosa E, et al. Clarification concerning amoxicillin skin testing. J Allergy Clin Immunol 2011;128:685 [author reply: 686].
65. Macy E, Ngor E. Recommendations for the management of beta-lactam intolerance. Clin Rev Allergy Immunol 2013. [Epub ahead of print].
66. Torres M, Ariza A, Mayorga C, et al. Clavulanic acid can be the component in amoxicillin-clavulanic acid responsible for immediate hypersensitivity reactions. J Allergy Clin Immunol 2010;125:502–5.e2.
67. Romano A, Gueant-Rodriguez R, Viola M, et al. Diagnosing immediate reactions to cephalosporins. Clin Exp Allergy 2005;35:1234–42.
68. Yoon S, Park S, Kim S, et al. Validation of the cephalosporin intradermal skin test for predicting immediate hypersensitivity: a prospective study with drug challenge. Allergy 2013;68:938–44.
69. Dickson S, Salazar K. Diagnosis and management of immediate hypersensitivity reactions to cephalosporins. Clin Rev Allergy Immunol 2013;45:131–42.
70. Somech R, Weber EA, Lavi S. Evaluation of immediate allergic reactions to cephalosporins in non-penicillin-allergic patients. Int Arch Allergy Immunol 2009;150:205–9.
71. Antunez C, Blanca-Lopez N, Torres MJ, et al. Immediate allergic reactions to cephalosporins: evaluation of cross-reactivity with a panel of penicillins and cephalosporins. J Allergy Clin Immunol 2006;117:404–10.
72. Romano A, Gaeta F, Valluzzi R, et al. Diagnosing hypersensitivity reactions to cephalosporins in children. Pediatrics 2008;122:521–7.
73. Garcia Nunez I, Barasona Villarejo MJ, Algaba Marmol MA, et al. Diagnosis of patients with immediate hypersensitivity to beta-lactams using retest. J Investig Allergol Clin Immunol 2012;22:41–7.
74. Parker PJ, Parrinello JT, Condemi JJ, et al. Penicillin resensitization among hospitalized patients. J Allergy Clin Immunol 1991;88:213–7.
75. Pichichero M, Pichichero D. Diagnosis of penicillin, amoxicillin, and cephalosporin allergy: reliability of examination assessed by skin testing and oral challenge. J Pediatr 1998;132:137–43.

76. Torres MJ, Sanchez-Sabate E, Alvarez J, et al. Skin test evaluation in nonimmediate allergic reactions to penicillins. Allergy 2004;59:219–24.
77. Goldberg A, Confino-Cohen R. Skin testing and oral penicillin challenge in patients with a history of remote penicillin allergy. Ann Allergy Asthma Immunol 2008;100:37–43.
78. Solensky R, Earl H, Gruchalla R. Lack of penicillin resensitization in patients with a history of penicillin allergy after receiving repeated penicillin courses. Arch Intern Med 2002;162:822–6.
79. Macy E, Burchette R. Oral antibiotic adverse reactions after penicillin skin testing: multi-year follow-up. Allergy 2002;57:1151–8.
80. Torres M, Blanca M, Fernandez J, et al. Diagnosis of immediate allergic reactions to beta-lactam antibiotics. Allergy 2003;58:961–72.
81. Co Minh H, Bousquet P, Fontaine C, et al. Systemic reactions during skin tests with beta-lactams: a risk factor analysis. J Allergy Clin Immunol 2006;177:466–8.
82. Atanaskovic-Markovic M, Velickovic T, Gavrovic-Jankulovic M, et al. Immediate allergic reactions to cephalosporins and penicillins and their cross-reactivity in children. Pediatr Allergy Immunol 2005;16:341–7.
83. Ponvert C, Perrin Y, Bados-Albiero A, et al. Allergy to betalactam antibiotics in children: results of a 20-year study based on clinical history, skin and challenge tests. Pediatr Allergy Immunol 2011;22:411–8.
84. Romano A, Gaeta F, Valluzzi R, et al. Diagnosing nonimmediate reactions to cephalosporins. J Allergy Clin Immunol 2012;129:1166–9.
85. Borch J, Bindslev-Jensen C. Full-course drug challenge test in the diagnosis of delayed allergic reactions to penicillin. Int Arch Allergy Immunol 2011;155:271–4.
86. Demoly P, Romano A, Botelho C, et al. Determining the negative predictive value of provocation tests with beta-lactams. Allergy 2010;65:327–32.
87. Hjortlund J, Mortz C, Skov P, et al. Diagnosis of penicillin allergy revisited: the value of case history, skin testing, specific IgE and prolonged challenge. Allergy 2013;68:1057–64.
88. Iglesias Cadarso A, Saez Jimenez S, Vidal Pan C, et al. Aztreonam-induced anaphylaxis. Lancet 1990;336:746–7.
89. de la Fuente Prieto R, Armentia Medina A, Sanchez Palla P, et al. Urticaria caused by sensitization to aztreonam. Allergy 1993;48:634–6.
90. Perez Pimiento A, Gomez Martinez M, Minguez Mena A, et al. Aztreonam and ceftazidime: evidence of in vivo cross allergenicity. Allergy 1998;53:624–5.
91. Chen Z, Baur X, Kutscha-Lissberg F, et al. IgE-mediated anaphylactic reaction to imipenem. Allergy 2000;55:92–3.
92. Romano A, Gueant-Rodriguez R, Viola M, et al. Cross-reactivity among drugs: clinical problems. Toxicology 2005;209:169–79.
93. Romano A, Viola M, Gueant-Rodriguez R, et al. Imipenem in patients with immediate hypersensitivity to penicillins. N Engl J Med 2006;354:2835–7.
94. Romano A, Viola M, Gueant-Rodriguez R, et al. Brief communication: tolerability of meropenem in patients with IgE-mediated hypersensitivity to penicillins. Ann Intern Med 2007;146:266–9.
95. Romano A, Gaeta F, Valluzzi R, et al. IgE-mediated hypersensitivity to cephalosporins: cross-reactivity and tolerability of penicillins, monobactams, and carbapenems. J Allergy Clin Immunol 2010;126:994–9.
96. Pichichero ME, Casey JR. Safe use of selected cephalosporins in penicillin-allergic patients: a meta-analysis. Otolaryngol Head Neck Surg 2007;136:340–7.
97. Atanaskovic-Markovic M. Educational case series: beta-lactam allergy and cross-reactivity. Pediatr Allergy Immunol 2011;22:770–5.

98. Romano A, Gueant-Rodriguez R, Viola M, et al. Cross-reactivity and tolerability of cephalosporins in patients with immediate hypersensitivity to penicillins. Ann Intern Med 2004;141:16–22.

99. Blanca-Lopez N, Andreu I, Torres Jaen M. Hypersensitivity reactions to quinolones. Curr Opin Allergy Clin Immunol 2011;11:285–91.

100. Blanca-Lopez N, Ariza A, Dona I, et al. Hypersensitivity reactions to fluoroquinolones: analysis of the factors involved. Clin Exp Allergy 2013;43:560–7.

101. Manfredi M, Severino M, Testi S, et al. Detection of specific IgE to quinolones. J Allergy Clin Immunol 2004;113:155–60.

102. Aranda A, Mayorga C, Ariza A, et al. In vitro evaluation of IgE-mediated hypersensitivity reactions to quinolones. Allergy 2011;66:247–54.

103. Ball P. Adverse drug reactions: implications for the development of fluoroquinolones. J Antimicrob Chemother 2003;51(Suppl 1):21–7.

104. Iannini P, Mandell L, Felmingham J, et al. Adverse cutaneous reactions and drugs: a focus on antimicrobials. J Chemother 2006;18:127–39.

105. Schmid D, Depta J, Pichler W. T cell-mediated hypersensitivity to quinolones: mechanisms and cross-reactivity. Clin Exp Allergy 2006;36:59–69.

106. Seitz C, Brocker E, Trautmann A. Diagnostic testing in suspected fluoroquinolone hypersensitivity. Clin Exp Allergy 2009;39:1738–45.

107. Araujo L, Demoly P. Macrolides allergy. Curr Pharm Des 2008;14:2840–62.

108. San Pedro de Saenz B, Gomez A, Quiralte J, et al. FDE to macrolides. Allergy 2002;57:55–6.

109. Benahmed S, Scaramuzza C, Messaad D, et al. The accuracy of the diagnosis of suspected macrolide antibiotic hypersensitivity: results of a single-blinded trial. Allergy 2004;59:1130–3.

110. Mori F, Barni S, Pucci N, et al. Sensitivity and specificity of skin tests in the diagnosis of clarithromycin allergy. Ann Allergy Asthma Immunol 2010;104:417–9.

111. Pascual C, Crespo J, Quiralte J, et al. In vitro detection of specific IgE antibodies to erythromycin. J Allergy Clin Immunol 1995;95:668–71.

112. Kruppa A, Scharffetter-Kochanek K, Krieg T, et al. Immediate reaction to roxithromycin and prick test cross-sensitization to erythromycin and clarithromycin. Dermatology 1998;196:335–6.

113. Swamy N, Laurie S, Ruiz-Huidobro E, et al. Successful clarithromycin desensitization in a multiple macrolide-allergic patient. Ann Allergy Asthma Immunol 2010;105:489–90.

114. Milkovic-Kraus S, Macan J, Kanceljak-Macan B. Occupational allergic contact dermatitis from azithromycin in pharmaceutical workers: a case series. Contact Dermatitis 2007;56:99–102.

115. Seitz C, Brocker E, Trautmann A. Suspicion of macrolide allergy after treatment of infectious diseases including Helicobacter pylori: results of allergological testing. Allergol Immunopathol (Madr) 2011;39:193–9.

116. Zawodniak A, Lochmatter P, Beeler A, et al. Cross-reactivity in drug hypersensitivity reactions to sulfasalazine and sulfamethoxazole. Int Arch Allergy Immunol 2010;153:152–6.

117. Schnyder B, Pichler W. Allergy to sulfonamides. J Allergy Clin Immunol 2013;131:256–7.e1-5.

118. Gruchalla R. 10. Drug allergy. J Allergy Clin Immunol 2003;111:S548–59.

119. van der Klauw M, Wilson J, Stricker B. Drug-associated anaphylaxis: 20 years of reporting in The Netherlands (1974-1994) and review of the literature. Clin Exp Allergy 1996;26:1355–63.

120. Empedrad R, Darter A, Earl H, et al. Nonirritating intradermal skin test concentrations for commonly prescribed antibiotics. J Allergy Clin Immunol 2003;112:629–30.
121. Gruchalla R, Sullivan T. Detection of human IgE to sulfamethoxazole by skin testing with sulfamethoxazoyl-poly-L-tyrosine. J Allergy Clin Immunol 1991;88:784–92.
122. Shapiro L, Knowles S, Weber E, et al. Safety of celecoxib in individuals allergic to sulfonamide: a pilot study. Drug Saf 2003;26:187–95.
123. Kavadas FD, Kasprzak A, Atkinson AR. Antibiotic skin testing accompanied by provocative challenges in children is a useful clinical tool. Allergy Asthma Clin Immunol 2013;9:22.
124. Tornero P, De Barrio M, Baeza M, et al. Cross-reactivity among p-amino group compounds in sulfonamide fixed drug eruption: diagnostic value of patch testing. Contact Dermatitis 2004;51:57–62.
125. Gilbert DN. Mandell, Douglas and Bennett's Principles and Practice of Infectious Diseases. Philadelphia: Churchill Livingstone Elsevier; 2010.
126. Romano A, Viola M, Di Fonso M, et al. Anaphylaxis to streptomycin. Allergy 2002;57:1087–8.
127. Connolly M, McAdoo J, Bourke J. Gentamicin-induced anaphylaxis. Ir J Med Sci 2007;176:317–8.
128. Dyck E, Vadas P. Anaphylaxis to topical bacitracin. Allergy 1997;52:870–1.
129. Sharif S, Goldberg B. Detection of IgE antibodies to bacitracin using a commercially available streptavidin-linked solid phase in a patient with anaphylaxis to triple antibiotic ointment. Ann Allergy Asthma Immunol 2007;98:563–6.
130. Gall R, Blakley B, Warrington R, et al. Intraoperative anaphylactic shock from bacitracin nasal packing after septorhinoplasty. Anesthesiology 1999;91:1545–7.
131. Lee Y, Cho Y, Han M. Anaphylaxis due to ribostamycin. Allergy 2004;59:1134–5.
132. Gehrig K, Warshaw E. Allergic contact dermatitis to topical antibiotics: epidemiology, responsible allergens, and management. J Am Acad Dermatol 2008;58:1–21.
133. Liippo J, Lammintausta K. Positive patch test reactions to gentamicin show sensitization to aminoglycosides from topical therapies, bone cements, and from systemic medication. Contact Dermatitis 2008;59:268–72.
134. Notman M, Phillips E, Knowles S, et al. Clindamycin skin testing has limited diagnostic potential. Contact Dermatitis 2005;53:335–8.
135. Seitz C, Brocker E, Trautmann A. Allergy diagnostic testing in clindamycin-induced skin reactions. Int Arch Allergy Immunol 2009;149:246–50.
136. Scala E, Giani M, Pirrotta L, et al. Multiple drug allergy syndrome: severe anaphylactic reaction due to topical rifamycin SV in a patient with hypersensitivity to ciprofloxacin. Int J Dermatol 2001;40:603–4.
137. Ebo D, Verheecke G, Bridts C, et al. Perioperative anaphylaxis from locally applied rifamycin SV and latex. Br J Anaesth 2006;96:738–41.
138. Buergin S, Scherer K, Hausermann P, et al. Immediate hypersensitivity to rifampicin in 3 patients: diagnostic procedures and induction of clinical tolerance. Int Arch Allergy Immunol 2006;140:20–6.
139. Cardot E, Tillie-Leblond I, Jeannin P, et al. Anaphylactic reaction to local administration of rifamycin SV. J Allergy Clin Immunol 1995;95:1–7.
140. Erel F, Karaayvaz M, Deveci M, et al. Severe anaphylaxis from rifamycin SV. Ann Allergy Asthma Immunol 1998;81:257–60.
141. Anne' S, Middleton EJ, Reisman R. Vancomycin anaphylaxis and successful desensitization. Ann Allergy 1994;73:402–4.
142. Bernedo N, Gonzalez I, Gastaminza G, et al. Positive patch test in vancomycin allergy. Contact Dermatitis 2001;45:43.

Hypersensitivity Reactions to Nonsteroidal Anti-Inflammatory Drugs

Maria Jose Torres, MD, PhD[a], Esther Barrionuevo, MD[a],
Marek Kowalski, MD, PhD[b,c], Miguel Blanca, MD, PhD[a,*]

KEYWORDS

- Nonsteroidal anti-inflammatory drugs • Hypersensitivity • Clinical diagnosis
- Allergic • Nonallergic • Management

KEY POINTS

- Nonsteroidal anti-inflammatory drugs are the most frequent drugs involved in hypersensitivity drug reactions.
- The mechanisms involved can be specific (immunologic), whether mediated by immunoglobulin E or T cells or by activation of pathways that release vasoactive mediators.
- Five major well-defined clinical entities are currently recognized, although overlapping may exist.
- The diagnosis is mostly based on clinical history and a drug-provocation test.
- Management consists of drug eviction, providing alternatives such as paracetamol and cyclooxygenase-2 inhibitors and, when needed, desensitization.

INTRODUCTION

Nonsteroidal anti-inflammatory drugs (NSAIDs) are among the medicines most frequently prescribed worldwide, many of which are available over the counter.[1] NSAIDs induce a wide variety of adverse reactions that are classified as type A (predictable and usually related to the effects of the drug) and type B (unpredictable and related to the individual response).[2] This review deals with type B drug hypersensitivity reactions (DHR), mediated by immunologic (allergic) or nonspecific pharmacologic mechanisms (nonallergic).[3] NSAIDs are of great concern because they are the drugs most commonly involved in DHR.[4–7]

The authors have nothing to disclose.
This review was supported by grants from Carlos III National Health Institute RD12/0013/0001 (RIRAAF network), PI10/01598, PI12/02247, and PI13/02598.
[a] Allergy Unit, University Hospital-IBIMA, Malaga 29008, Spain; [b] Department of Immunology Rheumatology and Allergy, Medical University of Lodz, Lodz, Poland; [c] Department of Immunology, Rheumatology & Allergy, Chair of Clinical Immunology and Microbiology, Medical University of Lodz, 251 Pomorska Street Blg 5, Lodz 92213, Poland
* Corresponding author. Allergy Unit, University Hospital-IBIMA, Plaza Hospital Civil s/n, Malaga 29008, Spain.
E-mail address: mblancago@gmail.com

CLASSIFICATION

NSAIDs have different chemical structures that share the capacity for inhibiting cyclo-oxygenase (COX) enzymes (COX-1 and COX-2) (**Table 1**). The mechanism for inducing DHR is related to the release of vasoactive mediators (histamine, prostaglandins, and sulfidopeptide leukotrienes [LTs])[5] or is due to their recognition as xenobiotics, inducing immunoglobulin E (IgE) or T-cell responses.[4]

The authors use the nomenclature for DHR proposed by the European Academy of Allergy and Clinical Immunology (EAACI),[3] based on the timing of reactions (acute or delayed), clinical pattern of symptoms (respiratory and/or cutaneous and/or anaphylaxis), and the presence or absence of cross-tolerance to other chemically unrelated NSAIDs.[5,6] Cross-reactive types (1, 2, and 3) involve nonallergic mechanisms while single-drug–induced types (4 and 5) involve allergic, putative IgE, and T-cell–mediated mechanisms (**Table 2**).[8–10] In addition, the presence of underlying chronic inflammatory disease of the skin (chronic spontaneous urticaria [CSU]) and of the respiratory tract (asthma/chronic rhinosinusitis [CRS]) should be considered. This phenotype-based classification allows the use of a simple history-based algorithm for diagnosis (**Fig. 1**) and indicates putative underlying mechanisms.[7]

EPIDEMIOLOGY

NSAIDs are usually reported to be the second most important group of drugs involved in DHRs after antibiotics, although recent studies indicate that they are in fact the principal group.[11–13] The prevalence of self-reported DHR to NSAIDs has been shown to be 1.9%, with acetylsalicylic acid (ASA; aspirin) and ibuprofen being the most frequent

Table 1
Examples of NSAIDs according to capacity for COX enzyme inhibition

Nonselective COX inhibitors	Salicylic acid derivatives	Acetylsalicylic acid	
	Indoleacetic acids	Indomethacin	
	Heteroaryl acetic acids	Diclofenac	
	Arylpropionic acids	Ibuprofen	
	Enolic acids	Piroxicam	
	Para-aminophenol derivatives	Paracetamol	
	Alkanones	Nabumetone	
	Anthranilic acids	Mefenamic acid	
Selective COX-2 inhibitors	Diaryl-substituted pyrazoles	Celecoxib	

From Cornejo-Garcia JA, Blanca-Lopez N, Doña I, et al. Hypersensitivity reactions to non-steroidal anti-inflammatory drugs. Curr Drug Metab 2009;10:973; with permission.

Table 2
Type of reactions and clinical manifestations induced by NSAIDs

Type of Reaction	Clinical Manifestation	Timing of Reaction	Underlying Disease	Cross-Reactivity	Putative Mechanism	
NSAID-exacerbated respiratory disease	Bronchial obstruction, dyspnea, and/or nasal congestion/ rhinorrhea	Acute (usually immediate to several hours after exposure)	Asthma/rhinosinusitis	Cross-reactive	Nonallergic	COX-1 inhibition
NSAID-exacerbated cutaneous disease	Wheals and/or angioedema		Chronic urticaria			COX-1 inhibition
NSAID-induced urticaria/angioedema	Wheals and/or angioedema		No underlying chronic diseases			Unknown, probably COX-1 inhibition
Single NSAID–induced urticaria/angioedema or anaphylaxis	Wheals/angioedema/ anaphylaxis		No underlying chronic diseases	Not cross-reactive	Allergic	IgE mediated
Single NSAID–induced delayed reactions	Various symptoms and organs involved (eg, fixed drug eruption, SJS/TEN, nephritis)	Delayed onset (usually more than 24 h after exposure)	No underlying chronic diseases			T-cell mediated

Abbreviations: SJS, Stevens-Johnson syndrome; TEN, toxic epidermal necrolysis.

From Kowalski ML, Asero R, Bavbek S, et al. Classification and practical approach to the diagnosis and management of hypersensitivity to nonsteroidal anti-inflammatory drugs. Allergy 2013;68:1221; with permission.

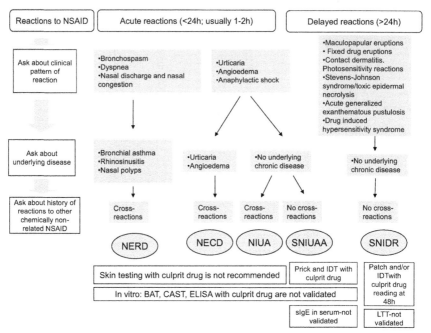

Fig. 1. Five major groups of clinical entities induced by NSAIDs with a practical approach for their identification. BAT, basophil activation test; CAST, cellular allergy stimulation test; ELISA, enzyme-linked immunosorbent assay; IDT, intradermal test; LTT, lymphocyte transformation test; NECD, NSAID-exacerbated cutaneous disease; NERD, NSAID-exacerbated respiratory disease; NIUA, NSAID-induced urticaria/angioedema; sIgE, specific IgE; SNIDR, single NSAID–induced delayed reactions; SNIUAA, single NSAID–induced urticaria/angioedema or anaphylaxis. (*From* Kowalski ML, Asero R, Bavbek S, et al. Classification and practical approach to the diagnosis and management of hypersensitivity to nonsteroidal anti-inflammatory drugs. Allergy 2013;68:1228; with permission.)

culprits.[14] The prevalence of NSAID DHRs in the general population ranges from 0.6% to 5.7%, depending on the population studied, the type of reaction, and the criteria used for diagnosis.[15] In fact, 55% of all patients labeled as NSAID-hypersensitive according to their clinical history tolerated NSAIDs following drug-provocation testing (DPT).[14]

Considering the different entities, the prevalence of NSAID-exacerbated respiratory disease (NERD) varies from 4.3% to 20%.[16–18] The presence of CRS with nasal polyps, severe asthma, and female gender are all associated with higher prevalence.[19,20] Moreover, a history of CRS and nasal polyposis are independent predictors for NERD.[21] Although this entity has been more extensively studied, the most frequent DHRs are those involving the skin,[22] appearing in 0.07% to 0.3% of the general population.[23,24] NSAIDs may be an aggravating factor for 10% to 30% of patients with CSU,[6] and this effect is dose-dependent and related to CSU activity. This entity is known as NSAID-exacerbated cutaneous disease (NECD). Finally, NSAID-induced urticaria/angioedema (NIUA) affects up to 60% of all patients with DHR to NSAIDs.[22]

The prevalence of immunologically mediated DHR to NSAIDs ranges from 0.1% to 3.6% of subjects treated with NSAIDs,[25,26] and represents up to 30% of all NSAID-induced DHRs in Spain.[22] Single-NSAID-induced urticarial/angioedema or anaphylaxis (SNIUAA) is the most frequent entity after NIUA, with pyrazolones, ibuprofen, diclofenac, ASA, and paracetamol the NSAIDs most often involved.[8,27–29] In a population-based case-cohort study, penicillins, analgesics, and NSAIDs were the drugs with the highest relative risk of inducing anaphylaxis.[25] However, SNIUAA seems to have decreased in the last decade, probably because of the lower consumption of pyrazolones.[10] The prevalence of single NSAID-induced delayed hypersensitivity reactions (SNIDR) is not known, the most frequently reported being exanthemas, fixed drug eruptions, contact dermatitis, and photosensitivity reactions. NSAIDs can also induce severe organ-specific (eg, cutaneous, kidney, liver) allergic reactions.

PATHOPHYSIOLOGY

As proposed by Szczeklik and colleagues,[30] the mechanism of NERD is not immunologic, but related to COX inhibition and prostaglandin synthesis. In fact, only NSAIDs that are strong or moderate inhibitors of COX-1 (an enzyme that converts arachidonic acid [AA] to prostaglandins and thromboxanes) can induce these reactions, whereas selective COX-2 inhibitors are well tolerated. Inhibition of COX-1 by ASA or other NSAIDs, in conjunction with an intrinsic regulatory defect (probably prostaglandin E deficiency), triggers a biochemical cascade involving the generation of LTs and the release of mast-cell–derived and eosinophil-derived mediators.[31] Intrinsic abnormalities of basal AA metabolism are characteristic of NERD and include the impaired generation of protective prostaglandin E_2 and lipoxins, downregulation of COX-2 and E-prostanoid receptor subtype 2 accompanied by overproduction of LTs, and increased expression of LT receptor 1.[32–34] More recently, it has been documented that platelet-adherent leukocyte interaction may drive the production of LTs in these patients.[35] The pathogenesis of chronic eosinophilic inflammation in the airway mucosa and in nasal polyps in NERD patients does not result from an exposure to NSAIDs, but may be related to underlying AA metabolism abnormalities; the role of viral infections or *Staphylococcus aureus* enterotoxin have also been suggested (**Fig. 2**).[36,37]

Because cross-responses also exist in NECD, a mechanism similar to that of NERD has been proposed.[38] There are similarities in the eicosanoid profile, with an increase in urine LT E_4 excretion associated with the clinical manifestations.[39] A further indication is the protective effect of LT-receptor antagonists.[40,41] Whether this can be also applied to NIUA is a matter of debate that needs further research.[42]

For selective DHRs, the time interval between NSAID administration and the appearance of symptoms suggest mechanisms mediated by IgE (SNIUAA) or T cells (SNIDR).[43,44]

GENETICS

Previous studies of the genetic basis of NSAID hypersensitivity have consisted in the evaluation of single-nucleotide polymorphisms (SNPs). Most studies have included patients with NERD, following a candidate gene approach based on biological plausibility,[45,46] and associations have been found for SNPs in genes related to LT synthesis/receptors[47–52] and prostaglandin and thromboxane pathways.[53–55] The number of variants analyzed is limited, and the associations inconsistently replicated. Regarding NIUA, 3 SNPs in genes coding for members of the AA pathway (rs7220870 in *ALOX15*, rs8004654 in *PTGDR*, and rs320095 in *CYSLTR1*) were found to be associated in 2 unrelated Spanish populations.[56] The potential participation of other pathways in NIUA has been highlighted by the association with the missense polymorphism rs10156191 in diamine oxidase, a key enzyme in histamine homeostasis.[57]

Genome-wide association studies (GWAS) represent an alternative to candidate gene approaches, with the first study conducted in a Korean population of NERD

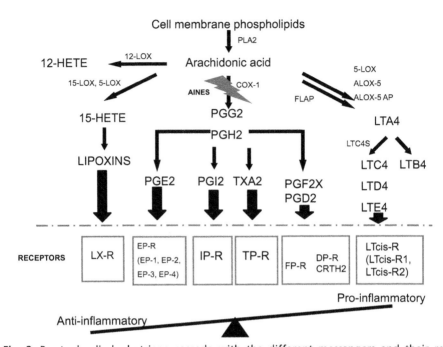

Fig. 2. Prostaglandin-leukotriene cascade with the different messengers and their receptors. ALOX-5 (arachidonate 5-lipoxygenase), ALOX-5 AP (5-lipoxygenase-activating protein), COX-1 (cyclooxygenase-1), CRTH2 (chemoattractant receptor-homologous molecule expressed on T helper type 2 cells, a second prostaglandin D2 receptor), DP-R (prostaglandin D receptor), EP-R (prostaglandin E receptor), EP-1 (prostaglandin E2 receptor subtype 1), EP-2 (prostaglandin E2 receptor subtype 2), EP-3 (prostaglandin E2 receptor subtype 3), EP-4 (prostaglandin E2 receptor subtype 4), FLAP (5-lipoxygenase-activating protein), FP-R (prostaglandin F receptor), IP-R (prostaglandin I receptor), LTA4 (leukotriene A4), LTC4S (leukotriene C4 synthase), LTC4 (leukotriene C4), LTB4 (leukotriene B4), LTD4 (leukotriene D4), LTE4 (leukotriene E4), LTcis-R (cysteinyl leukotriene receptor), LTcis-R1 (cysteinyl leukotriene receptor 1), LTcis-R2 (cysteinyl leukotriene receptor 2), LX-R (lipoxin receptor), PLA2 (phospholipase A2), PGG2 (prostaglandin G2), PGH2 (prostaglandin H2), PGE2 (prostaglandin E2), PGI2 (prostaglandin I2), PGF2X (prostaglandin F2X), PGD2 (prostaglandin D2), TP-R (thromboxane receptor), TXA2 (thromboxane A2), 5-LOX (5-lipoxyg aenase), 12-HETE (12-hydroxyeicosatretraenoic acid), 12-LOX (12-lipoxygenase), 15-HETE (12-hydroxyeicosatretraenoic acid), 15-LOX (15-lipoxygenase).

patients.[58] The nonsynonymous variant rs7572857 (Gly74Ser) in the centrosomal protein of the 68-kDa gene (*CEP68*) was associated with changes in forced expiratory volume in 1 second (FEV_1).[58] In another study, the rs1042151 (Met105Val) SNP in the *HLA-DPB1* gene showed the most significant association with NERD susceptibility.[59] However, the role of human leukocyte antigen (HLA) alleles in hypersensitivity to NSAIDs needs further clarification. Concerning NIUA, a recent article comparing 2 ethnically distinct populations found suggestive associations after meta-analysis (*HLF*, *RAD51L1*, *COL24A1*, *GalNAc-T13*, and *FBXL7*), some of which are related to second-messenger pathways.[60]

Despite recent research into the genetics of hypersensitivity to NSAIDs, the effects of gene variants cannot fully explain disease susceptibility. An important issue is missing heritability and the contribution of rare variants, which cannot be identified by current GWAS technologies. Further studies should integrate data from the 1000

Genomes Project, deep sequencing, and transcriptomics. This approach will enhance the understanding of the underlying mechanisms and improve the management of these patients.

CLINICAL MANIFESTATIONS

This section describes the 5 major clinical entities recognized in the new nomenclature proposed by EAACI.[6]

NSAID-Exacerbated Respiratory Disease

In a subset of patients with asthma, NSAIDs induce symptoms such as bronchocon-striction, usually accompanied by rhinorrhea and/or nasal congestion, within 2 hours after drug exposure.[61,62] Classically "the aspirin tetrad" consists of CRS, complicated by polyps, severe bronchial asthma, and cross-intolerance to other NSAIDs.

Although NERD presents a heterogeneous phenotype, patients usually suffer from a moderate or severe form of asthma requiring chronic treatment with moderate to high doses of inhaled glucocorticosteroids, and associated with a high risk of exacerbation.[63] Almost all patients have nasal and sinus symptoms related to polypoid hypertrophy of the mucosa of the nasal cavity and paranasal sinuses.[64] The course of CRS is protracted with recurrence after polypectomy.

NSAID-Exacerbated Cutaneous Disease

Subjects with CSU may develop wheals and/or angioedema after administration of NSAIDs.[65] As with NERD, the response is related to the potency of COX-1 inhibition and also to the basal activity of the CSU.[66] Symptoms usually appear in a time interval of 1 to 6 hours, although this can vary from a few minutes to many hours. The morphology of the lesions is variable, from erythematous plaques to confluent and migratory wheals, which can be accompanied by angioedema. Although there are no prospective studies on the evolution of NECD, CSU may subside and patients can become tolerant to NSAIDs.[67] As with CSU,[68] the association between atopy, allergic rhinitis, bronchial asthma, and NECD is not clear,[67–69] and further studies are required.

NSAID-Induced Urticaria/Angioedema

NIUA refers to the presence of urticaria and/or angioedema after the intake of different NSAIDs in patients without underlying CSU, with symptoms subsiding following drug withdrawal. Symptoms usually vary from mild to moderate, although anaphylaxis can occur.[22] Severity and persistence of symptoms may be related to a prolonged metabolism of histamine.[57] The association of urticaria/angioedema or isolated angioedema is more common than in NECD.[68] The time interval between NSAID intake and the appearance of symptoms is usually less than 1 hour, but can extend to 6 hours or longer.[22]

Although there is some debate as to whether these patients can convert to NECD over time,[68] a recent study has shown that after 12 years of follow-up the percentage of subjects developing CSU was not different from patients with SNIUAA or healthy controls.[69]

NIUA shows a strong association with atopy, particularly sensitization to house dust mite allergens,[22,70–72] which is strongest for younger patients with angioedema.[13] Concerning food allergy, some preliminary data in adults have shown that the prevalence is not higher than in controls.[73] However, more studies need to be conducted for a better definition of these associations.

Single NSAID–Induced Urticaria/Angioedema or Anaphylaxis

This entity consists of anaphylaxis, urticaria, and/or angioedema appearing soon after the intake of a single NSAID (usually within 1 hour), with good tolerance to other NSAIDs including strong COX-1 inhibitors.[8] SNIUAA have been reported to occur in up to 30% of all cases of hypersensitivity reactions to NSAIDs in a Spanish cohort.[22] The drugs more frequently involved are pyrazolone derivatives, followed by ibuprofen, diclofenac, ASA, and paracetamol.[74–84] These culprits may vary from country to country according to patterns of prescription and consumption.[8] A retrospective evaluation of hospitalizations in allergy services in the Netherlands found that 17% of hospitalizations were related to NSAID hypersensitivity, 30% of which were attributed to diclofenac, and the most common reaction was anaphylaxis.[75]

Single NSAID–Induced Delayed Hypersensitivity Reactions

These reactions are the least frequent and include a wide range of entities affecting mainly the skin, such as exanthema and fixed drug eruption. In some instances they are accompanied by fever or the involvement of other organs. The most frequent exanthemas are maculopapular, and are most often triggered by ibuprofen and naproxen[85] in addition to pirazolones.[86,87] The type of urticarial reaction is difficult to distinguish from those occurring in acute reactions.[85,88] Contact dermatitis and photosensitivity are common, and most often triggered by ketoprofen and diclofenac.[89–92] Fixed drug eruption and acute generalized exanthematous pustulosis may also occur.[93–96] Severe reactions such as Stevens-Johnson syndrome or Lyell syndrome are infrequent.[97]

SNIDRs are induced by a single NSAID, and the patient will show good tolerance to other chemically unrelated NSAIDs. These reactions have a delayed onset, 24 hours or more after exposure, and are mediated by a specific T-cell mechanism.[66,98]

MIXED REACTIONS

Mixed reactions occur when patients with a clinical history of respiratory symptoms also develop extrapulmonary manifestations such as urticaria, angioedema, stomachache, and, in some instances, full anaphylaxis.[20,26,99] In addition, 10% of the patients with NECD may develop airway manifestations.[100] In terms of prevalence, in one study in Spain, patients with manifestations involving both the skin and the airways represented 18% of all nonallergic NSAID hypersensitivity patients, making mixed reactions the second most frequent entity after NIUA.[22]

Mixed reactions can be confused with SNIUAA whereby several organs may be involved, including both skin and respiratory airways. The time course of the initiation of symptoms, which is faster in SNIUAA, may suggest whether a true IgE-mediated response is being dealt with.[7] Confusion may also occur when both airway and skin manifestations are present, but only the latter is induced by NSAIDs, as occurs in asthmatic or rhinitis patients who develop urticaria after NSAID administration despite no worsening of respiratory symptoms.[101]

INTERACTIONS

It is well known that in some instances, patients with food allergy may develop anaphylaxis if they have previously taken NSAIDs; this situation arises with both inhalant and food allergens. Sánchez-Borges and colleagues[102,103] have reported that systemic reactions for patients with food allergy contaminated with mites may occur if they simultaneously take NSAIDs. The reason for this interaction is complex, although it has been proposed that *Dermatophagoides pteronyssinus* and

Dermatophagoides farinae can inhibit COX-1 activity[102] or favor the release of LTs.[104] Further investigations have been suggested.[105]

Other studies have shown the influence of NSAIDs on mast-cell activation after food and/or exercise.[106,107] A possible explanation is that ASA may upregulate the allergic response to food allergens.[108] Another proposal is that ASA and potentially other NSAIDs may increase the gastrointestinal permeability, leading to an increase in the general circulation of the allergen components and thus facilitating the systemic response.[107,109]

Interactions between NSAIDs and hormonal factors may also occur. For example, premenstrual urticaria or anaphylaxis may occur following NSAID intake in patients with an otherwise good tolerance.[110,111] The mechanism for this association is as yet unknown.

DIAGNOSTIC APPROACH

The diagnosis of NSAID hypersensitivity is based on clinical history, which is essential to establishing whether a patient reacts to multiple NSAIDs (nonallergic) or a single drug (allergic). For nonallergic patients neither skin nor laboratory tests are of value; however, for patients experiencing allergic reactions, skin tests and some in vitro tests can be of benefit, albeit with limitations.

The reliability of clinical history depends on several variables, including type and duration of symptoms, time interval between drug intake and appearance of symptoms, response to treatment, and, possibly, the time interval between the reported adverse drug reaction and the allergologic examination.[5–7,22]

Skin Testing

The usefulness of skin testing with certain drugs, such as pyrazolones, has been reported in SNIUAA, although sensitivity is not optimal and the risk of systemic responses exists.[112] Skin testing with aspirin polylysine has not been able to show the presence of IgE antibodies[113,114] and has led to negative results with diclofenac.

In SNIDR, although skin tests have not been sufficiently standardized for clinical practice, they can be useful. Patch testing can confirm drug imputability, especially with noninjectable NSAIDs and for contact dermatitis. Photopatch tests are indicated for NSAID-induced photoallergic or phototoxic reactions.[115] Intradermal skin test with delayed reading at 24 to 48 hours has been mainly used for pyrazolones.[86]

In Vitro Tests

Although specific IgE antibodies have been reported in patients with SNIUAA to ASA,[116] ibuprofen,[117] propyphenazone,[28] and diclofenac[118] by individual study groups, commercial immunoassays are not available. With ASA, a prototype for detecting specific IgE antibodies has been reported using 2 different conjugation procedures.[116] Studies with the pyrazolone derivative propyphenazone conjugated with human serum albumin have shown the presence of specific IgE antibodies by both enzyme-linked immunosorbent assay and immunoblotting.[28]

The basophil activation test has been considered to be a reasonable method when reactions are mediated by IgE, with sensitivity for pyrazolones exceeding 50% and 90% specificity.[29] Although this sensitivity is not optimal, it provides a good alternative, especially in severe reactions. This test has also been used for evaluating NSAID cross-reactivity, with heterogeneous results in the sensitivity and, more importantly, very low specificity because of the high rate of false-positive responses.[119,120] Some investigators reported the value of this test in subjects with immediate reactions.[121,122]

Similar problems exist for other tests such as the cellular leukotriene release assay, the clinical application of which has yet to be validated.[19] Further studies are necessary to determine the role of other basophil markers or even other cells involved in the pathogenesis of NSAID hypersensitivity.

Aspirin specifically triggers 15-hydroxyeicosatetraenoic acid (15-HETE) generation in nasal polyp epithelial cells and peripheral blood leukocytes (PBL) from NERD patients, which suggests the presence of a specific abnormality of the 15-lipooxygenase pathway in these patients.[123] Accordingly, measurement of 15-HETE release from PBL following in vitro ASA challenge has been proposed for confirmation of a clinical history-based diagnosis in NERD patients, but more studies are needed to confirm the discriminative value of this test.

Drug-Provocation Test

A DPT can be used to confirm the diagnosis when there are no alternatives, or can be used to find a safe NSAID once the diagnosis has been confirmed. This latter approach is used to identify selective responders and provide safe alternatives, usually COX-2 inhibitors and weak COX-1 inhibitors in those with nonallergic hypersensitivity. This procedure must be performed by experienced personnel in a clinical setting where a rapid and adequate treatment can be administered if needed. Several protocols exist with different time intervals and total cumulative dose. If the DPT is performed with different NSAIDs, an interval of at least 1 week between each drug administration should be considered.[5,6]

A DPT should follow existing guidelines.[5,6] This procedure is not risk-free, and is contraindicated in patients with a FEV_1 lower than 1.5 L or a FEV_1 variability with placebo greater than 20%, pregnancy, infectious diseases, psychiatric disorders, uncontrolled asthma, severe cutaneous reactions such as Stevens-Johnson syndrome or Lyell syndrome, anaphylactic shock, and organ-specific reactions.

For nonimmunologic reactions (NERD, NECD, and NIUA), clinical history may be consistent enough to establish the diagnosis. In NERD, oral ASA challenge is the gold standard to confirm the diagnosis,[42] with local intranasal or bronchial provocation with lysine-ASA used as alternatives.[124] For NECD, oral ASA challenge may also be needed, but the response may be related to the activity of the CSU.

DPT is the only available method for diagnosing patients with nonimmunologic reactions with skin symptoms (NECD and NIUA).[125,126] If a patient has developed a reaction with 2 or 1 NSAIDs, an ASA DPT should be considered to establish the diagnosis.[22,125] If the DPT is positive and tolerance to paracetamol or COX-2 inhibitors is not known, a DPT with these drugs must be also considered.[126] There are several cases whereby NIUA is manifested as anaphylactic reactions, and caution must be exercised.

In patients with a suspicion of immunologically mediated reactions, the first approach is to look for history of tolerance to other strong COX-1 inhibitors. If this is not known, a DPT with another, chemically nonrelated strong COX-1 inhibitor should be performed, and if this is positive, subjects are considered cross-intolerants and therefore the selective response is ruled out. This procedure is contraindicated in severe reactions such as Stevens-Johnson syndrome and Lyell syndrome.

TREATMENT

Patients with nonallergic hypersensitivity require comprehensive management, which includes education on NSAID avoidance and the use of alternative drugs.[5,6]

In NERD patients, ASA tolerance can be induced by repeated administration of increasing oral doses of ASA, a procedure known as desensitization. Once a patient can tolerate 600 mg of ASA he or she is considered desensitized and can then take this drug on a daily basis indefinitely, without further adverse respiratory reactions.[127] Of interest, the ASA-tolerance state can be also achieved without provoking symptoms, by a slow, gradual increase in ASA dosing (silent desensitization).[128] Administration of ASA (300–1300 mg/d) after desensitization results in improvements in both upper and lower airway symptoms, and may lead to a significant reduction in hospitalization, emergency room visits, or the need for nasal/sinus surgery.[129–131] The clinical benefit, which is usually seen within the first weeks after desensitization, can be maintained during several years of treatment with ASA.[6,132] However, not all NERD patients demonstrate an improvement in the clinical course of the airway disease following ASA after desensitization, and an a priori identification of those patients who would benefit from ASA treatment is not possible at this stage of clinical practice. Further understanding of the mechanism of ASA desensitization may allow for more effective selection of patients benefiting from such treatment.[133] Desensitization to ASA may be also achieved in patients with other forms of hypersensitivity to NSAIDs (eg, NIUA), and has been used at lower doses (ranging from 75 to 150 mg) for chronic treatment with ASA of coronary heart disease or rheumatoid diseases in NSAID-hypersensitive patients.

In patients with allergic hypersensitivity, the treatment recommended is avoidance of the culprit NSAID and those chemically related. Patients can tolerate other non–chemically-related NSAIDs independently of the COX-1 inhibitory capacity.

REFERENCES

1. Roberts LJ, Morrow JD. Analgesic-antipyretic and antiinflammatory agents and drugs employed in the treatment of gout. In: Hardman JG, Limbird LL, Goodman Gilman A, editors. The pharmacological basis of therapeutics. 10th edition. New York: McGraw-Hill; 2001. p. 687–731 Drug Allergy.
2. Celik GE, Pichler WJ, Adkinson NF. Drug allergy. In: Adkinson NF, Brochner BS, Busse WW, et al, editors. Allergy, principles and practice. 7th edition. Philadelphia: Elsevier; 2007. p. 1205–26.
3. Johansson SG, Hourihane JO, Bousquet J, et al. A revised nomenclature for allergy. An EAACI position statement from the EAACI nomenclature task force. Allergy 2001;56:813–24.
4. Cornejo-Garcia JA, Blanca-Lopez N, Doña I, et al. Hypersensitivity reactions to non-steroidal anti-inflammatory drugs. Curr Drug Metab 2009;10:971–80.
5. Kowalski ML, Makowska JS, Blanca M, et al. Hypersensitivity to nonsteroidal anti-inflammatory drugs (NSAIDs)—classification, diagnosis and management: review of the EAACI/ENDA and GA2LEN/HANNA. Allergy 2011;66:818–29.
6. Kowalski ML, Asero R, Bavbek S, et al. Classification and practical approach to the diagnosis and management of hypersensitivity to nonsteroidal anti-inflammatory drugs. Allergy 2013;68:1219–32.
7. Ayuso P, Blanca-Lopez N, Doña I, et al. Advanced phenotyping in hypersensitivity drug reactions to NSAIDs. Clin Exp Allergy 2013;43:1097–109.
8. Canto MG, Andreu I, Fernandez J, et al. Selective immediate hypersensitivity reactions to NSAIDs. Curr Opin Allergy Clin Immunol 2009;9:293–7.
9. Stevenson DD, Sánchez-Borges M, Szczeklik A. Classification of allergic and pseudoallergic reactions to drugs that inhibit cyclooxygenase enzymes. Ann Allergy Asthma Immunol 2001;87:177–80.
10. Kowalski ML, Stevenson DD. Classification of reactions to nonsteroidal antiinflammatory drugs. Immunol Allergy Clin North Am 2013;33:135–45.

11. Doña I, Blanca-Lopez N, Torres MJ, et al. Drug hypersensitivity reactions: response patterns, drug involved, and temporal variations in a large series of patients. J Investig Allergol Clin Immunol 2012;22:363–71.

12. Messaad D, Sahla H, Benahmed S, et al. Drug provocation tests in patients with a history suggesting an immediate drug hypersensitivity reaction. Ann Intern Med 2004;140:1001–6.

13. Zambonino MA, Torres MJ, Muñoz C, et al. Drug provocation tests in the diagnosis of hypersensitivity reactions to non-steroidal anti-inflammatory drugs in children. Pediatr Allergy Immunol 2013;24:151–9.

14. Gomes E, Cardoso MF, Praca F, et al. Self-reported drug allergy in a general adult Portuguese population. Clin Exp Allergy 2004;34:1597–601.

15. Hedman J, Kaprio J, Poussa T. Prevalence of asthma, aspirin intolerance, nasal polyposis and chronic obstructive pulmonary disease in a population-based study. Int J Epidemiol 1999;28:717–22.

16. Schubert B, Grosse Perdekamp MT, Pfeuffer P, et al. Nonsteroidal anti-inflammatory drug hypersensitivity: fable or reality? Eur J Dermatol 2005;15:164–7.

17. Jenkins C, Costello J, Hodge L. Systematic review of prevalence of aspirin induced asthma and its implications for clinical practice. BMJ 2004;328:434.

18. Kasper L, Sladek K, Duplaga M, et al. Prevalence of asthma with aspirin hypersensitivity in the adult population of Poland. Allergy 2003;58:1064–6.

19. Bavbek S, Dursun B, Dursun E, et al. The prevalence of aspirin hypersensitivity in patients with nasal polyposis and contributing factors. Am J Rhinol Allergy 2011;25:411–5.

20. Szczeklik A, Nizankowska E, Duplaga M. Natural history of aspirin-induced asthma. AIANE Investigators. European Network on Aspirin-Induced Asthma. Eur Respir J 2000;16:432–6.

21. Bavbek S, Yilmaz I, Celik G, et al. Prevalence of aspirin-exacerbated respiratory disease in patients with asthma in Turkey: a cross-sectional survey. Allergol Immunopathol 2012;40:225–30.

22. Doña I, Blanca-Lopez N, Cornejo-García JA, et al. Characteristics of subjects experiencing hypersensitivity to non-steroidal anti-inflammatory drugs: patterns of response. Clin Exp Allergy 2011;41:86–95.

23. Sánchez-Borges M, Capriles-Hulett A, Caballero-Fonseca F. NSAID-induced urticaria and angioedema: a reappraisal of its clinical management. Am J Clin Dermatol 2002;3:599–607.

24. Erbagci Z. Multiple NSAID intolerance in chronic idiopathic urticaria is correlated with delayed, pronounced and prolonged autoreactivity. J Dermatol 2004;31:376–82.

25. Van der Klauw MM, Stricker BH, Herings RM, et al. A population based case-cohort study of drug-induced anaphylaxis. Br J Clin Pharmacol 1993;35:400–8.

26. Berkes EA. Anaphylactic and anaphylactoid reactions to aspirin and other NSAIDs. Clin Rev Allergy Immunol 2003;24:137–48.

27. Chaudhry T, Hissaria P, Wiese M, et al. Oral drug challenges in non-steroidal anti-inflammatory drug-induced urticaria, angioedema and anaphylaxis. Intern Med J 2012;42:665–71.

28. Himly M, Jahn-Schmid B, Pittertschatscher K, et al. IgE-mediated immediate-type hypersensitivity to the pyrazolone drug propyphenazone. J Allergy Clin Immunol 2003;111:882–8.

29. Gómez E, Blanca-Lopez N, Torres MJ, et al. Immunoglobulin E-mediated immediate allergic reactions to dipyrone: value of basophil activation test in the identification of patients. Clin Exp Allergy 2009;39:1217–24.

30. Szczeklik A, Gryglewski RJ, Czerniawska-Mysik G. Relationship of inhibition of prostaglandins biosynthesis by analgesics to asthma attacks in aspirin -sensitive patients. Br Med J 1975;1:67–9.
31. Park HS, Kowalski ML, Sánchez-Borges M. Hypersensitivity to aspirin and other non-steroidal antiinflammatory drugs. In: Franklin Adkinson N Jr, Brochner BS, Busse WW, et al, editors. Middleton's allergy principles and practice. Philadelphia: Elsevier; 2013. p. 1296–309.
32. Adkinson NF, Brochner BS, Busse WW, et al. Differential metabolism of arachidonic acid in nasal polyp epithelial cells cultured from aspirin-sensitive and aspirin-tolerant patients. Am J Respir Crit Care Med 2000;161(2 Pt 1):391–8.
33. Pierzchalska M, Szabó Z, Sanak M, et al. Deficient prostaglandin E2 production by bronchial fibroblasts of asthmatic patients, with special reference to aspirin-induced asthma. J Allergy Clin Immunol 2003;111:1041–8.
34. Yamaguchi H, Higashi N, Mita H, et al. Urinary concentrations of 15-epimer of lipoxin A(4) are lower in patients with aspirin-intolerant compared with aspirin-tolerant asthma. Clin Exp Allergy 2011;41:1711–8.
35. Laidlaw TM, Kidder MS, Bhattacharyya N, et al. Cysteinyl leukotriene overproduction in aspirin-exacerbated respiratory disease is driven by platelet-adherent leukocytes. Blood 2012;119:3790–8.
36. Pérez-Novo CA, Kowalski ML, Kuna P, et al. Aspirin sensitivity and IgE antibodies to *Staphylococcus aureus* enterotoxins in nasal polyposis: studies on the relationship. Int Arch Allergy Immunol 2004;133:255–60.
37. Yoo HS, Shin YS, Liu JN, et al. Clinical significance of immunoglobulin E responses to staphylococcal superantigens in patients with aspirin-exacerbated respiratory disease. Int Arch Allergy Immunol 2013;162:340–5.
38. Szszeklik A, Nizankowska E, Sanak M. Hypersensitivity to aspirin and non-steroidal antiinflmmatory drugs. In: Adkinson NF, Brochner BS, Busse WW, et al, editors. Allergy, principles and practice. 7th edition. Philadelphia: Elsevier; 2007. p. 1227–46.
39. Mastalerz L, Setkowicz M, Sanak M, et al. Hypersensitivity to aspirin: common eicosanoid alterations in urticaria and asthma. J Allergy Clin Immunol 2004; 113:771–5.
40. Asero R. Leukotriene receptor antagonists may prevent NSAID-induced exacerbations in patients with chronic urticaria. Ann Allergy Asthma Immunol 2000;85: 156–7.
41. Perez C, Sánchez-Borges M, Capriles E. Pretreatment with montelukast blocks NSAID-induced urticaria and angioedema. J Allergy Clin Immunol 2001;108:1060–1.
42. Campo P, Ayuso P, Salas M, et al. Mediator release after nasal aspirin provocation supports different phenotypes in subjects with hypersensitivity reactions to NSAIDs. Allergy 2013;68:1001–7.
43. Mayorga C, Torres MJ, Fernandez J, et al. Cutaneous symptoms in drug allergy: what have we learnt? Curr Opin Allergy Clin Immunol 2009;9:431–6.
44. Pichler WJ, Yawalkar N, Britschgi M, et al. Cellular and molecular pathophysiology of cutaneous drug reactions. Am J Clin Dermatol 2002;3:229–38.
45. Duroudier NP, Tulah AS, Sayers I. Leukotriene pathway genetics and pharmacogenetics in allergy. Allergy 2009;64(6):823–39.
46. Kim SH, Ye YM, Palikhe NS, et al. Genetic and ethnic risk factors associated with drug hypersensitivity. Curr Opin Allergy Clin Immunol 2010;10:280–90.
47. Sanak M, Pierzchalska M, Bazan-Socha S, et al. Enhanced expression of the leukotriene C(4) synthase due to overactive transcription of an allelic variant associated with aspirin-intolerant asthma. Am J Respir Cell Mol Biol 2000;23:290–6.

48. Kawagishi Y, Mita H, Taniguchi M, et al. Leukotriene C4 synthase promoter polymorphism in Japanese patients with aspirin-induced asthma. J Allergy Clin Immunol 2002;109:936–42.

49. Choi JH, Park HS, Oh HB, et al. Leukotriene-related gene polymorphisms in ASA-intolerant asthma: an association with a haplotype of 5-lipoxygenase. Hum Genet 2004;114:337–44.

50. Kim JM, Park BL, Park SM, et al. Association analysis of N-acetyl transferase-2 polymorphisms with aspirin intolerance among asthmatics. Pharmacogenomics 2010;11:951–8.

51. Pillai SG, Cousens DJ, Barnes AA, et al, Investigators of the GAIN Network. A coding polymorphism in the CYSLT2 receptor with reduced affinity to LTD4 is associated with asthma. Pharmacogenetics 2004;14:627–33.

52. Park JS, Chang HS, Park CS, et al. Association analysis of cysteinyl-leukotriene receptor 2 (CYSLTR2) polymorphisms with aspirin intolerance in asthmatics. Pharmacogenet Genomics 2005;15:483–92.

53. Kim SH, Choi JH, Park HS, et al. Association of thromboxane A2 receptor gene polymorphism with the phenotype of acetyl salicylic acid-intolerant asthma. Clin Exp Allergy 2005;35:585–90.

54. Kim SH, Kim YK, Park HW, et al. Association between polymorphisms in prostanoid receptor genes and aspirin-intolerant asthma. Pharmacogenet Genomics 2007;17:295–304.

55. Park BL, Park SM, Park JS, et al. Association of PTGER gene family polymorphisms with aspirin intolerant asthma in Korean asthmatics. BMB Rep 2010; 43:445–9.

56. Cornejo-García JA, Jagemann LR, Blanca-López N, et al. Genetic variants of the arachidonic acid pathway in non-steroidal anti-inflammatory drug-induced acute urticaria. Clin Exp Allergy 2012;42:1772–81.

57. Agúndez JA, Ayuso P, Cornejo-García JA, et al. The diamine oxidase gene is associated with hypersensitivity response to non-steroidal anti-inflammatory drugs. PLoS One 2012;7:e47571.

58. Kim JH, Park BL, Cheong HS, et al. Genome-wide and follow-up studies identify CEP68 gene variants associated with risk of aspirin-intolerant asthma. PLoS One 2010;5:e13818.

59. Park BL, Kim TH, Kim JH, et al. Genome-wide association study of aspirin-exacerbated respiratory disease in a Korean population. Hum Genet 2013; 132:313–21.

60. Cornejo-García JA, Liou LB, Blanca-López N, et al. Genome-wide association study in NSAID-induced acute urticaria/angioedema in Spanish and Han Chinese populations. Pharmacogenomics 2013;14:1857–69.

61. Szczeklik A, Stevenson DD. Aspirin-induced asthma: advances in pathogenesis, diagnosis, and management. J Allergy Clin Immunol 2003;111: 913–21.

62. Bochenek G, Kuschill-Dziurda J, Szafraniec K, et al. Certain subphenotypes of aspirin-exacerbated respiratory disease distinguished by latent class analysis. J Allergy Clin Immunol 2014;133:98–103.

63. Pawliczak R, Lewandowska-Polak A, Kowalski ML. Pathogenesis of nasal polyps: an update. Curr Allergy Asthma Resp 2005;6:463–71.

64. Kowalski ML, Ptasinska A, Bienkiewicz B, et al. Aspirin-triggered 15-HETE generation in peripheral blood leukocytes is a sensitive and specific and Aspirin Sensitive Patients Identification Test (ASPITest). Allergy 2005;60: 1139–45.

65. Asero R, Bavbek S, Blanca M, et al. Clinical management of patients with a history of urticaria/angioedema induced by multiple NSAIDs: an expert panel review. Int Arch Allergy Immunol 2013;160:126–33.
66. Torres MJ, Mayorga C, Blanca M. Nonimmediate allergic reactions induced by drugs: pathogenesis and diagnostic tests. J Investig Allergol Clin Immunol 2009;19:80–90.
67. Brunetti L, Francavilla R, Miniello VL, et al. High prevalence of autoimmune urticaria in children with chronic urticaria. J Allergy Clin Immunol 2004;114:922–7.
68. Asero R. Multiple nonsteroidal anti-inflammatory drug induced cutaneous disease: what differentiates patients with and without underlying chronic spontaneous urticaria. Int Arch Allergy Immunol 2013;163:114–8.
69. Doña I, Blanca-López N, Torres MJ, et al. NSAID-induced urticaria/angioedema does not evolve into chronic urticaria: a 12-year follow-up study. Allergy 2013; 69(4):438–44. http://dx.doi.org/10.1111/all.12335.
70. Sánchez-Borges M, Suárez-Chacón R, Capriles-Hulett A, et al. An update on oral anaphylaxis from mite ingestion. Ann Allergy Asthma Immunol 2005;94: 216–20.
71. Sánchez-Borges M, Suárez-Chacón R, Capriles-Hulett A, et al. Pancake syndrome (oral mite anaphylaxis). World Allergy Organ J 2009;2:91–6.
72. Sánchez-Borges M, Capriles-Hulett A, Capriles-Behrens E, et al. A new triad: sensitivity to aspirin, allergic rhinitis, and severe allergic reaction to ingested aeroallergens. Cutis 1997;59:311–4.
73. Gómez F, Doña I, Blanca-López N, et al. Food allergy is not a risk factor in cross-intolerance to nsaids for induction of symptoms [abstract]. J Allergy Clin Immunol 2013;131:167.
74. Gala G, Blanco R, Quirce S, et al. Diclofenac-induced urticaria with aspirin tolerance. Allergy 1998;53:623–4.
75. van Puijenbroek EP, Egberts AC, Meyboom RH, et al. Different risks for NSAID-induced anaphylaxis. Ann Pharmacother 2002;36:24–9.
76. Klote MM, Smith LJ. A case of anaphylaxis to naproxen. Allergy 2005;60:260–1.
77. Scala E, Giani M, Pirrotta L, et al. Selective severe anaphylactic reaction due to ketorolac tromethamine without nonsteroidal anti-inflammatory drug intolerance. J Allergy Clin Immunol 2001;107:557.
78. Kvedariene V, Bencherioua AM, Messaad D, et al. The accuracy of the diagnosis of suspected paracetamol (acetaminophen) hypersensitivity: results of a single-blinded trial. Clin Exp Allergy 2002;32:1366–9.
79. Stricker BH, Meyboom RH, Lindquist M. Acute hypersensitivity reactions to paracetamol. Br Med J (Clin Res Ed) 1985;29:938–9.
80. Leung R, Plomley R, Czarny D. Paracetamol anaphylaxis. Clin Exp Allergy 1992; 22:831–3.
81. Ownby DR. Acetaminophen-induced urticaria and tolerance of ibuprofen in an eight-year-old child. J Allergy Clin Immunol 1997;99(1 Pt 1):151–2.
82. Vidal C, Pérez-Carral C, González-Quintela A. Paracetamol (acetaminophen) hypersensitivity. Ann Allergy Asthma Immunol 1997;79:320–1.
83. Quiralte J, Blanco C, Castillo R, et al. Anaphylactoid reactions due to nonsteroidal antiinflammatory drugs: clinical and cross-reactivity studies. Ann Allergy Asthma Immunol 1997;78:293–6.
84. Schuster C, Wüthrich B. Anaphylactic drug reaction to celecoxib and sulfamethoxazole: cross reactivity or coincidence? Allergy 2003;58:1072.
85. Nettis E, Giordano D, Colanardi MC, et al. Delayed-type hypersensitivity rash from ibuprofen. Allergy 2003;58:539–40.

86. Macias E, Ruiz A, Moreno E, et al. Usefulness of intradermal test and patch test in the diagnosis of nonimmediate reactions to metamizol. Allergy 2007;62:1462–4.

87. Bernedo N, Audicana MT, Uriel O, et al. Metamizol as a cause of postoperative erythroderma. Contact Dermatitis 2004;50:317–8.

88. Sánchez-Borges M, Capriles-Hulett A, Caballero-Fonseca F. Cutaneous hypersensitivity reactions to inhibitors of cyclooxygenase-2. Results of 307 oral provocation tests and review of the literature. Allergy Clin Immunol Int-J World Allergy Org 2007;19:44–9.

89. Cantisani C, Grieco T, Faina V, et al. Ketoprofen allergic reactions. Recent Pat Inflamm Allergy Drug Discov 2010;4:58–64.

90. Lynde CB, Pierscianowski TA, Pratt MD. Allergic contact dermatitis caused by diclofenac cream. CMAJ 2009;181:925–6.

91. Devleeschouwer V, Roelandts R, Garmyn M, et al. Allergic and photoallergic contact dermatitis from ketoprofen: results of (photo) patch testing and follow-up of 42 patients. Contact Dermatitis 2008;58:159–66.

92. Montoro J, Rodríguez M, Díaz M, et al. Photoallergic contact dermatitis due to diclofenac. Contact Dermatitis 2003;48:115.

93. Lee AY. Fixed drug eruptions. Incidence, recognition, and avoidance. Am J Clin Dermatol 2000;1:277–85.

94. Brahimi N, Routier E, Raison-Peyron N, et al. A three-year-analysis of fixed drug eruptions in hospital settings in France. Eur J Dermatol 2010;20:461–4.

95. Bellini V, Stingeni L, Lisi P. Multifocal fixed drug eruption due to celecoxib. Dermatitis 2009;20:174–6.

96. Gonzalo-Garijo MA, Pérez-Calderón R, De Argila D, et al. Metamizole-induced acute generalized exanthematous pustulosis. Contact Derm 2003;49:47–8.

97. Mockenhaupt M, Viboud C, Dunant A, et al. Stevens-Johnson syndrome and toxic epidermal necrolysis: assessment of medication risks with emphasis on recently marketed drugs. The EuroSCAR-study. J Invest Dermatol 2008;128:35–44.

98. Gomez E, Blanca M, Torres MJ, et al. Immunologic evaluation of drug allergy. Allergy Asthma Immunol Res 2012;4:251–63.

99. Quiralte J, Blanco C, Castillo R, et al. Intolerance to nonsteroidal antiinflammatory drugs: results of controlled drug challenges in 98 patients. J Allergy Clin Immunol 1996;98:678–85.

100. Zembowicz A, Mastalerz I, Setkowicz M, et al. Histological spectrum of cutaneous reactions to aspirin in chronic idiopathic urticaria. J Cutan Pathol 2004;31:323–9.

101. Caimmi S, Caimmi D, Bousquet PJ, et al. How can we classify NSAID hypersensitivity reactions?. Validation from a large database. Int Arch Allergy Immunol 2012;159:306–12.

102. Sánchez-Borges M, Fernández-Caldas E, Capriles-Hulett A, et al. Mite induced inflammation: more than allergy. Allergy Rhinol (Providence) 2012;3:e25–9.

103. Sánchez-Borges M, Ouellet M, Percival M, et al. Inhibition of human cyclooxygenase-1 by Dermatophagoides allergenic extracts. J Allergy Clin Immunol 2005;115:S51.

104. Barret NA, Maekawa A, Rahman OM, et al. Dectin-2 recognition of house dust mite triggers cysteinyl leukotriene generation by dendritic cells. J Immunol 2009;182:1119–28.

105. Sato M, Kuwahara Y, Matsuyama S, et al. 2-Formyl-3-hydrobenzyl formate (Rhizoglyphiny formate), a novel salicylaldehyde analog from the house dust mite *Dermatophagoides pteronyssinus* (Astigmata, pyroglyphidae). Biosci Biotechnol Biochem 1993;57:1299–301.

106. Fukunaga A, Shimizu H, Tanaka M, et al. Limited influence of aspirin intake on mast cell activation in patients with food-dependent exercise-induced anaphylaxis: comparison using skin prick and histamine release tests. Acta Derm Venereol 2012;92:480–3.
107. Cardona V, Luengo O, Garriga T, et al. Co-factor-enhanced food allergy. Allergy 2012;67:1316–8.
108. Harada S, Horikawa T, Ashida M, et al. Aspirin enhances the induction of type I allergic symptoms when combined with food and exercise in patients with food-dependent exercise-induced anaphylaxis. Br J Dermatol 2001;145: 336–9.
109. Matsuo H, Morimoto K, Akaki T, et al. Exercise and aspirin increase levels of circulating gliadin peptides in patients with wheat-dependent exercise-induced anaphylaxis. Clin Exp Allergy 2005;35:461–6.
110. Vrieze A, Postma DS, Kerstjens H, et al. Perimenstrual asthma: a syndrome without known cause or cure. J Allergy Clin Immunol 2003;112:271–82.
111. Martinez-Moragón E, Plaz V, Serrano J, et al. Near-fatal asthma related to menstruation. J Allergy Clin Immunol 2004;113:242–4.
112. Carmona MJ, Blanca M, Garcia A, et al. Intolerance to piroxicam in patients with adverse reactions to nonsteroidal anti-inflammatory drugs. J Allergy Clin Immunol 1992;90:873–9.
113. de Weck AL. Immunochemical effects of aspirin anhydride, a contaminant of commercial acetyl salicylic acid preparations. Int Arch Allergy Immunol 1971; 41:393–5.
114. Phils JA, Perelmutter L. IgE mediated and nonmediated allergic type reactions to aspirin. Acta Allergol 1974;29:474–6.
115. Hasan T, Jansen CT. Photopatch test reactivity: effect of photoallergen concentration and UVA dosing. Contact Dermatitis 1996;34:383–6.
116. Blanca M, Perez E, Garcia JJ, et al. Angioedema and IgE antibodies to aspirin: a case report. Ann Allergy 1989;62:295–8.
117. Bluth MH, Beleza P, Hajee F, et al. IgE-mediated hypersensitivity after ibuprofen administration. Ann Clin Lab Sci 2007;37:362–5.
118. Harrer A, Lang R, Grims L, et al. Diclofenac hypersensitivity: antibody responses to the parent drug and relevant metabolites. PLoS One 2010;5:e13707.
119. Celik G, Bavbeck S, Misirligicl Z, et al. Release of cysteinyl leukotrienes with aspirin stimulation and the effect of prostaglandin E2 on this release from peripheral blood leucocytes in aspirin-induced asthmatic patients. Clin Exp Allergy 2001;31:1615–22.
120. Bavbek S, Ikincioğullari A, Dursun AB, et al. Upregulation of CD63 or CD203c alone or in combination is not sensitive in the diagnosis of nonsteroidal anti-inflammatory drug intolerance. Int Arch Allergy Immunol 2009; 150:261–70.
121. Korosec P, Mavsar N, Bajrovic N, et al. Basophil responsiveness and clinical picture of acetylsalicylic acid intolerance. Int Arch Allergy Immunol 2011;155: 257–62.
122. De Weck AL, Sanz ML, Gamboa PM, et al. Nonsteroidal anti-inflammatory drug hypersensitivity syndrome. A multicenter study. I. Clinical findings and in vitro diagnosis. J Investig Allergol Clin Immunol 2009;19:355–69.
123. Lewandowska-Polak A, Jedrzejczak-Czechowicz M, Makowska JS, et al. Lack of association between aspirin-triggered 15-hydroxyeicosatetraenoic acid release and mast cell/eosinophil activation in nasal polyps from aspirin-sensitive patients. J Investig Allergol Clin Immunol 2011;21:507–13.

124. Lee RU, Stevenson DD. Aspirin-exacerbated respiratory disease: evaluation and management. Allergy Asthma Immunol Res 2011;3:3–10.

125. Blanca-Lopez N, Torres MJ, Doña I, et al. Value of the clinical history in the diagnosis of urticaria/angioedema induced by NSAIDs with cross-intolerance. Clin Exp Allergy 2013;43:85–91.

126. Doña I, Blanca-López N, Jagemann LR, et al. Response to a selective COX-2 inhibitor in patients with urticaria/angioedema induced by nonsteroidal anti-inflammatory drugs. Allergy 2011;66:1428–33.

127. Szmidt M, Grzelewska-Rzymowska I, Kowalski ML, et al. Tolerance to acetylsalicylic acid (ASA) induced in ASA-sensitive asthmatics does not depend on initial adverse reaction. Allergy 1987;42:182–5.

128. Berges-Gimeno MP, Simon RA, Stevenson DD. Long-term treatment with aspirin desensitization in asthmatic patients with aspirin-exacerbated respiratory disease. J Allergy Clin Immunol 2003;111:180–6.

129. Lee JY, Simon RA, Stevenson DD. Selection of aspirin dosages for aspirin desensitization treatment in patients with aspirin-exacerbated respiratory disease. J Allergy Clin Immunol 2007;119:157–64.

130. Comert S, Celebioglu E, Yucel T, et al. Aspirin 300 mg/day is effective for treating aspirin-exacerbated respiratory disease. Allergy 2013;68:1443–51.

131. Kowalski ML, Grzelewska-Rzymowska I, Szmidt M, et al. Clinical efficacy of aspirin in "desensitised" aspirin-sensitive asthmatics. Eur J Respir Dis 1986; 69:219–25.

132. Burnett T, Katial R, Alam R. Mechanisms of aspirin desensitization. Immunol Allergy Clin North Am 2013;33:223–36.

133. Woessner KM, Simon RA. Cardiovascular prophylaxis and aspirin "allergy". Immunol Allergy Clin North Am 2013;33:263–74.

Local and General Anesthetics Immediate Hypersensitivity Reactions

 CrossMark

Gerald W. Volcheck, MD[a], Paul Michel Mertes, MD, PhD[b],*

KEYWORDS

- Anesthetics • Allergy • Anaphylaxis • Perioperative • Skin tests

KEY POINTS

- Immediate hypersensitivity reactions can occur with the use of anesthesia and are associated with significant morbidity and mortality.
- Evaluation of anaphylactic reactions in the anesthesia setting can be complex because of the large number of medications administered in the same time frame.
- Neuromuscular blocking agents, antibiotics, and latex are the most common causes of anesthesia-associated allergic reactions, though multiple medications and products may be causative.
- All patients with a history of an anesthesia-related hypersensitivity reaction should have an allergy evaluation to identify the cause.
- Allergy evaluation of an anesthesia-related hypersensitivity reaction may include skin tests, intradermal tests, challenges, in vitro specific–immunoglobulin E testing, or basophil activation test.

Hypersensitivity reactions occurring during anesthesia are rare but can rapidly evolve into life-threatening anaphylaxis, although rapid recognition and treatment of such reactions can prevent much of the morbidity and mortality that would otherwise occur.[1] Unfortunately, screening tests to prevent anaphylaxis during anesthesia are unlikely to have a significant impact on reducing the incidence of these reactions.[2] This incidence can be reduced by preventing subsequent reactions in patients with a history of anaphylaxis or with major undiagnosed or undocumented adverse events during previous anesthesia.[3]

It is important for the investigating physician to be aware that the perioperative setting represents a pharmacologically unique situation, during which patients are

The authors have nothing to disclose.
[a] Division of Allergic Diseases, Mayo Medical School, Mayo Clinic, 200 First Street Southwest, Rochester, MN 55905, USA; [b] Department of Anesthesia and Intensive Care, University Hospital of Strasbourg, Nouvel Hôpital Civil, 1 Place de l'Hôpital - BP 426, 67091 Strasbourg Cedex, France
* Corresponding author.
E-mail address: paul-michel.mertes@chru-strasbourg.fr

Immunol Allergy Clin N Am 34 (2014) 525–546
http://dx.doi.org/10.1016/j.iac.2014.03.004   immunology.theclinics.com

exposed to multiple foreign substances that have the potential to produce a variety of predictable and unpredictable adverse reactions. As a consequence, anesthetists are more likely to witness and manage immediate hypersensitivity reactions than other physicians. However, some of the clinical features of anaphylaxis can also be mimicked by other complications of anesthesia, such as hypotension and vasodilation resulting from anesthesia induction, difficulty in tracheal intubation, inadequate depth of anesthesia, hypovolemia, and hemorrhage. Investigation can be challenging, as patients are exposed to many coadministered drugs and agents that have all been associated with anaphylaxis. However, most reactions are accounted for by a relatively small number of agents.[4]

OVERVIEW OF INTRAOPERATIVE ANAPHYLAXIS
Terminology

The surveillance of perioperative anaphylaxis represents a statistical challenge because these reactions are rare, random, and there is no clear relationship between risk and repeated anesthetic use. Another weakness of any review of epidemiologic studies on the subject is the lack of a consensus definition and the heterogeneous use of terms in the literature.

Initially, the term *anaphylaxis* was used only for immunoglobulin E (IgE)–mediated reactions, whereas the term *anaphylactoid* was used for a reaction occurring via a non–IgE-dependent mechanism. However, anesthesiologists usually have little understanding of which drug is actually causing the anaphylactic reaction when several drugs are simultaneously administered as well as of the underlying mechanism.[5] Therefore, a new definition has been proposed by the European Academy for Allergy and Clinical Immunology whereby all reactions are described as anaphylaxis and subdivided into allergic (IgE or IgG mediated)[6] or nonallergic anaphylaxis only after diagnostic investigation.[7]

Incidence

Several series from different countries have estimated the incidence of clinical anaphylaxis during anesthesia to be between 1 in 1250 and 10,000.[8] Despite the reported variations, probably reflecting differences in clinical practice and reporting systems, the proportion of IgE-mediated reactions seems to be relatively similar between countries, ranging from 50% to 60%.[1,9–15] However, substantial variability regarding the different drugs or agents involved is reported, reactions involving neuromuscular blocking agents (NMBAs) being more frequent in several countries,[4,10,12,13,16] whereas allergic reactions involving antibiotics or chlorhexidine seem to be more frequent in the United States[9] and in Denmark,[17] respectively.

Mortality

Despite the fact that these reactions are witnessed and occur in a monitored setting, an unfavorable outcome may occur even when they are appropriately treated. A perioperative mortality rate of 4.76% has been recorded for all causative drugs in Japan[18] and a 4% rate in the United States.[19] According to the Yellow Card Scheme, overall mortality was even higher in the United Kingdom (9%).[20] These high rates contrast strongly with the low rate of 0% to 1.4% recently reported for Western Australia (2000–2009).[21] There are several reasons for high mortality from anaphylactic reactions despite trained staff being present in the operating room and despite short management delays. These reasons include patient frailty caused by the underlying condition prompting surgery, especially emergency surgery; the intrinsic cardiopulmonary depressive effects of anesthetics; a short reaction time caused by the massive dose of allergen administered intravenously; and a reputedly more severe reaction on administration of drugs, such as NMBAs or intravenous antibiotics.[22]

Clinical Presentation

Anaphylaxis may occur at any time during anesthesia and may progress slowly or rapidly. The end-organ effects of the variety of mediators resulting from effector cells activation produce the clinical syndrome of anaphylaxis. True allergic reactions require immune-mediated release of mediators. In contrast, other mechanisms can release the vasoactive substances that produce this clinical syndrome. Almost every organ and system may be affected, although patients' medical history may influence both the nature and severity of the clinical symptoms. Asthmatic patients are more likely to have significant bronchospasm,[23] whereas patients with preexisting cardiac disease or those taking β-adrenoceptor blockers are more likely to develop severe hypotension and shock.[24]

The route of administration and the nature of the allergen will affect the clinical course of the reaction. Ninety percent of reactions appear at anesthesia induction, or at the end of the procedure, within minutes or seconds after the intravenous injection of an offending agent, such as antibiotics, NMBAs, aprotinin, or analgesics. However, reactions may be delayed up to 4 hours when a labile blood product is incriminated.[25] Reactions resulting from infiltration of dyes[26,27] or of mucous membrane or skin exposure to latex or disinfectants tends to lead to reactions of slower onset.[28–30]

The clinical diagnosis is presumptive, although essential, because anaphylaxis may progress within minutes to become life threatening. The signs and symptoms differ to some extent from those of anaphylaxis not associated with anesthesia. All early symptoms usually observed in awake patients, such as malaise, pruritus, dizziness, and dyspnea, are absent in anesthetized patients, whereas most individual symptoms of anaphylaxis have a more common cause; diagnosis will often be made only after other likely causes have been excluded. In addition, in mild cases, spontaneous recovery may be observed even in the absence of any specific treatment. Under such circumstances, the lack of a proper diagnosis and appropriate allergy assessment may lead to fatal reexposure.[3]

Urticaria and angioedema, symptoms highly evocative of the onset of anaphylaxis, may be missed because patients are draped. Moreover, clinical features may occur in isolation, such as a sudden cardiac arrest without any other clinical signs; the absence of cutaneous symptoms does not exclude the diagnosis of anaphylaxis. The attending anesthesiologist can easily misdiagnose hypotension secondary to colloids administered to treat hypotension resulting from sympathetic blockade associated with spinal or epidural anesthesia or from intraoperative hemorrhage.

An acute coronary vasospasm, or Kounis syndrome, resulting from cardiac mast cell activation can also be erroneously attributed to a preexisting coronary artery disease.[31]

Drug Allergy Work-up

The diagnosis of perioperative anaphylaxis begins with a detailed symptom history, and a time frame between the injection of the incriminated drugs and the onset of the reaction is very helpful. The diagnostic strategy is based on laboratory tests performed on samples taken during and shortly after the reaction and on allergy tests carried out days to weeks later, which mainly include skin tests, specific IgE assays, and basophil activation tests. Early tests are mainly designed to determine whether or not an allergic mechanism is involved, whereas later testing attempts to identify the responsible drug and potential safe alternatives.

None of the available diagnostic tests is absolutely accurate. False-positive test results may cause unnecessary avoidance of a safe drug, whereas false-negative or equivocal results may severely undermine correct secondary prevention. Therefore, in the event of discrepancies between history and skin tests, challenge tests (when possible) and/or in vitro tests must be used to increase the overall sensitivity of the diagnostic procedure.

Tryptase and histamine

Tryptase levels acquired at the time of the reaction can be helpful. Mast cells activated during an IgE-mediated hypersensitivity reaction release proteases such as tryptase as well as stored histamine and newly generated vasoactive mediators. Because in human basophils, tryptase content is 300- to 700-fold less than in mast cells, tryptase levels in serum are used as a marker for systemic mast cell activation. Although it can be marginally elevated in different situations, an increased serum tryptase concentration in an acute setting strongly suggests an allergic mechanism. There is no consensus in the literature as to the cutoff point that should be used to consider a tryptase result as elevated.[32] A level greater than 25 μg/L^{-1} has been proposed when a single measurement is performed,[24] but lower cutoff values ranging between 8.23 and 11.4 μg/L have been proposed to increase tryptase sensitivity.[33] However, the use of a cutoff value without taking baseline levels into account is not always appropriate, as baseline levels higher than the cutoff point established can be found in some comorbidities, such as systemic mastocytosis. Therefore, the measurement of basal tryptase is now recommended[24]; a 2-fold increase compared with the basal level is considered significant.[32] Nevertheless, a normal tryptase level does not completely rule out anaphylaxis. Increased tryptase levels in postmortem sera suggest systemic anaphylaxis as a cause of death.[34]

Histamine measurement at the time of the reaction has also been proposed in the literature. Concentrations are maximal almost immediately and decrease thereafter with a half-life of about 20 minutes. Therefore, circulating levels should be assayed within the first hour of a reaction; in mild cases, only early measurements may be increased. Histamine has a greater sensitivity than tryptase[32] but does not allow to distinguish IgE-mediated from non–IgE-mediated reactions. Histamine assays should not be measured during pregnancy (particularly closer to delivery) and in patients receiving high doses of heparin because of a high rate of false-negative results caused by accelerated histamine degradation.

Skin testing

Skin prick test (SPT) and intradermal test (IDT) with immediate readings are the most commonly used procedures for investigation of immediate hypersensitivity reactions, although their reliability somewhat depends on which class of drug is being tested. The sensitivity of skin tests seems to be moderate to high for immediate hypersensitivity reactions to most perioperative drugs. Several factors may contribute to the variability of skin test results, including the individual's biologic responsiveness, the technique used to perform the test, the reagents (stability, vehicle, allergen concentration, purity), and the method used to grade skin reactions. Therefore, a validated protocol should be used; recent guidelines have been published in an effort to standardize the concentrations to be used (**Table 1**).[24,35]

Control tests using saline (negative control) and codeine or histamine (positive control) must accompany skin tests to determine whether or not the skin is able to release

Table 1
Maximal concentrations normally nonreactive for SPT and IDT

Available Agents	SPT			IDT	
	Conc (mg/mL^{-1})	Dilution	Cmax (mg/mL^{-1})	Dilution	Cmax (mg/mL^{-1})
NMBAs					
Atracurium	10.0	1/10	1.0	1/1000	0.01
Cis-atracurium	2.0	Undiluted	2.0	1/100	0.02
Mivacurium	2.0	1/10	0.2	1/1000	0.002
Pancuronium	2.0	Undiluted	2.0	1/10	0.2
Rocuronium	10.0	Undiluted	10.0	1/200	0.05
Vecuronium	4.0	Undiluted	4.0	1/10	0.4
Suxamethonium	50.0	1/5	10.0	1/500	0.1
Hypnotics					
Etomidate	2.0	Undiluted	2.0	1/10	0.2
Midazolam	5.0	Undiluted	5.0	1/10	0.5
Propofol	10.0	Undiluted	10.0	1/10	1.0
Thiopental	25.0	Undiluted	25.0	1/10	2.5
Ketamine	100.0	1/10	10.0	1/100	1.0
Opioids					
Alfentanil	0.5	Undiluted	0.5	1/10	0.05
Fentanyl	0.05	Undiluted	0.05	1/10	0.005
Sufentanil	0.005	Undiluted	0.005	1/10	0.0005
Remifentanil	0.05	Undiluted	0.05	1/10	0.005
Morphine	10.0	1/10	1.0	1/1000	0.01
Local anesthetics					
Bupivacaine	2.5	Undiluted	2.5	1/10	0.25
Lidocaine	10.0	Undiluted	10.0	1/10	1.0
Mepivacaine	10.0	Undiluted	10.0	1/10	1.0
Ropivacaine	2.0	Undiluted	2.0	1/10	0.2

Abbreviations: Cmax, maximal concentration; Conc, concentration.
Adapted from Mertes PM, Malinovsky JM, Jouffroy L, et al. Reducing the risk of anaphylaxis during anesthesia: 2011 updated guidelines for clinical practice. J Investig Allergol Clin Immunol 2011;21(6):447; with permission.

histamine and react to it. Immediate reactions (wheal and erythema) are read at 15 to 20 minutes. An SPT is considered positive when the diameter of the wheal is at least equal to half of that produced by the positive control and at least 3 mm larger than the negative control. For IDT, 0.02 to 0.05 mL of solution is injected into the dermis in order to create a postinjection wheal of up to 4 mm in diameter. An IDT is considered positive when the diameter of the wheal is at least twice the injection wheal. Skin tests should be performed 4 to 6 weeks after the reaction. If necessary, they can be performed earlier.[36] This practice, however, increases the risk of false-negative results; only positive results are taken into account.[37] Early assessment does not replace the one performed after a period of 4 to 6 weeks.[24]

Specific IgE immunoassays
Allergen-specific IgE immunoassays are also important complementary tests in the diagnosis of perioperative immediate hypersensitivity reactions. Quantification of

drug-specific IgE (sIgE) relies on the detection of a drug-carrier-antibody complex. Basically, the drug or the hapten is coupled with a solid phase, which is incubated with the patients' serum. The amount of sIgE bound is subsequently detected with a secondary antihuman IgE antibody labeled formerly with a radioisotope radioimmunoassay and nowadays with an enzyme with colorimetric reading (enzyme-linked immunosorbent assay [ELISA]) or with fluorescence reading (FEIA).

The search for specific IgE in serum mainly concerns NMBAs, thiopental, latex, β-lactams, chlorhexidine, ethylene oxide, and pholcodine (PHO). These tests can be performed either in conjunction with skin tests or in the event of discrepancies between evocative history and negative skin tests.

Basophil activation test

Historically, activation of basophils was analyzed by the measurement of cysteinyl leukotriene or histamine release ex vivo.[38,39] These techniques are progressively replaced by flow cytometry (Basophil activation test [BAT]) used to quantify the shift in expression of basophilic activation markers (CD63 and CD203c) after challenge with a specific allergen using specific antibodies conjugated with a fluorochrome or a dye.[40]

Cellular assays do not allow differentiating between IgE-dependent and IgE-independent basophil activation but might constitute a unique tool in the diagnosis of IgE-independent hypersensitivity reactions. In addition, they may be of particular interest for the diagnosis of IgE-mediated anaphylaxis to compounds that are skin irritant when a specific IgE assay is unavailable. BAT is very useful when skin test results are difficult to interpret (eg, in patients with dermographism; extensive atopic skin lesions; or patients on medication with antihistamine effects, such as antidepressants and antihistamines, which cannot be stopped).[24] They also seem complementary to skin testing in the assessment of cross-reactivity between drugs.[41]

Challenge tests

Provocation testing represents a gold standard when investigating an immediate hypersensitivity reaction but has limited indications in perianesthetic anaphylaxis because of the pharmacologic effects of anesthetics. These tests can be performed with drugs or agents for which skin tests cannot be conducted or when skin tests are negative (local anesthetics, antibiotics, or, exceptionally, latex) or not validated (NSAIDs). Local anesthetics can be tested by subcutaneously injecting 0.5 to 2.0 mL of undiluted anesthetic solution (without epinephrine). The test is considered negative if no hypersensitivity reaction occurs within 30 minutes after the injection. Oral provocation tests are useful for the diagnosis of β-lactam hypersensitivity when skin tests are negative. These tests should be conducted under strict supervision and only in specialized centers with monitoring and resuscitation facilities.[24]

GENERAL ANESTHETICS
Neuromuscular Blocking Agents

Immune-mediated reactions

NMBAs represent the class of drugs most commonly implicated in perioperative anaphylaxis, although striking differences can be observed between countries. Reactions are almost exclusively IgE mediated. Delayed allergic reactions have been described on rare occasions and concern only suxamethonium.[42,43]

In one of the largest reports, perioperative anaphylaxis was evaluated over an 8-year period from 1997 to 2004 using a combined analysis of 3 different French databases. Among the 1816 patients with IgE–mediated reactions, the most common cause for these allergic events were NMBAs (58%, $n = 1067$).[4] Reactions have also been reported with a high frequency in Australia and New Zealand,[44] the United Kingdom,[16] and Norway.[12] They seem to be relatively frequent in Spain, accounting for 37% of the reactions observed,[10] but less frequent in Sweden[45] and Denmark.[17] Information about the incidence or agents implicated in perioperative anaphylaxis in the United States is very limited. NMBAs have been recently reported to be the offending agent in 11% of cases of perioperative anaphylaxis in a single-center study.[9]

Cross-reactivity

NMBAs are divalent ammonium compounds that bind to the α-subunit of the acetylcholine receptor at the neuromuscular junction. Structure-activity studies have long established that these substituted ammonium ions were the complementary allergenic sites involved in specific IgE recognition. This finding explains the frequent cross-reactivity between the different NMBAs observed in 60% to 70% of patients allergic to NMBAs identified by skin testing.[46–54] The patterns of cross-reactivity vary considerably between patients. Cross-reactivity to all NMBAs is unusual but seems to be more frequent when an aminosteroid NMBA is involved in the initial reaction rather than a benzylisoquinoline-derived NMBA.[1,55] The IgE recognition site of the molecule also depends on the molecular environment of the ammonium ion.[56,57]

This IgE recognition site and the molecular environment explains the heterogeneity of the cross-reactivity among patients but also part of the differences regarding the relative risk of allergic reactions between NMBAs that have been recognized in large epidemiologic surveys.[13,58,59] There is a broad consensus to consider succinylcholine as an agent with a high risk of anaphylaxis in the literature, whereas pancuronium and cis-atracurium are the NMBAs associated with the lowest incidence.[13,60] Regarding the relative risk of anaphylaxis to rocuronium, things are more controversial. An increased frequency of allergic reactions to rocuronium was initially reported in Norway[61] and rapidly confirmed in France.[22] Unfortunately, this created controversy. The rapid increase in the rate of rocuronium anaphylaxis in Australia from 1996 to 1999 was assumed to be a result of increased market share,[62] whereas, based on normalized market-share data provided by the manufacturer for 1996 to 1999 in the United Kingdom, the rate of rocuronium anaphylaxis was considered as similar to that of vecuronium and atracurium.[63] Within the same period of time, Bhananker and colleagues[64] reported a similar rate of reactions to rocuronium and vecuronium in the United States. More recently, this increased risk of allergic reactions has been confirmed in Australia, with a 4-fold increased risk with rocuronium when compared with vecuronium.[55]

Several hypotheses have been provided to explain the apparent increased risk of allergic reactions to succinylcholine and rocuronium. The flexibility of the chain between the ammonium ions and the distance between the substituted ammonium ions might be of importance to favor cross-linking of IgEs bound at the surface of effector cells. Therefore, flexible molecules, such as succinylcholine, are considered more potent in stimulating sensitized cells. Similarly, in the past, alcuronium was claimed to be a high risk for anaphylaxis. Alcuronium and rocuronium share the same propenyl ammonium group in their structure, which might be involved in their increased allergenicity. These considerations represent an important issue in the design of an ideal NMBA with a reduced risk of allergic reactions.

Origin of sensitization to NMBAs

In contrast to the immunologic dogma of previous exposure, a substantial proportion of patients with NMBA IgE-mediated anaphylaxis have never been exposed to a muscle relaxant before, suggesting that there must be environmental factors that play a role in cross-sensitizing patients against NMBAs.[65] Because compounds containing tertiary and/or quaternary ammonium groups occur widely in the human environment in drugs, cosmetics, and disinfectants, sensitization to NMBAs may occur via these sources. Although this hypothesis has long been considered as difficult to prove,[66] a recent study conducted in hairdressers has demonstrated a significant increase in IgE sensitization to NMBAs and quaternary ammonium ion compounds, suggesting that repetitive exposure to quaternary ammonium compounds used in hairdressing is a risk factor for NMBAs sensitization.[67] Another attractive hypothesis arises from the work published by Florvaag and Johansson[68] who provided repeated evidence for a connection between the consumption of PHO, an opioid antitussive, and IgE-mediated anaphylactic reactions to NMBA. They demonstrated that PHO, which is sold over the counter in many countries, is a strong inducer of an IgE antibody response that leads to sensitization of 20% to 25% of the exposed patients. However, PHO is monovalent for 2 non–cross-reacting epitopes, a quaternary ammonium ion and a non–quaternary ammonium epitope. Thus, PHO itself is not able to induce an allergic reaction in sensitized patients. However, the presence of the PHO-induced IgE to a quaternary ammonium ion will result in a 200- to 300-fold increased risk of anaphylaxis when these patients will be exposed to a bivalent NMBA during a general anesthesia. These results led to the withdrawal of PHO from the Norwegian market, resulting in the decrease of IgEs to quaternary ammonium ions in the population and in the number of reports of allergic reactions to NMBA.[69] A prospective case-control study designed to confirm this possible link between PHO exposure and sensitization to NMBAs will start in 2014 in France.

Nevertheless, immediate hypersensitivity reactions involving an NMBA are not always immune mediated. A direct nonspecific mast cell and basophil activation leading to histamine release has been reported with the use of ᴅ-tubocurarine, atracurium, mivacurium, and rapacuronium.[70] There is not always a clear correlation between circulating histamine levels and the resulting symptoms, particularly for bronchospasm.[71,72] Reactions resulting from direct histamine release are usually less severe than IgE-mediated reactions,[22,60] with the exception of a subset of patients who have been considered as super-responders to the histamine-releasing effect of NMBAs.[73]

NMBAs may also cross-react with nicotinic and muscarinic receptors responsible for actions at the extraneuromuscular junction cholinergic receptors level, causing peripheral autonomic and ganglionic effects. Rapacuronium was responsible for a high incidence of bronchospasm secondary to a higher affinity for M2 versus M3 muscarinic receptors,[74–76] leading to its withdrawal from the market in the United States.

Allergy testing

Skin tests in association with the clinical history remain the mainstay of the diagnosis of an IgE-mediated reaction (see **Table 1**). There has been some controversy concerning the advantages of either SPT or IDT,[77] and negative SPT should be followed by IDT. Because of the frequent but not systematic cross-reactivity, all available NMBAs should be tested using IDT.[2,13,65,78–81] This testing should help avoid future adverse reactions and provide documented advice for future anesthesia.[13,79,80,82] However, one should always remember that no diagnostic procedure is devoid of the risk of false-positive or false-negative results. Although rare, some cases of renewed allergic reactions following exposure to an NMBA considered to be safe have been reported in the literature.[83,84] Therefore, when administering an NMBA to sensitized patients with a negative skin test, one should bear in mind the risk-benefit ratio.

In some cases, when the clinical history is highly evocative of an allergic reaction to an NMBA but skin tests remain negative, quantification of specific IgE to quaternary ammonium ion will be of high interest to optimize the diagnosis of allergy. Several specific immunoassays have been developed, such as a choline chloride,[85] a p-aminophenyl phosphoryl choline,[86] and a morphine-based[87] and a rocuronium-based assay.[88] These tests are usually performed several weeks after the reaction but can be carried out at the time of the reaction.[80,89,90]

Promising results have also been recently provided in the literature by BAT. Although skin tests will remain the first choice for the diagnosis of sensitization to an NMBA and for the study of cross-sensitization, they could be of high interest in cases with negative skin tests and positive sIgE.[41] Indeed, in vitro sensitization to quaternary ammonium structures does not per se indicate the presence of an allergy to NMBAs; a high proportion of subjects with positive IgE assay in the absence of any history of allergic reactions to an NMBA have been reported in the literature.[45,91] Use of the BAT in the skin test negative, positive IgE assay patient may prevent any unnecessary avoidance of an NMBA.

Hypnotics

Allergic reactions incriminating these drugs are rare.

Reactions were quite frequent with thiopental accounting for 38% of the reactions in the United States.[92] Their incidence was estimated to be 1:30,000.[93] Recently, thiopental was involved in less than 1% of allergic reactions in France, as a result of its decreased use.[60] Although, most of the reactions were related to the ability of barbiturates to elicit direct leukocyte histamine release, true IgE-mediated anaphylactic reactions confirmed by skin tests and specific IgE assay have been described.[94,95]

Immediate hypersensitivity reactions may also be observed with propofol. They accounted for 2.5% of allergic reactions in the last French surveys.[22,60] Diagnosing these reactions may be difficult, and the possibility of false-positive results due to hydrophobic interaction has been reported with IgE immunoassays.[56] It has been suggested that propofol should be omitted in patients with allergy to eggs or soy because of the presence of lecithins in the propofol vehicle, but this has not been confirmed in daily practice.[24,96]

Reactions to midazolam, etomidate, or ketamine seem to be really rare[22,60]; there are no documented cases of inhalational agents causing anaphylaxis.

Opioids

Immediate hypersensitivity reactions caused by opioids are very rare. Morphine, codeine phosphate, or pethidine can induce direct nonspecific skin mast cell activation but not heart or lung mast cell and basophil activation. Therefore, reactions are usually limited to pruritus, urticaria, and mild hypotension; there is significant overreporting of allergy to opiates. However, there are rare reports of IgE antibodies to morphine and codeine being detected in patients with opiate-associated anaphylaxis.[97] Fentanyl and its derivatives do not induce nonspecific mediator release from mast cells. There is no evidence of cross-reactivity between the different opioid subclasses phenanthrenes (eg, morphine, codeine), phenylpiperedines (alfentanil, fentanyl, remifentanil, sufentanil, and meperidine), and diphenylheptanes (methadone and propoxyphene) in the literature[82]; but cross-reactivity between morphine and codeine is frequent. Morphine cross-reacts strongly with IgE antibodies from patients allergic to NMBAs via the tertiary methylamino group. Although morphine is monovalent and, thus, cannot elicit a clinical reaction in patients allergic to NMBA patients, this cross-reactivity is used in these patients to detect IgE against quaternary ammonium ions.[54]

Allergy to synthetic opioid can be investigated by skin testing (see **Table 1**).

The diagnosis of morphine allergy remains more challenging. Skin tests may be helpful; however, because morphine may induce direct histamine release, the maximal concentration recommended for skin testing should not be exceeded. In some cases, when the clinical history does not support the diagnosis of an immediate reaction to morphine, a challenge test can be considered.

LOCAL ANESTHETICS
Background

Local anesthetics stabilize neuronal membranes by inhibiting the ionic movement required for the transmission of neural impulses. Local anesthesia permits the surgeon to perform the surgical procedure in a safe, comfortable fashion for the patient. Local anesthetics are used in dentistry, ophthalmology, minor surgery, endoscopies and obstetrics. They are available in multiple forms including gels, ointments, sprays, solutions and injectable forms. The topical anesthetics seem to be relatively safe. Allergic contact dermatitis and tissue irritation can occur. Patch testing can be used to identify contact sensitivity to a topical local anesthetic. Although benzocaine is often used as a screening agent, when used alone, sensitivity to other topical local anesthetics can be missed, and a -caine mix has been recommended.[98] This discussion, though, focuses on injected local anesthetics. Local anesthetics have been refined over the years, but adverse reactions still occur. Differentiating between allergic and nonallergic adverse reactions can be difficult because of the overlap of symptoms and lack of availability of documentation of the initial reaction. True allergy to local anesthetics is thought to represent less than 1% of all reactions to local anesthetics.[99–101]

Types of Local Anesthetics

Local anesthetics may be classified as benzoic acid esters (group 1) or others, primarily amides (group 2) based on the linking chain between the lipophilic aromatic ring and the hydrophilic amine group (**Box 1**). Reactions to the benzoic acid esters are thought to be secondary to their metabolism via plasma esterases to para-aminobenzoic acid (PABA). Procaine (Novocain) was one of the commonly used benzoic acid esters. The benzoic acid esters often cross-react with each other but generally do not cross-react with the group 2 agents. The amides, which are not metabolized into the PABA molecule, are less sensitizing and do not generally cross-react with each other. Currently, most local anesthesia is performed using amides. Commonly used amides and their characteristics include the agents listed later.

Lidocaine is considered the prototype for amide local anesthetics. It is characterized by a rapid onset of action and intermediate duration of efficacy. It is metabolized by the liver and excreted by the kidneys with 10% unchanged and 80% as metabolites.

Mepivacaine has a reasonably rapid onset and medium duration of action. It is metabolized by the liver. Higher-concentration (4%) mepivacaine causes slight vasoconstriction providing it with a longer duration of action.

Prilocaine is a secondary amide that is metabolized in both liver and kidneys, Therefore, liver and renal diseases may change prilocaine kinetics. Methemoglobinemia may be a side effect when large doses are used and should be avoided in patients with sickle cell anemia, chronic anemia, and hypoxia and in patients taking high doses of acetaminophen or phenacetin.

Articaine is an amide with unique structures including a thiophene ring that enhances its lipid solubility and an additional ester group allowing hydrolysis in the

Box 1
Commonly used local anesthetics

Group 1 (esters)

  Benzocaine

  Butamben picrate

  Cocaine

  Procaine (Novocain)

  Tetracaine (Pontocaine)

Group 2 (primarily amides)

  Short acting

    Lidocaine (Xylocaine)

  Medium acting

    Mepivacaine (Carbocaine, Polocaine)

    Prilocaine (Citanest)

    Articaine (also contains ester group)

    Lidocaine with epinephrine

  Long acting

    Bupivacaine (Marcaine)

plasma as well as in the liver. This structure allows for less systemic toxicity, especially with repeated doses.[102]

Bupivacaine is 4 times more potent than lidocaine, mepivacaine, and prilocaine and has a longer duration of action than lidocaine. It is often administered when long-term pain control is needed, such as extraction of impacted third molars or surgical wound sites.[103] This agent has potential higher cardiotoxicity and should be used with caution in patients taking β-blockers or digoxin.

Epinephrine (1:100,000) may be added to a local anesthetic to cause vasoconstriction, resulting in an increased duration of action and less systemic absorption of the local anesthetic. The adverse effect associated with a local anesthetic is often secondary to the systemic absorption of epinephrine. It may cause palpitations, tachycardia, arrhythmia, hypertension, tremor, headache, and anxiety.

Adverse Reactions

Adverse reactions to local anesthetics that mimic allergy can have numerous causes, including anxiety (needle phobia, panic attacks, vasovagal syncope), intravascular administration of local anesthetic, intravascular absorption of epinephrine, overdosage of local anesthetic, toxic levels caused by a lack of metabolism, and intolerance. When evaluating patients with a reported allergy to a local anesthetic, it is imperative to obtain a detailed history of the reaction and when possible to include the following:

1. Type of procedure performed at time of reaction
2. Timing of administration of local anesthetic in relation to symptom development
3. Complete review of systems of the reaction
4. Type, amount, and concentration of the local anesthetic used
5. Whether the local anesthetic contained epinephrine
6. Patients' medical history, particularly kidney, liver, cardiac, and psychiatric history

This information coupled with a basic knowledge of the commonly used local anesthetics will help determine whether the reaction is likely allergic in nature or secondary to another cause. Although the focus here is on the local anesthetics, it is also important to note other concomitant agents or exposures, particularly antibiotics, NSAIDs, and latex.

Large Clinical Studies

A recent literature review of local anesthetic reactions identified 23 case series involving 2978 patients.[101] Twenty-nine of these patients had true IgE mediated reactions to local anesthetics resulting in a prevalence of 0.97%. The number of patients in the case series ranged from 20 to 386. There was significant variability in the protocols used for the investigations. Most investigators used a combination of skin tests and challenges to confirm (or rule out) the diagnosis and find alternative agents. Most studies used recommended vasoconstrictor-free (epinephrine) preparations with and without preservatives for testing and subsequent use. The local anesthetic involved in the initial reaction was often not used in the skin testing or challenge evaluation. In a review of 135 cases with alleged allergic reactions to local anesthetics, 83 cases (61%) did not include challenge to the culprit local anesthetic.[104] In an analysis of 197 reported episodes in 177 patients, challenge tests with an alternative agents were performed in the first 54 patients, though the remainder of the patients was challenged with the suspected local anesthetic.[105] In 236 patients evaluated by SPT and IDT, followed by subcutaneous challenge, none was tested or challenged with the suspected local anesthetic but rather to a different one. In this group, 22% of the patients reported initial symptoms compatible with immediate hypersensitivity, 11% with local swelling at the injection site, 27% described nonspecific symptoms, 15% delayed reactions, and 25% were referred because they were atopic but had no history of adverse reactions to local anesthetics.[106] Atlhough negative challenge to an unrelated local anesthetic is valuable/beneficial clinically in that it provides a treatment option, the risk of underestimating the true incidence of hypersensitivity to local anesthetics in these populations exists.

The type of patients studied could also impact the results of testing. Given that true local anesthetic allergy is rare, studying large number of patients without symptoms suggestive of an immediate hypersensitivity will further dilute the percentage of true positive test results. Harboe and colleagues[104] noted a considerable overlap in manifestations between test-positive and test-negative groups, though itch, urticaria, and documented hypotension (as opposed to local rash, palpitations, feeling of narrow throat, or feeling faint) were reported most/more frequently in cases with positive tests.

Testing to Local Anesthetics

IgE-mediated reactions to local anesthetics, particularly amides, are rare. Evaluation consists of SPT, IDT, and challenges. McClimon and colleagues[107] studied the predictive value of skin testing in the diagnosis of local anesthetic allergy. In their study of 178 patients, the negative predictive value was 97%, using undiluted preserved local anesthetic solution without epinephrine for SPT, 1:100 dilution for IDT, and subsequent challenge with 0.1 mL, 0.5 mL, and 1.0 mL of undiluted local anesthetic solution. Of the 227 skin tests performed, 220 were negative and 7 were positive. Based on the study criteria, 6 of the 220 patients had positive challenges that were confined to local skin reactions. Three of the patients with positive IDT subsequently had negative challenges to the same agent. This finding is similar to the overall finding of Bhole and colleagues[101] who noticed an overall higher positive rate with IDT when compared with positive reactions as determined by challenge tests. The evaluation of 28 patients with histories of reaction to local anesthetics, elicited positive SPT in 4 patients and positive IDT (at 1:10 dilution) in 10. Subsequent challenge, though, was negative for all.[108] Multiple skin test–positive results to local anesthetics are rarely seen among skin test–positive patients, only one in the McClimon and colleagues[107] study. In the large studies, patients were often tested only to a single nonculprit local anesthetic. Gonzalez-Delgado and colleagues[109] demonstrated the clinical utility of skin testing in a man with a clinical history of reaction to mepivacaine with positive skin test reactions to mepivacaine, lidocaine, and ropivacaine but negative reaction to bupivacaine. Bupivacaine was subsequently tolerated in a double-blind placebo-controlled challenge.

Only 3 cases of in vitro–specific IgE to local anesthetics have been reported in the literature.[110–112] In one instance, the patient had a history highly suggestive of an immediate hypersensitivity reaction to mepivacaine. Intradermal skin testing at 1:100 dilution was positive to mepivacaine and bupivacaine and positive to lidocaine at 1:10 dilution. Skin testing to prilocaine was negative. Mepivacaine induced the strongest inhibition of IgE binding, followed by bupivacaine, lidocaine, and prilocaine, respectively. The significantly weaker inhibition with prilocaine was clinically relevant and confirmed the negative skin test, as the patient subsequently used it for dental procedures without complication.[111] Stahl and colleagues[112] reported a patient with immediate hypersensitivity reaction to lidocaine followed one week later by another immediate hypersensitivity reaction to an unknown local anesthetic, resulting in another immediate hypersensitivity reaction. Subsequent skin testing was positive to tetracaine and challenges positive to lidocaine and articaine. ELISA testing showed parallel curves to both amides and esters, but the esters did not correlate with the amides. Inhibition study demonstrated possible cross-reactivity between tetracaine and articaine but not between tetracaine and mepivacaine, likely because of the dual amide and ester group found on articaine. This case was the first case demonstrating specific IgE to both amides and esters in the same patient.

Allergy to local anesthetics may be caused by methylparaben, paraben, or metabisulfite used as preservatives. Although preservative-free local anesthetics exist, they may not be easy to obtain. Methylparaben, a preservative commonly found in foods and cosmetics, is used as a preservative in multiuse local anesthetics. In 1984, the Food and Drug Administration mandated its removal from single-dose local anesthetic cartridges. Reactions to methylparaben in local anesthetics have been reported.[113] Sulfites are antioxidants used to stabilize epinephrine in local anesthetic solutions. They are not typically used when the local anesthetic does not contain epinephrine. Sulfites have been involved in non–IgE-mediated hypersensitivity reactions, particularly in patients with asthma. Because testing is very inconsistent, it is difficult to know the role sulfites may play in reactions attributed to a local anesthetic preparation.

These findings have raised the question of the most efficient way to evaluate local anesthetic allergy. Multiple skin tests at various dilutions and progressive multistep challenges can be time consuming and painful for patients. Based on recent data, proposals that came forth using preservative-containing, non–epinephrine-containing local anesthetics include the following:

1. SPT and IDT (concentrations not defined), if negative, a single subcutaneous challenge (as opposed to incremental); if positive, then skin test and challenge to an unrelated local anesthetic[101]
2. SPT, if negative, IDT with 0.04 mL of 1:100 dilution, if negative, 1 mL subcutaneous challenge; if skin test result positive, retest with pure local anesthetic solution without methylparaben or other preservative[114]

3. SPT, if negative, IDT with 1:100 dilution, if negative, subcutaneous challenge with 1:10 dilution 0.1 mL, followed by undiluted 0.1 mL, followed by undiluted 1.0 mL[104]

Whether to test the culprit local anesthetic or an alternative agent will depend on the expected future need of the specific local anesthetic, but testing the initial offending drug is favored in order to make a definite diagnosis. Based on their different properties, a specific local anesthetic may be preferable.

OTHER SUBSTANCES IMPLICATED IN THE SETTING OF ANESTHESIA
Antibiotics

Antibiotics are often administered in the anesthesia setting. The percentage of allergic reactions during anesthesia secondary to antibiotics varies depending on the study and particularly the reporting country. The Groupe d'Etudes des Reactions Anaphylactoides Peranesthesiques, a network of 40 French allergo-anesthesia outpatient clinics whose aim is to survey reactions during anesthesia, noted an increase in percentage of antibiotics responsible for anaphylaxis during anesthesia in France from 2% in 1984 to 1989 to 18% in 2005 to 2007.[11] In these studies, NMBAs continue to be the most common cause, though decreasing from 81% in 1984 to 1989 to 47% in 2005 to 2007. This finding contrasts with 2 recent reports from tertiary care centers in North America in which antibiotics were the most commonly identified cause of anaphylaxis in the anesthesia setting accounting for 50% and 47% of reactions.[9,115] Similarly in Spain, Lobera and colleagues[10] reported antibiotics accounting for 44% of allergic reactions during anesthesia. Penicillins and cephalosporins account for most anesthesia-related anaphylactic reactions secondary to antibiotics. Vancomycin and quinolones have also been incriminated in some cases, but it can be difficult to distinguish vancomycin allergy from the basophil degranulation causing the red-man syndrome. Although quinolones can be involved based on timing or subsequent challenge, there is no standardized skin test or specific IgE assay available for quinolones.

Latex

Latex is typically cited as one of the top 3 causes of anaphylaxis during anesthesia. IgE-mediated latex allergy has been well documented with recognized risk groups, including children undergoing numerous procedures, particularly those with spina bifida; adults requiring multiple procedures; health care workers; and individuals with a food allergy to latex fruits. Investigation of latex allergy is performed in the United States using latex glove extracts, though the latex protein content is not standardized, whereas in Europe, commercial extracts with excellent sensitivity are available. Specific IgE to latex (including IgE to specific latex components: Hev b1, b3, b6, b7, b8, b9, b10, b11) is also commercially available. Latex as the cause of anesthesia-related allergy has increased in France from 0.5% (in 1984–1989) to 20.0% in 2005 to 2007.[11] Identification of patients at risk and strategies to reduce latex exposure both environmentally (eg, latex-free gloves and equipment) and in the surgical setting have resulted in decreased reactions secondary to latex in other areas.[9,104]

NSAIDs

NSAIDs have been increasingly used in postsurgical and postprocedural settings. They are given orally or by injection. The types of reaction can vary from isolated cutaneous or respiratory symptoms to anaphylaxis. In the very rare setting of IgE-mediated NSAID anaphylaxis, patients often only react to one NSAID. Unfortunately, the mechanism is not always clear; both IgE-mediated and non–IgE-mediated reactions occur. Skin testing is not reliable. The basophil activation test on blood basophils shows potential, though more studies are needed.[116] When exploring NSAIDs hypersensitivity, drug provocation test is particularly useful.

Chlorhexidine

Chlorhexidine is a standard skin antiseptic and disinfectant. It is widely used in medical, procedural, and surgical settings. Sensitization to chlorhexidine can occur from home products, such as mouthwash, toothpaste, dressings, ointments, and over-the-counter disinfectant solutions. Systemic allergic reactions ranging from widespread urticaria to anaphylactic shock have been reported to chlorhexidine via topical skin application, ophthalmic wash solution, chlorhexidine bath, coated central venous catheter, and urethral gels. The largest group reported so far (including 12 allergic patients) sheds some light on the potential risk factors for chlorhexidine sensitization.[28] Most of the patients were male with a median age of 64 years, with nearly half of the reactions occurring during urologic surgeries or procedures. During these procedures, chlorhexidine exposure is enhanced by absorption through mucosal surfaces (urethra, bladder) and skin (incision, epidural), especially if the chlorhexidine is not dry before the initiation of the procedure. Chlorhexidine skin testing has been shown to be predictive of allergic sensitivity to chlorhexidine and to correlate with in vitro chlorhexidine sIgE testing.[117]

Dyes

Dyes have become increasingly recognized as a cause of allergic or anaphylactic reactions in the anesthesia setting. The triarylmethane dyes, patent blue V and isosulfan blue, share a similar structure and are commonly used for lymphatic mapping. It is thought exposure to blue dye in cosmetics and other everyday products contributes to sensitization. The mechanism of reaction to the dye in unclear, both direct mast cell and/or basophil activation and specific IgE sensitization have been described. Methylene blue, a smaller molecule, which differs structurally from the triarylmethane dyes, has also been associated with reactions. Sensitization to both patent blue and methylene blue has been reported.[26] Reactions to dyes are often delayed, occurring 30 minutes after injection, and can be prolonged. Although the mechanism is not always clear, the drug allergy work-up includes SPT and IDT. These tests can help identify the cause of a reaction and, in conjunction with negative testing, may identify a safe dye alternative.

Colloids

Colloids have rarely been implicated in anesthesia-related anaphylaxis. The incidence has been estimated to range from 0.03% to 0.22%.[118] Gelatins and dextrans are more commonly associated with reactions than albumin and hetastarch. Skin tests can be performed to identify IgE-mediated reaction to gelatin and hydroxyethyl starch. Specific IgE assays to gelatin can also be used.

Aprotinin

Aprotinin, a serine protease inhibitor, is used to prevent bleeding. It has been administered in intravenous form and as a component of biologic sealants. In 2007, the intravenous drug was withdrawn from the market. Currently, it is part of the fibrin glue combined with human coagulation factors used to aid hemostasis and sealing of tissue wounds. Prevalence of reactions to aprotinin is higher in patients with a history of previous exposure. A reexposure interval less than 6 months could be considered a relative contraindication to fibrin glue application.[119] SPT and IDT (up to 1:10 dilution) can be used for diagnosis.

Prevention

Preventive testing of patients to the most common elicitors of anesthesia-related anaphylaxis is not justified by current evidence. The primary risk factor is a history of a hypersensitivity reaction with previous anesthesia or a known allergy to one or more medications or products likely to be administered during the procedure. Unless already documented, all patients with such history should have a comprehensive evaluation, including skin testing and/or specific IgE testing and drug provocation tests to the potential culprit anesthetic agents and related compounds, before further administration of anesthetics. A strategy should be used to avoid these medications and those that are cross-reactive. Patients who are atopic, those with asthma or allergic rhinitis, or those who have a medication allergy to a drug not likely to be used during the course of anesthesia or procedure are not considered to be at a significantly increased risk for a hypersensitivity reaction.

For those with latex sensitivity, a latex-free environment should be available. Many centers have set up latex-free operating rooms and procedural areas. This set-up requires coordination among the surgical, medical, and anesthetic teams.

The role of pretreatment with H1-receptor antagonists and corticosteroids is not well defined. These medications may help decrease non-IgE histamine-mediated reactions. However, they do not reliably prevent IgE-mediated reactions. Avoidance of the allergen is the only true way to prevent an anaphylactic reaction.

REFERENCES

1. Mertes PM, Demoly P, Malinovsky JM. Hypersensitivity reactions in the anesthesia setting/allergic reactions to anesthetics. Curr Opin Allergy Clin Immunol 2012;12(4):361–8.
2. Fisher MM, Doig GS. Prevention of anaphylactic reactions to anaesthetic drugs. Drug Saf 2004;27(6):393–410.
3. Malinovsky JM, Decagny S, Wessel F, et al. Systematic follow-up increases incidence of anaphylaxis during adverse reactions in anesthetized patients. Acta Anaesthesiol Scand 2008;52(2):175–81.
4. Mertes PM, Alla F, Trechot P, et al. Anaphylaxis during anesthesia in France: an 8-year national survey. J Allergy Clin Immunol 2011;128(2):366–73.
5. Kroigaard M, Garvey LH, Menne T, et al. Allergic reactions in anaesthesia: are suspected causes confirmed on subsequent testing? Br J Anaesth 2005; 95(4):468–71.
6. Mancardi DA, Albanesi M, Jonsson F, et al. The high-affinity human IgG receptor FcγRI (CD64) promotes IgG-mediated inflammation, anaphylaxis, and antitumor immunotherapy. Blood 2013;121(9):1563–73.
7. Johansson SG, Bieber T, Dahl R, et al. Revised nomenclature for allergy for global use: report of the Nomenclature Review Committee of the World Allergy Organization, October 2003. J Allergy Clin Immunol 2004;113(5): 832–6.
8. Mertes PM, Tajima K, Regnier-Kimmoun MA, et al. Perioperative anaphylaxis. Med Clin North Am 2010;94(4):761–89, xi.
9. Gurrieri C, Weingarten TN, Martin DP, et al. Allergic reactions during anesthesia at a large United States referral center. Anesth Analg 2011;113(5): 1202–12.
10. Lobera T, Audicana MT, Pozo MD, et al. Study of hypersensitivity reactions and anaphylaxis during anesthesia in Spain. J Investig Allergol Clin Immunol 2008; 18(5):350–6.

11. Dong SW, Mertes PM, Petitpain N, et al. Hypersensitivity reactions during anesthesia. Results from the ninth French survey (2005-2007). Minerva Anestesiol 2012;78(8):868–78.
12. Harboe T, Guttormsen AB, Irgens A, et al. Anaphylaxis during anesthesia in Norway: a 6-year single-center follow-up study. Anesthesiology 2005;102(5): 897–903.
13. Fisher M, Baldo BA. Anaphylaxis during anaesthesia: current aspects of diagnosis and prevention. Eur J Anaesthesiol 1994;11(4):263–84.
14. Chong YY, Caballero MR, Lukawska J, et al. Anaphylaxis during general anaesthesia: one-year survey from a British allergy clinic. Singapore Med J 2008; 49(6):483–7.
15. Thienthong S, Hintong T, Pulnitiporn A. The Thai Anesthesia Incidents Study (THAI Study) of perioperative allergic reactions. J Med Assoc Thai 2005; 88(Suppl 7):S128–33.
16. Pepys J, Pepys EO, Baldo BA, et al. Anaphylactic/anaphylactoid reactions to anaesthetic and associated agents. Skin prick tests in aetiological diagnosis. Anaesthesia 1994;49(6):470–5.
17. Garvey LH, Roed-Petersen J, Menne T, et al. Danish Anaesthesia Allergy Centre - preliminary results. Acta Anaesthesiol Scand 2001;45(10):1204–9.
18. Mitsuhata H, Matsumoto S, Hasegawa J. The epidemiology and clinical features of anaphylactic and anaphylactoid reactions in the perioperative period in Japan. Masui 1992;41:1664–9.
19. Hepner DL, Castells MC. Anaphylaxis during the perioperative period. Anesth Analg 2003;97(5):1381–95.
20. Light KP, Lovell AT, Butt H, et al. Adverse effects of neuromuscular blocking agents based on yellow card reporting in the U.K.: are there differences between males and females? Pharmacoepidemiol Drug Saf 2006;15(3):151–60.
21. Gibbs NM, Sadleir PH, Clarke RC, et al. Survival from perioperative anaphylaxis in Western Australia 2000-2009. Br J Anaesth 2013;111(4):589–93.
22. Mertes PM, Laxenaire MC, Alla F. Anaphylactic and anaphylactoid reactions occurring during anesthesia in France in 1999-2000. Anesthesiology 2003; 99(3):536–45.
23. Fisher MM, Ramakrishnan N, Doig G, et al. The investigation of bronchospasm during induction of anaesthesia. Acta Anaesthesiol Scand 2009;53(8): 1006–11.
24. Mertes PM, Malinovsky JM, Jouffroy L, et al. Reducing the risk of anaphylaxis during anesthesia: 2011 updated guidelines for clinical practice. J Investig Allergol Clin Immunol 2011;21(6):442–53.
25. Mertes PM, Bazin A, Alla F, et al. Hypersensitivity reactions to blood components: document issued by the allergy committee of the French medicines and healthcare products regulatory agency. J Investig Allergol Clin Immunol 2011;21(3):171–8.
26. Mertes PM, Malinovsky JM, Mouton-Faivre C, et al. Anaphylaxis to dyes during the perioperative period: reports of 14 clinical cases. J Allergy Clin Immunol 2008;122(2):348–52.
27. Hunting AS, Nopp A, Johansson SG, et al. Anaphylaxis to patent blue V. I. Clinical aspects. Allergy 2010;65(1):117–23.
28. Garvey LH, Kroigaard M, Poulsen LK, et al. IgE-mediated allergy to chlorhexidine. J Allergy Clin Immunol 2007;120(2):409–15.
29. Laxenaire MC, Mouton C, Frederic A, et al. Anaphylactic shock after tourniquet removal in orthopedic surgery. Ann Fr Anesth Reanim 1996;15(2):179–84.

30. Nel L, Eren E. Peri-operative anaphylaxis. Br J Clin Pharmacol 2011;71(5): 647–58.
31. Kounis NG, Mazarakis A, Tsigkas G, et al. Kounis syndrome: a new twist on an old disease. Future Cardiol 2011;7(6):805–24.
32. Berroa F, Lafuente A, Javaloyes G, et al. The usefulness of plasma histamine and different tryptase cut-off points in the diagnosis of peranaesthetic hypersensitivity reactions. Clin Exp Allergy 2014;44(2):270–7.
33. Enrique E, Garcia-Ortega P, Sotorra O, et al. Usefulness of UniCAP-tryptase fluoroimmunoassay in the diagnosis of anaphylaxis. Allergy 1999;54(6):602–6.
34. Mayer DE, Krauskopf A, Hemmer W, et al. Usefulness of post mortem determination of serum tryptase, histamine and diamine oxidase in the diagnosis of fatal anaphylaxis. Forensic Sci Int 2011;212(1–3):96–101.
35. Brockow K, Garvey LH, Aberer W, et al. Skin test concentrations for systemically administered drugs – an ENDA/EAACI Drug Allergy Interest Group position paper. Allergy 2013;68(6):702–12.
36. Lafuente A, Javaloyes G, Berroa F, et al. Early skin testing is effective for diagnosis of hypersensitivity reactions occurring during anesthesia. Allergy 2013; 68(6):820–2.
37. Soetens F, Rose M, Fisher M. Timing of skin testing after a suspected anaphylactic reaction during anaesthesia. Acta Anaesthesiol Scand 2012;56(8):1042–6.
38. Mata E, Gueant JL, Moneret-Vautrin DA, et al. Clinical evaluation of in vitro leukocyte histamine release in allergy to muscle relaxant drugs. Allergy 1992;47(5): 471–6.
39. Assem E. Leukotriene C4 release from blood cells in vitro in patients with anaphylactoid reactions to neuromuscular blockers. Agents Actions 1993;38: C242–4.
40. Ebo DG, Bridts CH, Hagendorens MM, et al. Basophil activation test by flow cytometry: present and future applications in allergology. Cytometry B Clin Cytom 2008;74(4):201–10.
41. Leysen J, Bridts CH, De Clerck LS, et al. Allergy to rocuronium: from clinical suspicion to correct diagnosis. Allergy 2011;66(8):1014–9.
42. Scala E, Guerra EC, Giani M, et al. Delayed allergic reaction to suxamethonium driven by oligoclonal Th1-skewed CD4+CCR4+IFN-gamma+ memory T cells. Int Arch Allergy Immunol 2006;141(1):24–30.
43. Delgado J, Quiralte J, Castillo R, et al. Systemic contact dermatitis from suxamethonium. Contact Dermatitis 1996;35(2):120–1.
44. Fisher MM, Baldo BA. The incidence and clinical features of anaphylactic reactions during anesthesia in Australia. Ann Fr Anesth Reanim 1993;12(2):97–104.
45. Florvaag E, Johansson SG, Oman H, et al. Prevalence of IgE antibodies to morphine. Relation to the high and low incidences of NMBA anaphylaxis in Norway and Sweden, respectively. Acta Anaesthesiol Scand 2005;49(4):437–44.
46. de Weck AL. Immunochemical particularities of anaphylactic reactions to compounds used in anesthesia. Ann Fr Anesth Reanim 1993;12(2):126–30.
47. Baldo BA, Fisher MM. Substituted ammonium ions as allergenic determinants in drug allergy. Nature 1983;306(5940):262–4.
48. Baldo BA, Harle DG. Drug allergenic determinants. In: Baldo BA, editor. Molecular approaches to the study of allergens monographs in allergy, vol. 28. Basel (Switzerland): Karger; 1990. p. 11–51.
49. Laxenaire MC, Gastin I, Moneret-Vautrin DA, et al. Cross-reactivity of rocuronium with other neuromuscular blocking agents. Eur J Anaesthesiol Suppl 1995;11: 55–64.

50. Moneret-Vautrin DA, Gueant JL, Kamel L, et al. Anaphylaxis to muscle relaxants: cross-sensitivity studied by radioimmunoassays compared to intradermal tests in 34 cases. J Allergy Clin Immunol 1988;82(5 Pt 1):745–52.
51. Leynadier F, Dry J. Anaphylaxis to muscle-relaxant drugs: study of cross-reactivity by skin tests. Int Arch Allergy Appl Immunol 1991;94(1–4):349–53.
52. Fisher MM. Anaphylaxis to muscle relaxants: cross sensitivity between relaxants. Anaesth Intensive Care 1980;8(2):211–3.
53. Fisher MM. Cisatracurium and atracurium as antigens. Anaesth Intensive Care 1999;27(4):369–70.
54. Fisher MM, Baldo BA. Immunoassays in the diagnosis of anaphylaxis to neuromuscular blocking drugs: the value of morphine for the detection of IgE antibodies in allergic subjects. Anaesth Intensive Care 2000;28:167–70.
55. Sadleir PH, Clarke RC, Bunning DL, et al. Anaphylaxis to neuromuscular blocking drugs: incidence and cross-reactivity in Western Australia from 2002 to 2011. Br J Anaesth 2013;110(6):981–7.
56. Gueant JL, Mata E, Masson C, et al. Non-specific cross-reactivity of hydrophobic serum IgE to hydrophobic drugs. Mol Immunol 1995;32(4):259–66.
57. Gueant JL, Mata E, Namour F, et al. Criteria of evaluation and of interpretation of Sepharose drug IgE-RIA to anaesthetic drugs. Allergy 1999;54(Suppl 58):17–22.
58. Laxenaire MC. Epidemiology of anesthetic anaphylactoid reactions. Fourth multicenter survey (July 1994-December 1996). Ann Fr Anesth Reanim 1999; 18(7):796–809.
59. Galletly DC, Treuren BC. Anaphylactoid reactions during anaesthesia. Seven years' experience of intradermal testing. Anaesthesia 1985;40(4):329–33.
60. Mertes PM, Laxenaire MC. Anaphylactic and anaphylactoid reactions occurring during anaesthesia in France. Seventh epidemiologic survey (January 2001-December 2002). Ann Fr Anesth Reanim 2004;23(12):1133–43 [in French].
61. Guttormsen AB. Allergic reactions during anaesthesia - increased attention to the problem in Denmark and Norway. Acta Anaesthesiol Scand 2001;45(10):1189–90.
62. Rose M, Fisher M. Rocuronium: high risk for anaphylaxis? Br J Anaesth 2001; 86(5):678–82.
63. Watkins J. Incidence of UK reactions involving rocuronium may simply reflect market use. Br J Anaesth 2001;87(3):522.
64. Bhananker SM, O'Donnell JT, Salemi JR, et al. The risk of anaphylactic reactions to rocuronium in the United States is comparable to that of vecuronium: an analysis of food and drug administration reporting of adverse events. Anesth Analg 2005;101(3):819–22.
65. Mertes PM, Laxenaire MC. Adverse reactions to neuromuscular blocking agents. Curr Allergy Asthma Rep 2004;4(1):7–16.
66. Baldo BA, Fisher MM, Pham NH. On the origin and specificity of antibodies to neuromuscular blocking (muscle relaxant) drugs: an immunochemical perspective. Clin Exp Allergy 2009;39(3):325–44.
67. Dong S, Acouetey DS, Gueant-Rodriguez RM, et al. Prevalence of IgE against neuromuscular blocking agents in hairdressers and bakers. Clin Exp Allergy 2013;43(11):1256–62.
68. Florvaag E, Johansson SG. The pholcodine case. Cough medicines, IgE-sensitization, and anaphylaxis: a devious connection. World Allergy Organ J 2012;5(7):73–8.
69. Florvaag E, Johansson SG, Irgens A, et al. IgE-sensitization to the cough suppressant pholcodine and the effects of its withdrawal from the Norwegian market. Allergy 2011;66(7):955–60.

70. Doenicke AW, Czeslick E, Moss J, et al. Onset time, endotracheal intubating conditions, and plasma histamine after cisatracurium and vecuronium administration. Anesth Analg 1998;87(2):434–8.

71. Doenicke A, Moss J, Lorenz W, et al. Are hypotension and rash after atracurium really caused by histamine release? Anesth Analg 1994;78(5):967–72.

72. Cannon JE, Fahey MR, Moss J, et al. Large doses of vecuronium and plasma histamine concentrations. Can J Anaesth 1988;35(4):350–3.

73. Fisher M. Anaphylaxis to anaesthetic drugs. Novartis Found Symp 2004;257: 193–202 [discussion: 202–10, 276–85].

74. Jooste E, Zhang Y, Emala CW. Rapacuronium preferentially antagonizes the function of M2 versus M3 muscarinic receptors in guinea pig airway smooth muscle. Anesthesiology 2005;102(1):117–24.

75. Jooste EH, Sharma A, Zhang Y, et al. Rapacuronium augments acetylcholine-induced bronchoconstriction via positive allosteric interactions at the M3 muscarinic receptor. Anesthesiology 2005;103(6):1195–203.

76. Jooste E, Klafter F, Hirshman CA, et al. A mechanism for rapacuronium-induced bronchospasm: M2 muscarinic receptor antagonism. Anesthesiology 2003; 98(4):906–11.

77. McKinnon RP, Wildsmith JA. Histaminoid reactions in anaesthesia. Br J Anaesth 1995;74(2):217–28.

78. Mertes PM, Laxenaire M. Anaphylaxis during general anaesthesia. Prevention and management. CNS Drugs 2000;14(2):115–33.

79. Mertes PM, Laxenaire MC. Allergy and anaphylaxis in anaesthesia. Minerva Anestesiol 2004;70(5):285–91.

80. Mertes PM, Laxenaire MC, Lienhart A, et al. Reducing the risk of anaphylaxis during anaesthesia: guidelines for clinical practice. J Investig Allergol Clin Immunol 2005;15(2):91–101.

81. Moneret-Vautrin DA, Kanny G. Anaphylaxis to muscle relaxants: rational for skin tests. Allerg Immunol (Paris) 2002;34(7):233–40.

82. Ebo DG, Fisher MM, Hagendorens MM, et al. Anaphylaxis during anaesthesia: diagnostic approach. Allergy 2007;62(5):471–87.

83. Fisher MM, Merefield D, Baldo B. Failure to prevent an anaphylactic reaction to a second neuromuscular blocking drug during anaesthesia. Br J Anaesth 1999; 82(5):770–3.

84. Thacker MA, Davis FM. Subsequent general anaesthesia in patients with a history of previous anaphylactoid/anaphylactic reaction to muscle relaxant. Anaesth Intensive Care 1999;27(2):190–3.

85. Gueant JL, Mata E, Monin B, et al. Evaluation of a new reactive solid phase for radioimmunoassay of serum specific IgE against muscle relaxant drugs. Allergy 1991;46(6):452–8.

86. Guilloux L, Ricard-Blum S, Ville G, et al. A new radioimmunoassay using a commercially available solid support for the detection of IgE antibodies against muscle relaxants. J Allergy Clin Immunol 1992;90(2):153–9.

87. Laroche D, Chollet-Martin S, Leturgie P, et al. Evaluation of a new routine diagnostic test for immunoglobulin e sensitization to neuromuscular blocking agents. Anesthesiology 2011;114(1):91–7.

88. Ebo DG, Venemalm L, Bridts CH, et al. Immunoglobulin E antibodies to rocuronium: a new diagnostic tool. Anesthesiology 2007;107(2):253–9.

89. Laroche D, Lefrancois C, Gerard JL, et al. Early diagnosis of anaphylactic reactions to neuromuscular blocking drugs. Br J Anaesth 1992;69(6):611–4.

90. Guttormsen AB, Johansson SG, Oman H, et al. No consumption of IgE antibody in serum during allergic drug anaphylaxis. Allergy 2007;62(11):1326–30.

91. Porri F, Lemiere C, Birnbaum J, et al. Prevalence of muscle relaxant sensitivity in a general population: implications for a preoperative screening. Clin Exp Allergy 1999;29(1):72–5.

92. Moscicki RA, Sockin SM, Corsello BF, et al. Anaphylaxis during induction of general anesthesia: subsequent evaluation and management. J Allergy Clin Immunol 1990;86(3 Pt 1):325–32.

93. Clarke RS. Epidemiology of adverse reactions in anaesthesia in the United Kingdom. Klin Wochenschr 1982;60(17):1003–5.

94. Harle D, Baldo B, Fisher M. The molecular basis of IgE antibody binding to thiopentone. Binding of IgE from thiopentone-allergic and non-allergic subjects. Mol Immunol 1990;27:853–8.

95. Fisher M, Ross J, Harle D, et al. Anaphylaxis to thiopentone: an unusual outbreak in a single hospital. Anaesth Intensive Care 1989;17(3):361–5.

96. Murphy A, Campbell DE, Baines D, et al. Allergic reactions to propofol in egg-allergic children. Anesth Analg 2011;113(1):140–4.

97. Harle DG, Baldo BA, Coroneos NJ, et al. Anaphylaxis following administration of papaveretum. Case report: implication of IgE antibodies that react with morphine and codeine, and identification of an allergic determinant. Anesthesiology 1989;71:489–94.

98. Warshaw EM, Schram SE, Belsito DV, et al. Patch-test reactions to topical anesthetics: retrospective analysis of cross-sectional data 2001 to 2004. Dermatitis 2008;19:81–5.

99. Giovannitti JA, Bennett CR. Assessment of allergy to local anesthetics. J Am Dent Assoc 1979;98:701–6.

100. Schatz M, Fung DL. Anaphylactic and anaphylactoid reactions due to anesthetic agents. Clin Rev Allergy 1986;4:215–27.

101. Bhole MV, Manson AL, Seneviratne SL, et al. IgE-mediated allergy to local anaesthetics: separating fact from perception: a UK perspective. Br J Anaesth 2012;108(6):903–11.

102. Oertel R, Ebert U, Rahn R, et al. Clinical pharmacokinetics of articaine. Clin Pharmacokinet 1997;33(6):417–25.

103. Ogle OE, Mahjoubi G. Local anesthesia: agents, techniques and complications. Dent Clin North Am 2012;56:133–48.

104. Harboe T, Guttormsen AB, Aarebrot S, et al. Suspected allergy to local anesthetics: follow-up in 135 cases. Acta Anaesthesiol Scand 2010;54:536–42.

105. Gall H, Kaufmann R, Kalveram CM. Adverse reactions to local anesthetics: analysis of 197 cases. J Allergy Clin Immunol 1996;97:933–7.

106. Berkun Y, Ben-Zvi A, Levy Y, et al. Evaluation of adverse reactions to local anesthetics: experience with 236 patients. Ann Allergy Asthma Immunol 2003; 91:342–5.

107. McClimon B, Rank M, Li J. The predictive value of skin testing in the diagnosis of local anesthetic allergy. Allergy Asthma Proc 2011;32:95–8.

108. Wasserfallen JB, Frei PC. Long-term evaluation of usefulness of skin and incremental challenge tests in patients with history of adverse reaction to local anesthetics. Allergy 1995;50:162–5.

109. Gonzalez-Delgado P, Anton R, Soriano V, et al. Cross-reactivity among amide-type local anesthetics in a case of allergy to mepivacaine. J Investig Allergol Clin Immunol 2006;16(5):311–3.

110. Noormalin A, Shajnaz M, Rosmilah M, et al. IgE-mediated hypersensitivity to lignocaine; a case report. Trop Biomed 2005;22:179–83.
111. Venemalm L, Degerbecck F, Smith W. IgE-mediated reaction to mepivacaine. J Allergy Clin Immunol 2008;121:1058–9.
112. Stahl M, Gome R, Waibel K. Allergy to local anesthetics: specific IgE demonstration to both amides and esters in a single patient. Ann Allergy Asthma Immunol 2012;108:60–7.
113. Macy E, Schatz M, Zeiger RS. Immediate hypersensitivity to methylparaben causing false-positive results of local anesthetic skin testing or provocative dose testing. Permanente J 2002;6:17–21.
114. Macy E. Local anesthetic adverse reaction evaluations: the role of the allergist. Ann Allergy Asthma Immunol 2003;91:319–20.
115. Gonzalez-Estrada A, Pien LC, Lang DM. Perioperative anaphylaxis: antibiotics are the most common identifiable cause. Ann Allergy Asthma Immunol 2013; 111(5 Suppl 1):A3.
116. Sanz ML, Gamboa PM, Mayorga C. Basophil activation tests in the evaluation of immediate drug hypersensitivity. Curr Opin Allergy Clin Immunol 2009;9: 298–304.
117. Aalto-Korte K, Makinen-Kiljunen S. Symptoms of immediate chlorhexidine hypersensitivity in patients with a positive prick test. Contact Dermatitis 2006;55: 173–7.
118. Laxenaire MC, Charpenteir C, Feldman L. Anaphylactoid reactions to colloid plasma substitutes: incidence, risk factors, mechanisms. A French multicenter prospective study. Ann Fr Anesth Reanim 1994;13:301–10.
119. Oswald AM, Joly LM, Gury C, et al. Fatal intraoperative anaphylaxis related to aprotinin after local application of fibrin glue. Anesthesiology 2003;99:762–3.

Hypersensitivity to Contrast Media and Dyes

Knut Brockow, MD[a],*, Mario Sánchez-Borges, MD[b]

KEYWORDS

- Hypersensitivity • Radiocontrast media • Gadolinium-based contrast media • Dyes
- Fluorescein • Blue dyes • Diagnostic procedure • Management

KEY POINTS

- Increasing use leads to an increased incidence of hypersensitivity reactions to diagnostic contrast media and dyes.
- Immediate clinical manifestations are those of anaphylaxis and urticaria/angioedema, although with radiocontrast media nonimmediate exanthems also may occur.
- Skin tests (and possibly laboratory tests) are helpful for the confirmation of allergy and the exclusion of skin-test–positive alternative preparations for future procedures in those patients with positive test results.
- In all other patients, consideration of the necessity, premedication, selection of a preparation as structurally different as possible, and preparedness for emergency is recommended.

HYPERSENSITIVITY REACTIONS TO IODINATED RADIOCONTRAST MEDIA

Iodinated radiocontrast media (RCM) are concentrated solutions of tri-iodinated benzene derivatives used for diagnosis and treatment of vascular disease by enhancement of radiographic contrast. Although the risk of an adverse reaction after a single RCM administration is low, RCM are among the most common elicitors of anaphylaxis and exanthemas, owing to the administration of more than 75 million procedures per year worldwide.[1] Reactions may be classified into immediate (<1 hour) or nonimmediate (>1 hour after administration) hypersensitivity reactions, or toxic reactions related to the well-known toxicity of the compounds (eg, nephrotoxicity, neurotoxicity), or may also be caused by factors totally unrelated to RCM, such as chronic idiopathic urticaria (**Fig. 1**).[2] Four structurally different RCM (monomeric and dimeric, ionic and

Conflicts of Interest: None.
[a] Department of Dermatology and Allergy Biederstein, Technische Universität München, Biedersteiner Strasse 29, Munich 80802, Germany; [b] Allergy and Clinical Immunology Department, Centro Médico Docente La Trinidad, Clínica El Avila, 6a transversal de Altamira, piso 8, consultorio 803, Caracas 1060, Venezuela
* Corresponding author.
E-mail address: knut.brockow@lrz.tum.de

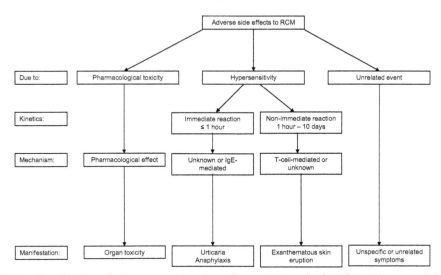

Fig. 1. Classification of adverse reactions to radiocontrast media (RCM). IgE, immunoglobulin E. (*Adapted from* Brockow K, Christiansen C, Kanny G, et al. Management of hypersensitivity reactions to iodinated contrast media. Allergy 2005;60:157; with permission.)

nonionic) are on the market, with nonionic monomers as the most commonly sold products, whereas ionic monomers for intravenous use have been withdrawn in most countries.

Incidence and Risk Factors

Immediate hypersensitivity reactions (IHRs) have been reported in 0.7% to 3% of patients receiving nonionic RCM, severe reactions in 0.02% to 0.04% of intravenous procedures, and fatal IHRs in 0.00001% to 0.0003% of contrast media applications.[3] Exanthematic nonimmediate hypersensitivity reactions (NIHR) affect 0.5% to 3% of RCM-exposed patients; higher frequencies have been reported, but seem to be less reliable.[1,4] There is a higher incidence of nonimmediate exanthemas associated with dimeric nonionic RCM.[5]

The main risk factor for IHR and NIHR is previous severe reactions.[6] Further less prominent predisposing factors reported were female gender, renal insufficiency, a history of doctor-diagnosed asthma, drug allergy, food allergy, contact allergy (for NIHRs), and interleukin-2 treatment (for NIHRs).[6–9] Repeated exposures to RCM increase the risk of IHRs.[10] An immediate reaction is not a risk factor for developing NIHR, and vice versa.[1]

Clinical Manifestations

The onset of IHR is rapid. About 70% occur within 5 minutes after injection, and 96% of severe reactions manifest within 20 minutes.[11,12] Pruritus and urticaria/angioedema occur in about 70% of patients with IHR.[3,13] Heat sensation, nausea, and vomiting may occur but also may be rather toxic reactions when not accompanied by other symptoms, such as abdominal pain and diarrhea. Severe reactions of the respiratory and cardiovascular systems are dyspnea, bronchospasm or tachycardia, and hypotension, sometimes with loss of consciousness.[1] Fatal reactions may occur.

Maculopapular exanthems occurring hours to several days after the RCM administration are typical NIHRs.[1] Other, less frequent manifestations of nonimmediate skin reactions include fixed drug eruption, erythema exsudativum multiforme, pompholyx, symmetric drug-related intertriginous and flexural exanthema, or drug-related eosinophilia with systemic symptoms (DRESS).[1] Nonimmediate RCM reactions typically are mild or moderate in severity. Exceptional, life-threatening, or fatal cases are associated with vasculitis, Stevens-Johnson syndrome, toxic epidermal necrolysis, or delayed anaphylactic reactions.[1,14]

Pathophysiology

For IHRs, an immunoglobulin E (IgE)-mediated allergic mechanism can be demonstrated only in a minority of cases. However, an alternative mechanism, such as a direct membrane effect possibly related to the osmolarity of the solution, an activation of the complement system, or direct bradykinin formation, has also never been convincingly shown to be present in vivo selectively in reactors.[15] IHRs are associated with histamine release from basophils and mast cells.[16] There are reports of high levels of tryptase in connection with severe or fatal reactions.[16,17] Positive immediate skin tests, the detection of contrast media–specific IgE in patients with IHRs, and positive basophil activation tests in a subgroup of patients support the principal concept of an IgE-mediated mechanism.[9,15,18]

NIHRs induced by RCM are T-cell mediated. Reported onset of skin eruptions 2 to 10 days after the first exposure, immunohistologic studies of exanthemas and positive skin-test sites showing a perivascular infiltrate of CD4$^+$ and CD8$^+$ T cells with expression of CD25, HLA-DR, CLA, and CD69, and positive delayed skin tests argue for a type IV allergic mechanism.[15] In addition, peripheral blood mononuclear cells from patients showed in vitro proliferation in the presence of the culprit RCM when added to the culture, and expressed an increase in different lymphocyte activation markers (eg, CD69, CD25, HLA-DR, CLA).[19,20] RCM-specific T-cell clones have been generated.[19]

It is interesting that no previous sensitization phase seems to be necessary in IHR and NIHR.[15] NIHR may occur after first contact with a single dose of RCM after 5 to 10 days.[21] Allergy to iodine does not play a major role in RCM hypersensitivity, as only exceptional patients reacted to a provocation test with Lugol solution.[22]

Diagnostic Methods

In IHRs, elevated histamine or tryptase in plasma and serum, respectively, in comparison with baseline, may confirm anaphylaxis to RCM.[23] Blood samples should be obtained as soon as possible for histamine and 1 to 2 hours after the onset of symptoms for tryptase. Further allergologic workup is recommended between 1 and 6 months after the reaction (**Table 1**).[23] Skin-prick test (SPT) with undiluted RCM is performed before intradermal tests (IDTs) with substances diluted 10-fold in sterile saline. Readings are done after 15 to 20 minutes. For NIHRs and unclear reactions, delayed readings of IDTs and patch tests are also done after 48 and 72 hours, and optionally at other time points such as at 24 or 96 hours in cases of local pruritus or erythematous plaques. Patch tests should be performed with undiluted substances. Because cross-reactivity is frequent, it is advised to test a panel of several different RCM in an attempt to find a skin-test–negative product for future RCM examinations.[23] In vitro tests, such as the basophil activation test, the lymphocyte transformation test, and the lymphocyte activation test, appear to be of value, as they are positive in previous reactors[14,24]; however, their sensitivity and specificity has not yet been firmly established. Provocation tests with progressive increases of the injected RCM dose over several days are useful to confirm a negative skin-test result in NIHRs.[25,26] This procedure has also been reported in IHRs without severe reactions by one European study group.[27] Because of the potential risk involved, provocation tests should be

Table 1
Skin-test concentrations recommended for iodinated radiocontrast media and gadolinium-based magnetic resonance contrast media

		Readings	
Test	Concentration[a]	Immediate Reaction	Nonimmediate Reaction[b]
Skin-prick test	Undiluted	20 min	20 min, 48 h, 72 h[c]
Intradermal test	1:10 diluted[d]	20 min	20 min, 48 h, 72 h[c]
Patch test	Undiluted		20 min, 48 h, 72 h[c]

[a] Undiluted radiocontrast media (with an iodine concentration of 300–320 mg/mL) or gadolinium-based magnet resonance contrast media.
[b] Only for radiocontrast media.
[c] The reading times are tentative: if the patient notices a positive reaction (pruritus, erythema) at the skin-test site at other time points, additional readings may be performed (eg, after 24 h or 96 h).
[d] For nonsevere nonimmediate radiocontrast media reactions, undiluted preparations may also be used.
Adapted from Brockow K. Immediate and delayed reactions to radiocontrast media: is there an allergic mechanism? Immunol Allergy Clin North Am 2009;29:453–68; with permission.

performed only in centers with experience in performing and monitoring these tests, and in immediate emergency treatment.[28]

Management

Radiologists should be trained in how to treat IHRs, and an observation period of 20 to 30 minutes after the administration of the RCM has been recommended.[29] It has been reported that many residents were not able to administer emergency treatment appropriately.[30,31]

Because of their very limited sensitivity and their specificity of approximately 95%, skin tests should not be used as a prescreening tool in patients without any previous reaction.[32] If a patient with a past hypersensitivity reaction needs a new contrasted examination, the culprit substance should not be administered without any allergy test.[23] In such patients, skin tests are recommended. In a patient with a positive reaction to the culprit substance, a panel of RCM should be tested to find a skin-test–negative product. In most cases with IHRs and in a proportion of patients with NIHRs, skin tests will remain negative and the proper mechanism will not be identified. In these cases, a structurally unrelated RCM should be considered for the next examination. In NIHR, a graded drug-provocation test with progressive increases of the RCM dose can confirm negative skin-test responses.[26,27] The prophylactic use of premedication in patients with previous IHRs and NIHRs is becoming more controversial, but is still commonly applied and recommended by certain investigators.[33] A combination of corticosteroids (eg, prednisolone) and antihistamines given before application are the most frequently used agents, if the culprit drug cannot be identified by skin tests. However, radiologists have to accept that severe breakthrough reactions are still possible in patients receiving premedication, if the same or a cross-reactive RCM has been used. Thus, physicians should not rely on the efficacy of premedication alone.

HYPERSENSITIVITY REACTIONS TO GADOLINIUM CONTRAST MEDIA

Gadolinium-based contrast media are paramagnetic macrocyclic or linear gadolinium-containing chelates used to highlight contrast for magnetic resonance imaging (MRI). In subjects with renal disease, they have been associated with a disease resembling scleromyxedema or scleroderma called nephrogenic systemic fibrosis. These non–allergy-like reactions are not further discussed in this article. IHRs to gadolinium-containing intravenous contrast media have been reported, but are less frequent in comparison with those after administration of RCM.

Incidence and Risk Factors

IHRs to gadolinium contrast media have been reported in approximately 0.07% of adults and 0.04% in children.[34,35] Of these, 74% were graded as mild, 19% as moderate, and 7% as severe.[34] There has been a report that abdominal MRI examinations would more frequently elicit IHRs (0.01%) in comparison with brain (0.005%) or spine examinations (0.003%).[36] Reported risk factors are similar to those of RCM and include previous reaction (30%), female gender, and concomitant allergies and asthma.[35] Controversy exists as to whether reaction rates depend on the structure of gadolinium-based substances, with higher reaction rates for gadoteridol and gadobenate dimeglumine, or if the evidence for this conclusion is as yet insufficient.[35–38]

Clinical Manifestations

The clinical manifestations of IHRs to gadolinium contrast media do not differ from those to iodinated RCM. The most common symptoms are urticaria (50%–90%) and nausea, whereas anaphylaxis is more seldom seen.[35,39] There is no report for NIHR.

Pathogenesis

As is the case for iodinated RCM, the mechanisms involved in IHRs to gadolinium contrast media have not been fully elucidated. However, specific positive skin tests in some of the examined patients point to a possible IgE-mediated mechanism.

Diagnostic Methods

Confirmation of an anaphylaxis by the history, the clinical picture, an increased level of tryptase or histamine during the acute episode, and skin tests using SPT with undiluted media in addition to IDT with 1:10-diluted gadolinium substances have been recommended.[40,41] It has been reported that IDTs with undiluted gadolinium preparations were irritative and unspecific.[40] The percentage of patients with positive skin tests remains unknown; however, if positive responses do appear they have been used to guide the selection of alternative gadolinium preparations to be used in the future.[42]

Management

In parallel with the management of iodinated RCM hypersensitivity, in patients with previous reactions to gadolinium preparations either the avoidance of gadolinium preparations and use of an iodinated RCM, or a combination of administration of a structurally different gadolinium preparation and skin testing to find a skin-test–negative product in those patients with positive skin test to the culprit, is recommended.[42] The value of premedication in patients without a positive skin test is unknown.[40]

HYPERSENSITIVITY REACTIONS TO DYES

Various natural and synthetic dyes are commonly used for diagnostic purposes in different medical conditions, especially in oncology, ophthalmology, and urology. Although hypersensitivity reactions to dyes are relatively uncommon, they can be severe and life-threatening. Moreover, owing to the increased frequency of dye use, more patients are at risk for these adverse reactions, therefore clinicians should be aware of them. This section discusses the most widely used dyes, including fluorescein, the so-called blue dyes (Patent blue V [PBV], Isosulfan blue [IB], Methylene blue [MB]), Indocyanine green (IG), and Indigo Carmine (IC).

Fluorescein

Sodium fluorescein is a low molecular weight, highly water-soluble compound with fluorescent properties used for the study of chorioretinal diseases (**Fig. 2**). It allows sequential visualization of blood flow simultaneously through retinal, choroidal, and iris tissues. It has also been used in neurosurgery to identify the excision range of a brain tumor.[43]

Incidence and risk factors
The general incidence of adverse reactions to intravenous fluorescein has been estimated as 5%, with 0.05% being severe reactions.[44] However, other investigators have reported variable rates ranging between 3% and 20%.[45,46] In patients who underwent fluorescein angiography for the first time, Lira and colleagues[47] reported urticaria in 1.06%, bronchospasm in 0.38%, and laryngeal edema in 0.1%. Urticaria occurs in 0.5% to 1.2%[44,48,49] and respiratory distress in 0.02% to 0.1% of patients.[48,50] Reactions to orally administered fluorescein are observed in 1% to 2%.[51,52]

Risk factors for IHRs to fluorescein are previous reactions to colloidal plasma substitutes,[44,53] a history of dye allergy, diabetes, systemic arterial hypertension,[44,54] and a history of allergy.[47]

Clinical manifestations
Mild reactions (nausea, vomiting, pruritus, sneezing, vasovagal disorders, inadvertent arterial injection) are observed in 2% to 10%, moderate reactions (urticaria, other skin eruptions, syncope, thrombophlebitis, pyrexia, local tissue necrosis, muscular paralysis) in 1.5%,[47] and severe reactions in 0.05% of patients. Cardiovascular shock, myocardial infarction, laryngeal edema, bronchospasm, and tonic-clonic seizures are regarded as severe reactions.[44] Death occurred in 1 of every 200,000 patients.[55,56] One case of a patient with bullous pemphigoid induced by fluorescein has been published.[57]

Pathogenesis
The mechanisms involved in IHRs to fluorescein have not been fully elucidated. The following have been proposed[48]: (1) nonallergic histamine release; (2) IgE-mediated immediate hypersensitivity[48,49]; (3) complement activation; (4) disturbances of arachidonic acid metabolism; (5) vasovagal phenomena; (6) anxiety-related medullary sympathetic discharge; (7) direct vasospastic toxic effect; (8) contamination during the

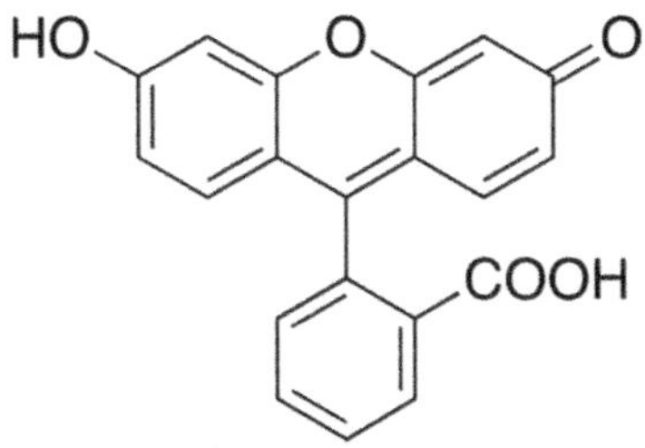

Fig. 2. Chemical structure of fluorescein.

manufacturing process; (9) destruction of the vascular endothelium through Factor XII and the coagulation system[49,58]; (10) combinations of the above.

Diagnostic methods

Elevated serum levels of tryptase and histamine during the reaction confirm the diagnosis of anaphylaxis.[49,59] Because the pathogenesis of IHR to fluorescein has not been clarified, there is no clear consensus among investigators regarding how to confirm hypersensitivity to this dye. The following have been used:

1. Skin tests: prick test with fluorescein 20% and IDT at 2%.[60] López-Sáez and colleagues[61] used IDTs at 1:1000, 1:100, and 1:10 dilutions. Some investigators have suggested that skin tests have high sensitivity and negative predictive value,[60] but there are not enough cases from which to draw any firm conclusions.
2. Intravenous provocation test.[60]
3. Conjunctival provocation. Trindade-Porto and colleagues[62] suggested that whenever skin tests are negative, a conjunctival provocation test should be performed.

Management

Various approaches for the management of high-risk patients with fluorescein hypersensitivity have been used, including pharmaceutical prophylaxis with antihistamines[60] or a combination of antihistamines and corticosteroids, fluorescein desensitization,[63,64] switch to oral fluorescein angiography, and the use of other alternative techniques such as optical coherence tomography. Some investigators consider that antihistamine prophylaxis has low efficacy,[60] and antihistamines and corticosteroids are not always effective.[56,65]

Ellis and colleagues[65] proposed that antihistamines might have a place in prophylaxis against side reactions to intravenous fluorescein in patients with a history of allergies, allergic reactions to drugs, or previous reactions to fluorescein.

Patent Blue V

PBV and IB belong to the group of triarylmethane synthetic dyes (**Fig. 3**). These dyes basically share the same sodium or calcium salt of diethylammonium hydroxide inner salt, differ in the position of the substituted sulfonate, and are selectively absorbed into the lymphatics, bound to albumin, and excreted into the urine and bile. Both are used for demonstrating sequential lymphatic dissemination of melanoma into sentinel nodes, identification of sentinel nodes in breast cancer, to identify lymphatics for lymphovenular anastomosis, in fistulography, and for determination of cardiac output. PBV and IB are also used as food additives, in the manufacture of textiles, cosmetics, plastics, and paper, and in agriculture.[66] PBV is also known as Acid blue 3, Disulfine blue, and food additive E131.[67]

Incidence and risk factors

The incidence of IHRs to PBV is reported at 0.88%, with grade I reactions (minor) at 0.48%, grade II (moderate) at 0.32%, and grade III (severe) at 0.08%,[68,69] although higher incidence rates of anaphylaxis have been reported.[70–73]

Risk factors for IHRs to PBV are exposure to tryphenylmethane dyes from textiles, cosmetics, print shops, farms, pharmaceutical plants, food-processing plants, and plaque-disclosing agents in dentistry.

Clinical manifestations

Symptoms usually are observed after 5 to 45 minutes of PBV injection.[74] Cutaneous manifestations include large blue/green hives coalescing to form huge welts, the so-called blue urticaria, that has been regarded as pathognomonic of a reaction to

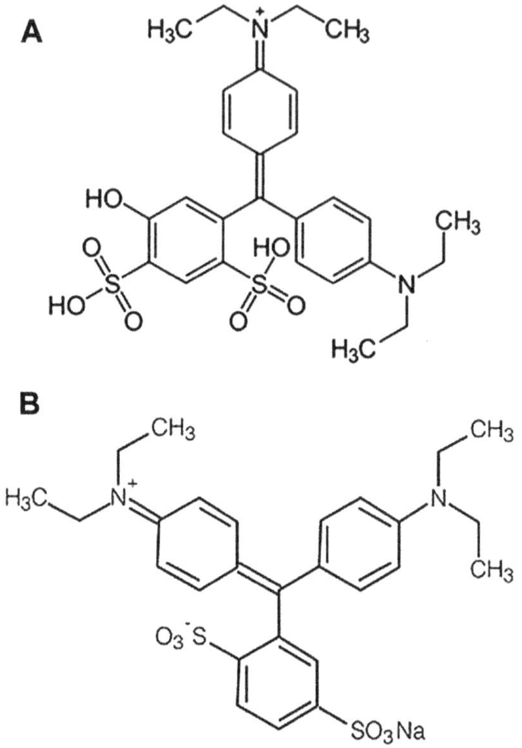

Fig. 3. Chemical structure of triarylmethane dyes. (A) Patent blue V. (B) Isosulfan blue.

PBV; blue-colored periorbital angioedema, urticaria, pruritus, erythema, and angioedema of arms and hands. Other symptoms include shock, bronchospasm, nasal congestion, and gastrointestinal symptoms. Biphasic reactions can occur,[70,75,76] and a poor response to ephedrine and intravenous fluids and the need for adrenaline because of sustained release of the dye through lymph nodes have been reported.[74]

Pathogenesis
Although reactions to PBV could be due to direct mast-cell or basophil activation, evidence for IgE-mediated reactions to PBV has been obtained from the following observations: (1) positive SPTs with PBV[74]; (2) passive transfer of the sensitivity[77]; (3) positive CD-sens test indicating high basophil allergen threshold sensitivity[78]; (4) detection of specific IgE to PBV by enzyme-linked immunosorbent assay.[79] It is postulated that PBV may be the hapten cross-linking specific IgE antibodies after binding to a carrier.

Diagnostic methods
Increased serum levels of tryptase and histamine during reactions to PBV suggest mast cell/basophil activation and confirm the diagnosis of anaphylaxis.[74,80] SPTs with undiluted PBV and IDTs with 1:1000 to 1:10 dilutions are recommended.[74,80,81] Measurement of specific IgE in the serum[79] and basophil activation test[82] can be helpful, although those are available only in a few centers.

Owing to the strong structural homology between PBV and IB, there is strong cross-reactivity among both dyes. Because MB is structurally not related to these dyes no cross-reactions are expected (see **Fig. 3**), but have been described.[80]

Management

Various approaches have been proposed to prevent reactions to PBV, including the reduction of the amount of dye to be administered[83]; the use of MB as alternative dye after a skin test; lymphatic mapping with radiocolloid (technetium-labeled nanocolloidal albumin); and preoperative prophylaxis with chlorpheniramine, hydrocortisone, and famotidine.[84,85] However, although pharmacologic prophylaxis seems to attenuate the severity, it does not reduce the overall incidence of IHRs to blue dyes.

Isosulfan Blue

IB is the sodium salt of PBV, also called Sulfan blue, Food blue 3, Patent blue VF, Patent blue violet, and acid blue 1 (see **Fig. 3**). This dye is used for lymphatic mapping in the context of sentinel lymph node biopsy in patients with melanoma, breast, bladder, cervical, and endometrial cancer, and as a coloring agent in textiles, cosmetics, detergents, paints, inks, antifreeze, cold remedies, laxatives, and suppositories.

Incidence and risk factors

Hypersensitivity reactions to IB are observed in 0.9% to 1.9% of cases.[66,74,76,86–88] Severe reactions are observed in 0.5% to 1.1%,[66,76] and anaphylaxis in 0.2% to 1.1%.[89] Allergy to sulfonamides does not constitute a risk factor for reactions to IB.[66]

Clinical manifestations

Symptoms start 15 to 49 minutes after exposure[66] and include anaphylactic shock requiring vasopressor support,[70,90] blue urticaria, facial angioedema, pruritus, generalized macular rash, hypoxemia, and wheezing. Biphasic reactions may occur.[70,75,76,91]

Pathogenesis

Sensitization occurs through exposure to a cross-reacting antigen contained in everyday products. There is evidence suggesting that reactions to IB are mediated by specific IgE[69] whereby IB would act as a hapten that weakly binds to serum proteins, but there is the possibility that some reactions are antibody-independent with direct mast cell and basophil membrane activation, or activation of the alternative complement pathway. As previously mentioned, IB and PBV show extensive cross-reactivity.

Diagnostic methods

Increased serum levels of tryptase and histamine are present in acute reactions to IB.[92–94] SPT and IDT with IB dilutions of 1:10,000 to 1:100 confirm sensitivity to the dye.

Management

The approach for managing patients hypersensitive to IB is similar to that used in patients with reactions to PBV and include the use of smaller volumes of the dye,[83] the utilization of MB as an alternative for sentinel lymph node localization,[80,95,96] and preoperative medication with antihistamines, and corticosteroids to reduce the severity of anaphylactic reactions, although this pretreatment would not prevent the occurrence of the reaction.[95]

Methylene Blue

MB is a polyaromatic cationic dye of the phenothiazine group, also known as CAS No. 61-73-4, anhydrous methylene blue, CAS No. 7220-79-3, or MB trihydrate. Its structure is unrelated to the triarylmethane dyes (PBV and IB) (**Fig. 4**). MB is a tracer that has been used for detecting urinary tract and digestive fistulas, assessment of tubal

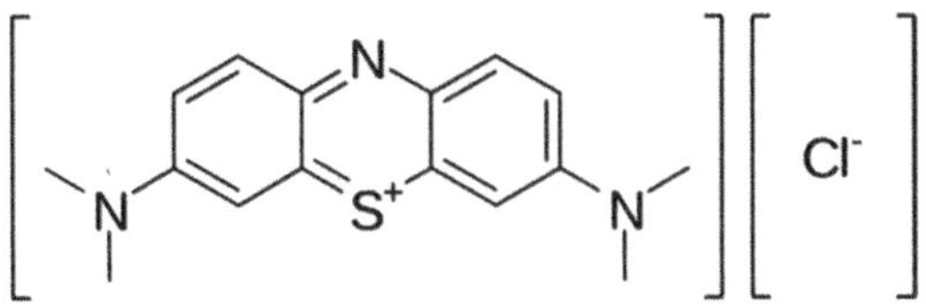

Fig. 4. Chemical structure of Methylene blue.

permeability or sentinel lymph node biopsies, the treatment of hypotension during septic shock, and for treating anaphylaxis. In lower doses it is used for the treatment of methemoglobinemia.

Treatment of fresh frozen plasma with MB is used for pathogen inactivation, a photodynamic process preventing viral RNA and DNA replication.

Incidence and risk factors
MB rarely induces hypersensitivity, and is generally regarded as a safer alternative to triarylmethane dyes for satellite node mapping.[89] MB does not cross-react with PBV and IB, although concomitant sensitizations have been described.[80]

Clinical manifestations
MB rarely induces anaphylaxis, but occasionally peripheral arterial desaturation, facial angioedema, generalized urticaria, hypotension, and tachycardia have been reported.[97–99] On the other hand, skin necrosis and ulceration have been associated with MB injection.[100–103] Other adverse effects induced by MB include burning pain, blue macules, bluish skin discoloration, fetal congenital anomalies,[104–106] spinal cord necrosis,[107] pulmonary edema,[108] and acute generalized exanthematous pustulosis.[109]

MB-treated fresh frozen plasma has also been reported to induce severe allergic reactions,[110] although this observation has not been confirmed by other investigators.[111]

Pathogenesis
Anaphylaxis to MB is mediated by IgE, accompanied in 75% of cases by an increase in serum tryptase, and in 66% by an increase in histamine. Acute generalized exanthematous pustulosis is mediated by drug-specific T cells.

MB intercalates into viral nucleic acid, and subsequent illumination generates singlet oxygen radicals, leading to guanosine oxidation and destruction of the viral nucleic acid. The combination of MB and illumination alters plasma proteins, resulting in the production of neoantigens.[112]

Diagnostic methods
Skin IDTs with MB 1% diluted from 10^{-4} to 10^{-2} have been proposed for the confirmation of MB allergic hypersensitivity.[80] **Table 2** summarizes the concentrations of dyes for skin testing in patients with suspected allergy. The basophil activation test is an alternative investigational diagnostic method.[99,110]

Management
MB does not cross-react with PBV and IB,[70,97,113] and therefore constitutes an alternative dye, especially for satellite lymph node localization in patients who have reacted to triarylmethane dyes.

Table 2
Skin-test concentrations for dyes commonly used for medical purposes

Dye	Skin-Prick Tests	Intradermal Tests	Patch Tests
Fluorescein	Undiluted	1:10	Undiluted
Patent blue V	Undiluted	1:10	—
Isosulfan blue	1:1000 to 1:100	1:1000 to 1:100	—
Methylene blue	Undiluted	1:10,000 to 1:100	—

Indocyanine Green

IG is a tricarbocyanine organic dye with less than 5% iodine (see **Fig. 4**; **Fig. 5**). This dye has been used for the diagnosis of conditions affecting the choroidal vasculature, and the study of cardiac output and hepatic function.

Incidence and risk factors

IHRs to IG are rarely observed. In one study, severe reactions were present in 0.05% to 0.07%,[114,115] moderate reactions in 0.2%, and mild reactions in 0.15%.[114] One death during cardiac catheterization with IG has been published.[116]

Su and colleagues[117] studied the incidence of IHR to the simultaneous intravenous injection of fluorescein and IG for fundus angiography. IHRs were observed in 28 of 396 patients with drug allergy (7.2%) and in 145 of 3426 without allergy history (4.2%) ($P = .008$), while patients with an allergy history also showed more severe reactions.

Clinical manifestations

Nausea, light-headedness, disorientation, irregular pulse, shallow respiration, diaphoresis, cyanosis, hypotension, incontinence, pruritus, and wheezing are the most frequent symptoms of IHRs to IG,[118] whereas full-blown anaphylactic shock occurs less frequently.[118,119]

Pathogenesis

Mechanisms of IHRs to IG are unknown, and it has been hypothesized that anaphylaxis may be related to the iodine additive or the dye itself.

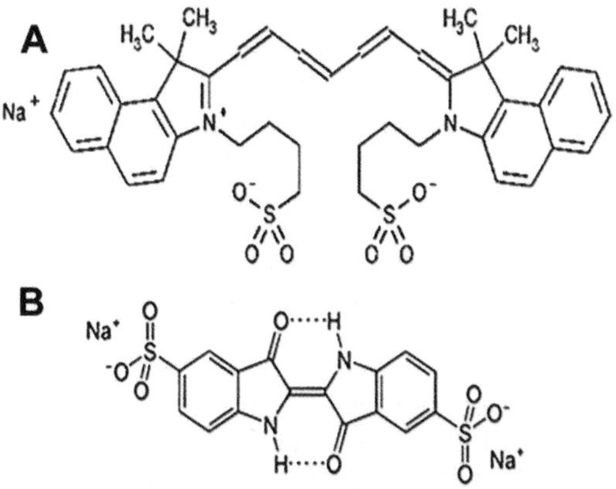

Fig. 5. Chemical structure of Indigo derivatives. (*A*) Indocyanine green. (*B*) Indigo carmine.

Diagnostic methods
No diagnostic methods have been described in the literature.

Management
In patients who have experienced an IHR to IG, avoidance of the dye is recommended.

Indigo Carmine

Indigo is produced by fermenting the *Indigofera tinctoria* plant, and has been used as a dye in denims, blue jeans, and other fabrics. Indigotine and IC are indigo derivatives widely used as synthetic coloring agents in the food and cosmetic industries (see **Figs. 4** and **5**).

Indigotine (FD&C blue dye No. 2) has been associated with respiratory occupational symptoms (cough, dyspnea, wheezing, and nasal congestion) and occupational asthma that was confirmed by means of bronchial provocation. IC (sodium indigotin disulfonate) is considered biologically inert and extremely safe, and it used medically for the evaluation of the lower urinary tract during cystoscopy.

Incidence and risk factors
IHRs to IC are very uncommon.[120] Allergy to sulfonamides has been suggested as a risk factor for IHRs to IC.[121]

Clinical manifestations
IC can rarely trigger severe life-threatening anaphylaxis and cardiac arrest.[122] Other clinical manifestations include urticaria, bradycardia, bronchospasm, and hypotension.[121,123]

Pathogenesis
The pathogenesis of IHRs to IC is currently unknown.

Diagnostic methods
No diagnostic methods have been described thus far.

Management
Avoidance of IC is recommended in patients who have had an IHR to the dye.

REFERENCES

1. Brockow K. Immediate and delayed cutaneous reactions to radiocontrast media. Chem Immunol Allergy 2012;97:180–90.
2. Brockow K, Ring J. Classification and pathophysiology of radiocontrast media hypersensitivity. Chem Immunol Allergy 2010;95:157–69.
3. Katayama H, Yamaguchi K, Kozuka T, et al. Adverse reactions to ionic and nonionic contrast media. A report from the Japanese Committee on the Safety of Contrast Media. Radiology 1990;175:621–8.
4. Webb JA, Stacul F, Thomsen HS, et al. Late adverse reactions to intravascular iodinated contrast media. Eur Radiol 2003;13:181–4.
5. Sutton AG, Finn P, Grech ED, et al. Early and late reactions after the use of iopamidol 340, ioxaglate 320, and iodixanol 320 in cardiac catheterization. Am Heart J 2001;141:677–83.
6. Namasivayam S, Kalra MK, Torres WE, et al. Adverse reactions to intravenous iodinated contrast media: an update. Curr Probl Diagn Radiol 2006;35:164–9.
7. Kobayashi D, Takahashi O, Ueda T, et al. Asthma severity is a risk factor for acute hypersensitivity reactions to contrast agents: a large-scale cohort study. Chest 2012;141:1367–8.

8. Choyke PL, Miller DL, Lotze MT, et al. Delayed reactions to contrast media after interleukin-2 immunotherapy. Radiology 1992;183:111–4.
9. Goksel O, Aydin O, Atasoy C, et al. Hypersensitivity reactions to contrast media: prevalence, risk factors and the role of skin tests in diagnosis—a cross-sectional survey. Int Arch Allergy Immunol 2011;155:297–305.
10. Fujiwara N, Tateishi R, Akahane M, et al. Changes in risk of immediate adverse reactions to iodinated contrast media by repeated administrations in patients with hepatocellular carcinoma. PLoS One 2013;8:e76018.
11. Brockow K, Romano A, Aberer W, et al. Skin testing in patients with hypersensitivity reactions to iodinated contrast media—a European multicenter study. Allergy 2009;64:234–41.
12. Idee JM, Pines E, Prigent P, et al. Allergy-like reactions to iodinated contrast agents. A critical analysis. Fundam Clin Pharmacol 2005;19:263–81.
13. Kalimo K, Jansen CT, Kormano M. Allergological risk factors as predictors of radiographic contrast media hypersensitivity. Ann Allergy 1980;45:253–5.
14. Brown M, Yowler C, Brandt C. Recurrent toxic epidermal necrolysis secondary to iopromide contrast. J Burn Care Res 2013;34:e53–6.
15. Brockow K. Immediate and delayed reactions to radiocontrast media: is there an allergic mechanism? Immunol Allergy Clin North Am 2009;29:453–68.
16. Laroche D, Aimone-Gastin I, Dubois F, et al. Mechanisms of severe, immediate reactions to iodinated contrast material. Radiology 1998;209:183–90.
17. Brockow K, Vieluf D, Puschel K, et al. Increased postmortem serum mast cell tryptase in a fatal anaphylactoid reaction to nonionic radiocontrast medium. J Allergy Clin Immunol 1999;104:237–8.
18. Pinnobphun P, Buranapraditkun S, Kampitak T, et al. The diagnostic value of basophil activation test in patients with an immediate hypersensitivity reaction to radiocontrast media. Ann Allergy Asthma Immunol 2011;106:387–93.
19. Lerch M, Keller M, Britschgi M, et al. Cross-reactivity patterns of T cells specific for iodinated contrast media. J Allergy Clin Immunol 2007;119:1529–36.
20. Torres MJ, Mayorga C, Cornejo-Garcia JA, et al. Monitoring non-immediate allergic reactions to iodine contrast media. Clin Exp Immunol 2008;152:233–8.
21. Bircher AJ, Brockow K, Grosber M, et al. Late elicitation of maculopapular exanthemas to iodinated contrast media after first exposure. Ann Allergy Asthma Immunol 2013;111:576–7.
22. Scherer K, Harr T, Bach S, et al. The role of iodine in hypersensitivity reactions to radio contrast media. Clin Exp Allergy 2010;40:468–75.
23. Brockow K, Christiansen C, Kanny G, et al. Management of hypersensitivity reactions to iodinated contrast media. Allergy 2005;60:150–8.
24. Kanny G, Pichler W, Morisset M, et al. T cell-mediated reactions to iodinated contrast media: evaluation by skin and lymphocyte activation tests. J Allergy Clin Immunol 2005;115:179–85.
25. Hasdenteufel F, Waton J, Cordebar V, et al. Delayed hypersensitivity reactions caused by iodixanol: an assessment of cross-reactivity in 22 patients. J Allergy Clin Immunol 2011;128:1356–7.
26. Torres MJ, Gomez F, Dona I, et al. Diagnostic evaluation of patients with nonimmediate cutaneous hypersensitivity reactions to iodinated contrast media. Allergy 2012;67:929–35.
27. Caimmi S, Benyahia B, Suau D, et al. Clinical value of negative skin tests to iodinated contrast media. Clin Exp Allergy 2010;40:805–10.
28. Aberer W, Bircher A, Romano A, et al. Drug provocation testing in the diagnosis of drug hypersensitivity reactions: general considerations. Allergy 2003;58:854–63.

29. Thomsen HS, Morcos SK. ESUR guidelines on contrast media. Abdom Imaging 2006;31:131–40.
30. Lightfoot CB, Abraham RJ, Mammen T, et al. Survey of radiologists' knowledge regarding the management of severe contrast material-induced allergic reactions. Radiology 2009;251:691–6.
31. Gaca AM, Frush DP, Hohenhaus SM, et al. Enhancing pediatric safety: using simulation to assess radiology resident preparedness for anaphylaxis from intravenous contrast media. Radiology 2007;245:236–44.
32. Kim SH, Jo EJ, Kim MY, et al. Clinical value of radiocontrast media skin tests as a prescreening and diagnostic tool in hypersensitivity reactions. Ann Allergy Asthma Immunol 2013;110:258–62.
33. Brockow K, Ring J. Anaphylaxis to radiographic contrast media. Curr Opin Allergy Clin Immunol 2011;11:326–31.
34. Dillman JR, Ellis JH, Cohan RH, et al. Frequency and severity of acute allergic-like reactions to gadolinium-containing i.v. contrast media in children and adults. AJR Am J Roentgenol 2007;189:1533–8.
35. Jung JW, Kang HR, Kim MH, et al. Immediate hypersensitivity reaction to gadolinium-based MR contrast media. Radiology 2012;264:414–22.
36. Prince MR, Zhang H, Zou Z, et al. Incidence of immediate gadolinium contrast media reactions. AJR Am J Roentgenol 2011;196:W138–43.
37. Davenport MS, Dillman JR, Cohan RH, et al. Effect of abrupt substitution of gadobenate dimeglumine for gadopentetate dimeglumine on rate of allergic-like reactions. Radiology 2013;266:773–82.
38. Idee JM, Gaillard S, Corot C. Gadolinium-bound contrast agents: no evidence-based data to support a relationship between structure and hypersensitivity reactions. Indian J Dermatol 2012;57:245.
39. Hunt CH, Hartman RP, Hesley GK. Frequency and severity of adverse effects of iodinated and gadolinium contrast materials: retrospective review of 456,930 doses. AJR Am J Roentgenol 2009;193:1124–7.
40. Galera C, Pur Ozygit L, Cavigioli S, et al. Gadoteridol-induced anaphylaxis—not a class allergy. Allergy 2010;65:132–4.
41. Hasdenteufel F, Luyasu S, Renaudin JM, et al. Anaphylactic shock after first exposure to gadoterate meglumine: two case reports documented by positive allergy assessment. J Allergy Clin Immunol 2008;121:527–8.
42. Moulin C, Said BB, Berard F. Tolerability of gadobenate dimeglumine in a patient with reported allergy to gadoterate meglumine. AJR Am J Roentgenol 2011;197:W1163.
43. Kuroiwa T, Kajimoto Y, Ohta T. Development of a fluorescein operative microscope for use during malignant glioma surgery: a technical note and preliminary report. Surg Neurol 1998;50(1):41–9.
44. Kwiterovich KA, Maguire MG, Murphy RP, et al. Frequency of adverse systemic reactions after fluorescein angiography. Results of a prospective study. Ophthalmology 1991;98(7):1139–42.
45. Patz A, Finkelstein D, Fine SL, et al. The role of fluorescein angiography in national collaborative studies. Ophthalmology 1986;93(11):1466–70.
46. Singerman LJ. Fluorescein angiography. Practical role in the office management of macular diseases. Ophthalmology 1986;93(9):1209–15.
47. Lira RP, Oliveira CL, Marques MV, et al. Adverse reactions of fluorescein angiography: a prospective study. Arq Bras Oftalmol 2007;70(4):615–8.
48. Yannuzzi LA, Rohrer KT, Tindel LJ, et al. Fluorescein angiography complication survey. Ophthalmology 1986;93(5):611–7.

49. Lacava AC, Leal EB, Caballero JC, et al. Angiografia fluoresceínica e suas complicações, relato de un caso de óbito. Rev Bras Oftalmol 1996;55(1): 59–62.
50. Karhunen U, Raitta C, Kala R. Adverse reactions to fluorescein angiography. Acta Ophthalmol (Copenh) 1986;64(3):282–6.
51. Hara T, Inami M, Hara T. Efficacy and safety of fluorescein angiography with orally administered sodium fluorescein. Am J Ophthalmol 1998;126(4):560–4.
52. Gómez-Ulla F, Gutiérrez C, Seoane I. Severe anaphylactic reaction to orally administered fluorescein. Am J Ophthalmol 1991;112(1):94.
53. Celik I, Duda D, Stinner B, et al. Early and late histamine release induced by albumin, hetastarch and polygeline: some unexpected findings. Inflamm Res 2003;52(10):408–16.
54. Zografos L. International survey on the incidence of severe or fatal complications which may occur during fluorescein angiography. J Fr Ophtalmol 1983; 6(5):495–506.
55. Hitosugi M, Omura K, Yokoyama T, et al. An autopsy case of fatal anaphylactic shock following fluorescein angiography: a case report. Med Sci Law 2004; 44(3):264–5.
56. Rohr AS, Pappano JE Jr. Prophylaxis against fluorescein-induced anaphylactoid reactions. J Allergy Clin Immunol 1992;90(3 Pt 1):407–8.
57. Demirci G, Demirci GT, Gulkilik G. Case report of bullous pemphigoid following fundus fluorescein angiography. Case Rep Ophthalmol 2010;1(1):1–4.
58. Anderson JA. Allergic reactions to drugs and biological agents. JAMA 1992; 268(20):2844–57.
59. Tanahashi S, Lida H, Dohi S. An anaphylactoid reaction after administration of fluorescein sodium during neurosurgery. Anesth Analg 2006;103(2):503.
60. Perez-Rodriguez E, Matheu-Delgado V, Sánchez-Machín I, et al. Reacciones adversas durante la administración de fluoresceína endovenosa. [Adverse reactions related with intravenous fluorescein]. Arch Soc Esp Oftalmol 2005; 80(8):441–2 [in Spanish].
61. López-Sáez MP, Ordoqui E, Tornero P, et al. Fluorescein-induced allergic reaction. Ann Allergy Asthma Immunol 1998;81(5 Pt 1):428–30.
62. Trindade-Porto C, Alonso-Llamazares A, Robledo T, et al. Fluorescein-induced adverse reaction. Allergy 1999;54(11):1230.
63. Nucera E, Schiavino D, Merendino E, et al. Successful fluorescein desensitization. Allergy 2003;58(5):45.
64. Knowles SR, Weber EA, Berbrayer CS. Allergic reaction to fluorescein dye: successful one-day desensitization. Can J Ophthalmol 2007;42(2):329–30.
65. Ellis PP, Schoenberger M, Rendi MA. Antihistamines as prophylaxis against side reactions to intravenous fluorescein. Trans Am Ophthalmol Soc 1980;78: 190–205.
66. Montgomery LL, Thorne AC, Van Zee KJ, et al. Isosulfan blue dye reactions during sentinel lymph node mapping for breast cancer. Anesth Analg 2002;95(2): 385–8.
67. Scherer K, Bircher AJ, Figueiredo V. Blue dyes in medicine—a confusing terminology. Contact Dermatitis 2006;54(4):231–2.
68. Tripathy S, Nair PV. Adverse drug reaction, patent blue V dye and anaesthesia. Indian J Anaesth 2012;56(6):563–6.
69. Keller B, Yawalkar N, Pichler C, et al. Hypersensitivity reaction against patent blue during sentinel lymph node removal in three melanoma patients. Am J Surg 2007;193(1):122–4.

70. Scherer K, Studer W, Figueiredo V, et al. Anaphylaxis to isosulfan blue and cross-reactivity to patent blue V: case report and review of the nomenclature of vital blue dyes. Ann Allergy Asthma Immunol 2006;96(3):497–500.
71. Barthelmes L, Goyal A, Newcombe RG, et al. Adverse reactions to patent blue V dye—the new start and almanac experience. Eur J Surg Oncol 2010;36(4): 399–403.
72. Kalimo K, Jansén CT, Kormano M. Sensitivity to patent blue dye during skin-prick testing and lymphography. A retrospective and prospective study. Radiology 1981;141(2):365–7.
73. Beenen E, de Roy van Zuidewijn DB. Patients blue on patent blue: an adverse reaction during four sentinel node procedures. Surg Oncol 2005;14(4):151–4.
74. Hunting AS, Nopp A, Johansson SG, et al. Anaphylaxis to patent blue V. I. clinical aspects. Allergy 2010;65(1):117–23.
75. Quiliquini A, Hogendijk S, Hauser C. Anaphylaxis to patent blue. Dermatology 1998;197(4):400.
76. Albo D, Wayne JD, Hunt KK, et al. Anaphylactic reactions to isosulfan blue dye during sentinel lymph node biopsy for breast cancer. Am J Surg 2001;182(4):393–8.
77. Pevny I, Bohndorf W. Group allergy due to patent blue sensitization. Med Klin 1972;67(20):698–702.
78. Johansson SG, Nopp A, Oman H, et al. Anaphylaxis to patent blue V. II. A unique IgE-mediated reaction. Allergy 2010;65(1):124–9.
79. Wöhrl S, Focke M, Hinterhuber G, et al. Near-fatal anaphylaxis to patent blue V. Br J Dermatol 2004;150(5):1037–8.
80. Mertes PM, Malinovsky JM, Mouton-Faivre C, et al. Anaphylaxis to dyes during the perioperative period: reports of 14 clinical cases. J Allergy Clin Immunol 2008;122(2):348–52.
81. Brockow K, Garvey LH, Aberer W, et al. Skin test concentrations for systemically administered drugs—an ENDA/EAACI Drug Allergy Interest Group position paper. Allergy 2013;68(6):702–12.
82. Ebo DG, Wets RD, Spiessens TK, et al. Flow-assisted diagnosis of anaphylaxis to patent blue. Allergy 2005;60(5):703–4.
83. King TA, Fey JV, Van Zee KJ, et al. A prospective analysis of the effect of blue-dye volume on sentinel lymph node mapping success and incidence of allergic reaction in patients with breast cancer. Ann Surg Oncol 2004;11(5):535–41.
84. Raut CP, Hunt KK, Akins JS, et al. Incidence of anaphylactoid reactions to iso-sulfan blue dye during breast carcinoma lymphatic mapping in patients treated with preoperative prophylaxis: results of a surgical prospective clinical practice protocol. Cancer 2005;104(4):692–9.
85. Daley MD, Norman PH, Leak JA, et al. Adverse events associated with the intra-operative injection of isosulfan blue. J Clin Anesth 2004;16(5):332–41.
86. Leong SP, Donegan E, Heffernon W, et al. Adverse reactions to isosulfan blue during selective sentinel lymph node dissection in melanoma. Ann Surg Oncol 2000;7(5):361–6.
87. Cimmino VM, Brown AC, Szocik JF, et al. Allergic reactions to isosulfan blue during sentinel node biopsy—a common event. Surgery 2001;130(3):439–42.
88. Lanitis S, Filippakis G, Sidhu V, et al. Atypical anaphylactic reaction to patent blue during sentinel lymph node biopsy for breast cancer. Ann R Coll Surg Engl 2008;90(4):338–9.
89. Kaufman G, Guth AA, Pachter HL, et al. A cautionary tale: anaphylaxis to isosul-fan blue dye after 12 years and 3339 cases of lymphatic mapping. Am Surg 2008;74(2):152–5.

90. Longnecker SM, Guzzardo MM, Van Voris LP. Life-threatening anaphylaxis following subcutaneous administration of isosulfan blue 1%. Clin Pharm 1985; 4(2):219–21.
91. Lee JM, Greenes DS. Biphasic anaphylactic reactions in pediatrics. Pediatrics 2000;106(4):762–6.
92. Sprung J, Tully MJ, Ziser A. Anaphylactic reactions to isosulfan blue dye during sentinel node lymphadenectomy for breast cancer. Anesth Analg 2003;96(4): 1051–3.
93. Laurie SA, Khan DA, Gruchalla RS, et al. Anaphylaxis to isosulfan blue. Ann Allergy Asthma Immunol 2002;88(1):64–6.
94. Quiney NF, Kissin MW, Tytler I. Anaphylactic reaction to isosulphan blue. Br J Anaesth 2003;90(1):105–6.
95. Simmons R, Thevarajah S, Brennan MB, et al. Methylene blue dye as an alternative to isosulfan blue dye for sentinel lymph node localization. Ann Surg Oncol 2003;10(3):242–7.
96. Raut CP, Daley MD, Hunt KK, et al. Anaphylactoid reactions to isosulfan blue dye during breast cancer lymphatic mapping in patients given preoperative prophylaxis. J Clin Oncol 2004;22(3):567–8.
97. Dewachter P, Mouton-Faivre C, Tréchot P, et al. Severe anaphylactic shock with methylene blue instillation. Anesth Analg 2005;101(1):149–50.
98. Jangjoo A, Forghani MN, Mehrabibahar M, et al. Anaphylaxis reaction of a breast cancer patient to methylene blue during breast surgery with sentinel node mapping. Acta Oncol 2010;49(6):877–8.
99. Dewachter P, Castro S, Nicaise-Roland P, et al. Anaphylactic reaction after methylene blue-treated plasma transfusion. Br J Anaesth 2011;106(5):687–9.
100. Salhab M, Al Sarakbi W, Mokbel K. Skin and fat necrosis of the breast following methylene blue dye injection for sentinel node biopsy in a patient with breast cancer. Int Semin Surg Oncol 2005;2:26.
101. Stradling B, Aranha G, Gabram S. Adverse skin lesions after methylene blue injections for sentinel lymph node localization. Am J Surg 2002;184(4):350–2.
102. Perry PM, Meinhard E. Necrotic subcutaneous abscesses following injections of methylene blue. Br J Clin Pract 1974;28(8):289–91.
103. Ruhlen JL. Tissue necrosis. Cutaneous and subcutaneous damage following extravasation of methylene blue. J Kans Med Soc 1982;83(5):260.
104. Nicolini U, Monni G. Intestinal obstruction in babies exposed in utero to methylene blue. Lancet 1990;336(8725):1258–9.
105. Porat R, Gilbert S, Magilner D. Methylene blue-induced phototoxicity: an unrecognized complication. Pediatrics 1996;97(5):717–21.
106. van der Pol JG, Wolf H, Boer K, et al. Jejunal atresia related to the use of methylene blue in genetic amniocentesis in twins. Br J Obstet Gynaecol 1992;99(2):141–3.
107. Sharr MM, Weller RO, Brice JG. Spinal cord necrosis after intrathecal injection of methylene blue. J Neurol Neurosurg Psychiatry 1978;41(4):384–6.
108. Trikha A, Mohan V, Kashyap L, et al. Pulmonary edema following intrauterine methylene blue injection. Acta Anaesthesiol Scand 1996;40(3):382–4.
109. Sener O, Kose Ö, Kartal Ö, et al. Acute generalized exanthematous pustulosis due to oral use of blue dyes. Korean J Intern Med 2011;26(3):360–3.
110. Mertes PM, Demoly P, Alperovitch A, et al. Methylene blue-treated plasma: an increased allergy risk? J Allergy Clin Immunol 2012;130(3):808–12.
111. Seltsam A, Mueller TH. Updated hemovigilance data do not show an increased risk of allergic reactions to methylene blue-treated plasma. J Allergy Clin Immunol 2013;131(4):1253–4.

112. D'Alessandro A, Zolla L. Proteomics for quality-control processes in transfusion medicine. Anal Bioanal Chem 2010;398(1):111–24.
113. Dewachter P, Mouton-Faivre C, Benhaijoub A, et al. Anaphylactic reaction to patent blue V after sentinel lymph node biopsy. Acta Anaesthesiol Scand 2006;50(2):245–7.
114. Hope-Ross M, Yannuzzi LA, Gragoudas ES. Adverse reactions due to indocyanine green. Ophthalmology 1994;101(3):529–33.
115. Obana A, Miki T, Hayashi K, et al. Survey of complications of indocyanine green angiography in Japan. Am J Ophthalmol 1994;118(6):749–53.
116. Benya R, Quintana J, Brundage B. Adverse reactions to indocyanine green: a case report and a review of the literature. Cathet Cardiovasc Diagn 1989; 17(4):231–3.
117. Su Z, Ye P, Teng Y, et al. Adverse reaction in patients with drug allergy history after simultaneous intravenous fundus fluorescein angiography and indocyanine green angiography. J Ocul Pharmacol Ther 2012;28(4):410–3.
118. Olsen TW, Lim JI, Capone A Jr, et al. Anaphylactic shock following indocyanine green angiography. Arch Ophthalmol 1996;114(1):97.
119. Wolf S, Arend O, Schulte K, et al. Severe anaphylactic reaction after indocyanine green fluorescence angiography. Am J Ophthalmol 1992;114(5):638–9.
120. Yusim Y, Livingstone D, Sidi A. Blue dyes, blue people: the systemic effects of blue dyes when administered via different routes. J Clin Anesth 2007;19(4): 315–21.
121. Graziano S, Hoyte L, Vilich F, et al. Life-threatening reaction to indigo carmine— a sulfa allergy? Int Urogynecol J Pelvic Floor Dysfunct 2005;16(5):418–9.
122. Gousse AE, Safir MH, Madjar S. Life-threatening anaphylactoid reaction associated with indigo carmine intravenous injection. Urology 2000;56(3):508.
123. Naitoh J, Fox BM. Severe hypotension, bronchospasm, and urticaria from intravenous indigo carmine. Urology 1994;44(2):271–2.

Adverse Events to Nontargeted and Targeted Chemotherapeutic Agents
Emphasis on Hypersensitivity Responses

Brian A. Baldo, PhD[a,b,*], Mauro Pagani, MD[c]

KEYWORDS

- Cancer drug hypersensitivities • Chemotherapeutic drug hypersensitivities
- Adverse events to cancer drugs • Monoclonal antibody adverse events
- Side effects of chemotherapeutic drugs • Monoclonal antibody hypersensitivities
- Diagnosis of chemotherapeutic drug hypersensitivities
- Desensitization to cancer drugs

KEY POINTS

- Nontargeted therapies can induce hypersensitivity reactions, some severe, in about 5% of treated patients.
- Hypersensitivity reactions are unpredictable, and it is not possible to identify patients at risk of developing such reactions.
- Diagnosis of these reactions is essential because the antineoplastic agents are, for the patients, often unique and irreplaceable.
- Prevention of hypersensitivity reactions is based on skin testing, premedication, and/or desensitization.
- Targeted therapies induce their own unique adverse effects: a lengthened QT interval, decreased left ventricular ejection fraction, and a distinct hand-foot skin reaction.
- Mucocutaneous reactions to epidermal growth factor receptor inhibitors include a papulopustular rash, xerosis, pigmentary changes, fissures, and paronychia.
- Diagnosis of hypersensitivities to small-molecule targeted therapies is hampered by a lack of suitable tests and/or their availability. Few desensitization protocols have been used so far.

Continued

Conflict of interest statement: No financial contribution or any other assistance was received by the authors in relation to the preparation and presentation of this work. No potential conflict of interest is, or has been, involved.

[a] Molecular Immunology Unit, Kolling Institute of Medical Research, Royal North Shore Hospital of Sydney, Sydney 2065, Australia; [b] Department of Medicine, University of Sydney, Sydney 2006, Australia; [c] Medicine Department, Pieve di Coriano Hospital, Azienda Ospedaliera C.Poma, Mantova, Italy
* Corresponding author. 11 Bent Street, Lindfield, New South Wales 2070, Australia.
E-mail address: babaldo@iinet.net.au

Immunol Allergy Clin N Am 34 (2014) 565–596
http://dx.doi.org/10.1016/j.iac.2014.04.003   immunology.theclinics.com
0889-8561/14/$ – see front matter © 2014 Elsevier Inc. All rights reserved.

Continued

- Monoclonal antibodies provoke all 4 types of hypersensitivities, including immune cytopenias, vasculitis, serum sickness, and pulmonary and cardiac events. Some successful desensitization protocols have been developed.

INTRODUCTION

The so-called chemotherapeutic drugs cause a wide variety of adverse events ranging from, for example, headache, mild gastrointestinal symptoms, cough, transient rash, and itching to severe cytopenias; anaphylaxis; lung, liver, cardiac, and neural toxicities; several reactions of the skin and mucous membranes; and rarely life-threatening bullous toxidermias.[1–3] Although only some of these myriad adverse reactions are true hypersensitivities, that is, reactions with a specific humoral and/or cellular immune component or basis, reactions are sometimes incorrectly described as hypersensitivities, whereas other true hypersensitivities go unrecognized.[1,3,4] Although the term *hypersensitivity* is widely used in immunology, allergy, and oncology and features prominently in reports of clinical trials, information released by regulatory agencies and pharmaceutical companies, a common definition of the term is frequently lacking across the disciplines. The word is often applied to reactions that clearly have no immune basis or when the underlying mechanism has not been established.[3] Now, with a rapidly growing number of drugs (already well in excess of 100) used for treatment of the numerous different cancers,[5] neglect by allergists and immunologists of the wide range of drug-induced adverse systemic and cutaneous reactions provoked by these agents needs to be recognized and remedied both at the levels of diagnosis and management.

Here the authors attempt to bring the problem of drug-induced adverse events so commonly seen during cancer therapy to the attention of allergists by outlining the extent, variety, and nature of reactions that may occur; classifying the drugs to permit understanding of the relationships and differences between them and the responses they provoke; highlighting the mechanistic basis of true drug-induced hypersensitivities while emphasizing the need for the acceptance of a common definition across all disciplines; and discussing the need for premedication treatments, desensitizations, and specialized diagnostic testing to identify the 4 types of hypersensitivities. In an attempt to logically organize for classification and presentation the large number and diverse nature of the small-molecule antineoplastic drugs, monoclonal antibodies (mAbs) and cytotoxic chimeric proteins, the different agents are firstly divided on a nontargeted and targeted basis and then considered as some individual examples from groups classified according to their mechanisms of action.[3,6,7]

NONTARGETED DRUGS

Hypersensitivity reactions to chemotherapeutic drugs have been documented for most cancer chemotherapies. They are considered to be uncommon, even though their real incidences are not well known.[8] In fact, most reactions are usually mild and are not reported by oncologists, so the problem is probably underestimated. However, hypersensitivity reactions represent a significant problem with certain agents, in particular platinum compounds, taxanes, L-asparaginase, epipodophyllotoxins, and procarbazine, whereas it is lower with others.[9] In this regard, chemotherapeutic agents may be divided into 3 groups represented by drugs with high, intermediate, or low potential to cause hypersensitivity reactions (**Table 1**). Reactions

Table 1
Chemotherapeutic drugs divided on the basis of their potential to cause hypersensitivity reactions

Drugs with High Potential	Drugs with Low Potential	Drugs with Occasional Potential
L-Asparaginase (*Escherichia coli*–derived, *Erwinia*-derived, pegasaparaginase)	Anthracyclines (daunorubicin, doxorubicin, epirubicin, mitoxantrone, idarubicin, valrubicin)	Bleomycin
Platinum compounds (carboplatin, cisplatin, oxaliplatin)	Mercaptopurine	Cyclophosphamide
Taxanes (paclitaxel, docetaxel)	Azathioprine	Vincristine
Epipodophyllotoxins (etoposide, teniposide)		Methotrexate
Procarbazine		Mitomycin C

can be caused by the parent compounds, their metabolites, or the solvent in which they are solubilized (eg, Cremophor EL [a polyethoxylated castor oil] for paclitaxel).

Risk Factors

Knowledge of the risk factors for the development of a hypersensitivity reaction to a chemotherapeutic drug is essential for the identification of at-risk patients. Risk factors, described by several researchers, include previous exposure, a personal history of allergies, route of administration, the preparation/additives of the drug, coincident medications, and concurrent autoimmune diseases[10]; but risks have been defined for only a few drugs, for example, a previous exposure to platinum salts[11] and intravenous administration for L-asparaginase.[12] **Table 2** summarizes the most relevant published studies of risk factors.

Table 2
Risk factors for hypersensitivity reactions to chemotherapy

No of Patients	Culprit Drug	Risk Factors	Author
	L-Asparaginase	Intravenous administration	Weiss,[12] 1992
15	Paclitaxel	History of bee-sting HSRs	Grosen et al,[13] 2000
83	Carboplatin	History of HSRs to drugs	Markman et al,[14] 2003
14	Paclitaxel	History of skin HSRs to drugs, obesity, postmenopausal status	Sendo et al,[15] 2005
68	Carboplatin	Carbo-free interval >12 mo History of HSRs to drugs	Schwartz et al,[16] 2007
15	Carboplatin	Carbo-free interval >23 mo History of HSRs	Gadducci et al,[11] 2008
45	Oxaliplatin	OHP-free interval >12 mo, age <60 y	Mori et al,[17] 2010
166	Carboplatin + paclitaxel	Age <70 y	Joly et al,[18] 2011
102	Docetaxel	Second line of chemotherapy	Syrigou et al,[19] 2011
22	Carboplatin + paclitaxel	History of systemic HSRs	Piovano et al,[20] 2012

Abbreviations: Carbo, carboplatin; HSRs, hypersensitivity reactions; OHP, oxaliplatin.

Clinical Pictures

Clinical manifestations are variable, and reactions are unpredictable. The symptoms involve the skin (rash, pruritus, urticaria, angioedema, palmar erythema, facial flushing), gastrointestinal tract (abdominal pain, nausea, diarrhea), respiratory tract (dyspnea, bronchospasm), and the system (alterations in blood pressure and heart rate). More severe reactions (always occurring during the infusion of chemotherapy) provoke chest pain; angina pectoris; anaphylaxis; and, in rare cases, even death.[10] Mild to moderate reactions can develop either during the treatment or in the 24 to 72 hours after the end of the administration of chemotherapy.

Pathogenesis

The mechanisms of the hypersensitivity reactions are not always intensively analyzed. Similar to other drug reactions and considering the results of some skin tests and in vitro analyses, the more severe acute reactions probably involve drug-specific immunoglobulin E (IgE) antibodies (eg, with the platinum compounds). Most mild reactions seem to be determined by other mechanisms, such as direct mast cell or basophil activation/degranulation or activation of the complement cascade.[21] In addition, cases of type II, III, or IV hypersensitivity reactions have been reported. **Table 3** shows examples of these 4 types of reactions.

Diagnosis

The correct identification and diagnosis of hypersensitivity reactions to cytostatic drugs play a crucial role in the treatment of neoplastic patients because, unlike other drugs (eg, antibiotics) that may be easily replaced and exchanged in case of adverse reactions, chemotherapeutic drugs are often uniquely complementary for a particular cancer and, therefore, essential for the treatment of the disease (**Box 1**). Therefore, if a hypersensitivity reaction occurs, the physician may have to decide between the benefit of continuing the treatment and the risk of, for example, a potential fatal anaphylactic reaction during the subsequent chemotherapy. Hence, the correct diagnosis of an allergic side effect to a cytostatic drug is crucial and cannot be postponed.

The diagnosis of hypersensitivity reactions to a drug is based on history, clinical manifestations, and if possible, skin tests, in vitro tests and provocation tests.[22] In neoplastic patients, anamnestic evaluation is complicated by many confounding factors: (1) patients often take a lot of drugs, for example, analgesics or antiemetics that may also provoke hypersensitivity reactions; (2) the neoplastic cells may cause, probably via the direct activation of mast cells, some clinical manifestations that mimic

Table 3
Immunopathogenetic mechanisms of hypersensitivity reactions

Type of HSR	Immunopathogenetic Mechanism	Symptoms	Example
I	IgE-mediated	Urticaria, angioedema, bronchospasm, anaphylaxis	L-asparaginase Platinum salts?
II	Cytolytic antibodies (IgG or IgM)	Hemolytic anemia	Oxaliplatin
III	Antigen-antibody immune complex	Vasculitis	Methotrexate
IV	Cell-mediated sensitized T lymphocytes	Contact dermatitis	Anthracyclines

Abbreviation: HSR, hypersensitivity reaction.

Box 1
Difficulties in the diagnosis of hypersensitivity reactions to chemotherapy

Anamnesis: Neoplastic patients take many drugs that can each provoke reactions, and some cancers increase the risk of allergic manifestations.

Skin tests: Skin tests are only useful for platinum salts. Their role for other drugs (L-asparaginase, paclitaxel, etoposide, procarbazine, cyclophosphamide, and so forth) is uncertain.

In vitro tests: Detection of drug-specific IgE is probably useful in cases of suspected hypersensitivity reactions to platinum salts. There are very little data for other classes of drugs.

---

hypersensitivity reactions; and (3) some epidemiologic studies have demonstrated that certain cancers are associated with an increased risk of allergies.[23,24] Therefore, the physician must obtain a careful clinical history, analyzing the characteristics and chronology of symptoms and their relationship to the intake of cytotoxic agents or other drugs. For example, hypersensitivity reactions to taxanes usually develop during the first or second infusion, whereas reactions to platinum salts occur after several doses of therapy, on average 6 to 7, suggesting that desensitization to the drug is needed.

The clinical history is also important because chemotherapy may often provoke non–IgE-mediated reactions and even non–immune-mediated reactions.[10] In the presumed immune-mediated reactions, prick and intradermal tests performed to detect drug-specific IgE are only useful for a few chemotherapeutic drugs, in particular platinum salts, but not for other drugs. The role of platinum drug–specific IgE antibodies in the development of hypersensitivity reactions to these agents, especially carboplatin and oxaliplatin, is well documented[10,25]; the finding of positive skin tests underlines an IgE-mediated mechanism. Indeed, skin tests are rather sensitive for the diagnosis of hypersensitivity reactions to platinum compounds with a sensitivity ranging from 75% to 100%.[25–31] The most reliable results are obtained with the intradermal test when reactions have developed during the infusion of the drug or within 2 hours of the end of therapy.[25] However, Madrigal-Burgaleta and colleagues[32] observed positive prick tests in 4 patients with well-documented hypersensitivity reactions to oxaliplatin. The patch test, helpful in the diagnosis of delayed reactions, does not seem to be useful in the diagnosis of allergies to cytostatic drugs.[25] In addition, some recent preliminary observations demonstrated the presence of specific IgE for carboplatin and oxaliplatin in the serum of allergic patients.[32,33] For other chemotherapeutic drugs, skin tests proved positive in some patients who reacted to paclitaxel,[34] cyclophosphamide,[35,36] L-asparaginase,[37] procarbazine,[38] and etoposide[39,40]; but the diagnostic and predictive value of these results remains uncertain. **Table 4** summarizes the concentrations of chemotherapeutic drugs used for skin testing. Apropos

---

Table 4
Recommended skin test concentrations for chemotherapeutic drugs

Drug	SPT	IDT	Comments
Carboplatin	10 mg/mL	1.0 mg/mL	—
Oxaliplatin	1 mg/mL	0.1 mg/mL	—
Cisplatin	1 mg/mL	0.1 mg/mL	—
Other drugs	Undiluted	1:10 dilution	Not all chemotherapeutic drugs have been tested

Abbreviations: IDT, intradermal test; SPT, skin prick test.

of this, some antineoplastic agents, namely, anthracyclines, vinblastine, vincristine, mitomycin C, and mechlorethamine, can determine severe local cutaneous reactions when accidentally touch the skin; therefore, skin tests should not be performed with these drugs.

Factors Influencing the Treatment in Case of Hypersensitivity Reactions

After an allergological work-up during which a severe hypersensitivity reaction to a chemotherapeutic drug is diagnosed, the oncologist and/or allergist must decide whether to stop the chemotherapy or continue it with the same drug or a substitute drug. The decision should be taken after carefully analyzing the factors related to the severity of the reaction, the characteristics of the patient, the type and stage of the disease, and the nature and details of the chemotherapy.

The National Cancer Institute has graded the severity of the reactions into 5 levels (**Table 5**).[41] Generally, grade 1 to 2 reactions allow the continuation of chemotherapy without modification. Grade 3 reactions may require the substitution of the culprit drug. If this is not possible, and there is robust evidence of efficacy, premedication with steroids and antihistamines and/or a reduction in the rate of infusion are recommended. In the case of grade 4 reactions, rechallenge should be avoided and the drug replaced, unless the treatment is curative. The application of a desensitization protocol should also be evaluated (**Box 2**).

Regarding the factors related to the disease and patients, the level of cancer progression, a poor performance status, important comorbidities, or the use of certain drugs (eg, beta-blockers for immediate hypersensitivity reactions) are relevant and may be important contraindications for the infusion of the culprit drug.

Regarding chemotherapy, the physician must evaluate if it is possible to replace the culprit drug with another belonging to a different class of cytostatic drugs or with another drug of the same class. For example, substitution of carboplatin with

Table 5	
Grading of hypersensitivity reactions according to National Cancer Institute's Criteria	
Grade	**Hypersensitivity Reactions**
1	Transient flushing or rash Drug fever 38°C (100.4°F) Intervention not indicated
2	Rash, flushing, urticaria, dyspnea, Drug fever 38°C (100.4°F) Intervention or infusion interruption indicated, responds promptly to symptomatic treatment (eg, antihistamines, nonsteroidal antiinflammatory drugs, narcotics), prophylactic medications indicated <24 h
3	Symptomatic bronchospasm with or without urticaria, allergy-related edema/angioedema, hypotension Prolonged (eg, not rapidly responsive to symptomatic medication and/or brief interruption of infusion), recurrence of symptoms following initial improvement, hospitalization indicated for clinical sequelae (eg, renal impairment, pulmonary infiltrates)
4	Anaphylaxis Life-threatening consequences, urgent intervention indicated
5	Death

Data from National Cancer Institute. Common Terminology Criteria for Adverse Events v4.03 (CTCAE). 2009. Available at: http://ctep.cancer.gov. Accessed October 30, 2013.

Box 2
Recommendations in case of hypersensitivity reactions to chemotherapy

Grade 1 to 2 reactions allow the continuation/pursuit of drug therapy without modification.

Grade 3 reactions may require the substitution of the culprit drug. If this is not possible and when there is a robust evidence of efficacy, premedication with steroids and antihistamines and/or reduction of the rate of infusion is recommended.

In case of *grade 4* reactions, rechallenge should be avoided and the drug replaced, unless the treatment is curative; in this case, the application of a desensitization protocol should be evaluated.

---

another platinum compound, cisplatin, may be limited (and guided) by cross-reactivity of the platinum-specific IgE antibodies.[42] Leguy-Seguin and colleagues[25] observed positive skin tests to oxaliplatin and carboplatin in 3 patients allergic to oxaliplatin and who had never been exposed to carboplatin. However, 8 allergic patients tolerated another platinum compound, which was skin test negative.[25] Thus, if skin tests are negative with another platinum agent, the alternative drug might be used.[25,43,44] For some drugs belonging to the same class (eg, the taxanes), which share the same therapeutic indications but may cross-react, docetaxel could potentially substitute for paclitaxel in cases of severe hypersensitivity reactions to the latter. For example, Lokich and Anderson[45] and Moon and colleagues[46] obtained good results on 6 patients; but Dizon and colleagues[47] and Sanchez-Munoz and colleagues[48] reported a cross-reactivity rate of 90% and 41%, respectively, for the 2 drugs, presumably because of their structural similarity. Generally, therefore, the substitution of one taxane by another is not recommended. In the case of hypersensitivity reactions to *Escherichia coli*–derived L-asparaginase, its substitution with the *Erwinia*-derived preparation or, better still, the pegylated (PEG) form, PEG-asparaginase, is usually safe, although about 15% of patients may develop allergic reactions to pegasparaginase.[49,50] Unfortunately, the availability of *Erwinia*-derived L-asparaginase and pegasparaginase is limited in many parts of the world, making premedication or desensitization protocols necessary alternatives. Following premedication with steroids and antihistamines and a desensitization protocol on 16 patients with previous allergic reactions to L-asparaginase, Soyer and colleagues[51] showed that chemotherapy could be completed in almost 70% of the patients. Hence, in countries with shortages of alternative asparaginase preparations, this approach might be a suitable option.

Prevention of Hypersensitivity Reactions to Nontargeted Drugs

To prevent allergic reactions, 3 possibilities are available: premedication, skin testing, and desensitization (**Box 3**).

Premedication with steroids and antihistamines, used worldwide in the schedules of chemotherapy with taxanes, has dramatically decreased the incidence of hypersensitivity reactions to 2% to 4% of cases.[12,21,52] Recent findings by Berger and colleagues[53] demonstrated that premedication was not mandatory after 2 doses of paclitaxel if patients did not previously develop hypersensitivity reactions. This observation is undoubtedly interesting, but more studies are necessary to confirm the results.

Another modality of treatment emerged from the clinical trials of Olson and colleagues[54] and Markman and colleagues.[55] Both groups of researchers readministered paclitaxel to patients who experienced hypersensitivity reactions to the drug on the same day the reaction occurred: 93% of the patients were able to complete the

> **Box 3**
> **Procedures for the prevention of hypersensitivity reactions to chemotherapy**
>
> 1. *Premedication* with steroids and antihistamines is indicated in case of administration of taxanes, whereas it is not useful to prevent hypersensitivity reactions caused by platinum salts.
>
> 2. *Skin tests* (prick and intradermal) play an important role in the prevention of reactions to platinum salts. They are especially effective for patients who are less than 70 years of age who received at least 4 doses of platinum salt and when the interval before readministration is greater than 12 months. Preventive skin tests are not indicated for other classes of chemotherapy.
>
> 3. *Desensitization* must be performed in cases of severe hypersensitivity reactions to a chemotherapeutic drug when the drug is irreplaceable and the therapy cannot be discontinued. Desensitization can be used for all drugs, but the widest experiences are with platinum compounds and the taxanes.

planned chemotherapy without reactions. The mechanism postulated by the researchers is that the first reactions depleted the mediators responsible for the symptoms. Premedication is said to be effective and has been recommended for the prevention of hypersensitivity reactions to pegasparaginase in adult patients,[56] but several researchers have observed that premedication is ineffective in preventing true IgE-mediated allergic reactions to platinum salts.[42,57–59]

Skin tests in between chemotherapy courses to predict a reaction have been analyzed for carboplatin and oxaliplatin. Markman and colleagues[60] demonstrated that intradermal tests with an undiluted solution of carboplatin (0.02 mL) performed 30 minutes before the chemotherapy were able to identify patients who could receive carboplatin safely with a negative predictive value of 98.5%. In addition, in a recent study,[61] 101 patients were submitted to skin testing with oxaliplatin. Two patients proved positive, whereas 5 developed hypersensitivity reactions despite a negative skin test finding (false-negative rate 5.05%). These patients underwent desensitization, and the planned schedule of chemotherapy was completed in 5 cases. Therefore, skin tests for carboplatin and oxaliplatin seem to be useful for the primary prevention of an allergic reaction to these drugs. They could be performed on patients after 5 cycles of chemotherapy containing carboplatin, especially when the therapy is readministered to neoplastic patients after an interval between the last and the new infusion of more than 12 months.

Desensitization is indicated for neoplastic patients who experience severe allergic reactions despite premedication, when the culprit drug is not replaceable, and/or in cases of positive skin tests to platinum compounds.[60] The aim of desensitization is to induce a transient tolerance that can be achieved in a relatively short period (on average 6 hours), permitting the safe reintroduction of a drug that provoked the hypersensitivity reactions.[62] In chemotherapy, most desensitization protocols involve platinum compounds or taxanes; but, theoretically, desensitizations to other cytostatic drugs could be attempted and might be successful with this procedure.[63,64] Clinical experience shows that desensitization is effective in IgE- and non–IgE-mediated immediate hypersensitivity reactions of any severity.[31] Many protocols have been described in the scientific literature, but the best evaluated one seems to be a 12-step procedure developed by Castells and colleagues[27] in which the patients receive the established dose for chemotherapy divided into 12 incremental steps. In brief, the drug is prepared in 3 solutions: the first contains a 100-fold dilution of the final target concentration; the second contains a 10-fold dilution; and the third is obtained by subtracting from the final total dose the cumulative dose presented in the first 2 solutions. Each solution is administered in 4 steps at increasing infusion rates. This protocol usually provokes adverse reactions, especially during the infusion of the third solution; but a temporary stop of the therapy and the parenteral administration of antihistamines and steroids usually permits the continuation of the therapy until completion. In a recent work, Patil and colleagues[65] identified 3 different groups of patients with hypersensitivity reactions, namely, skin test positive, skin test negative, and skin tests converters, in which skin test results converted to positive during desensitization after an initial negative result. Skin test–positive patients and converters were more likely to have hypersensitivity reactions during desensitization, whereas true-negative patients could subsequently complete the planned schedule of chemotherapy without desensitization. Desensitization is an effective and safe procedure; but it is also rather complex, involving a team of allergists, oncologists, nurses, and possibly anesthetists. Thus, it is normally used for life-saving and irreplaceable cytostatic drugs only. Lastly, desensitization protocols do not alter the effect of therapy. **Table 6** summarizes the different possible management approaches after hypersensitivity reactions to chemotherapeutic drugs.

TARGETED DRUGS

Specific targeting of tumor cells without inflicting collateral damage on normal healthy cells has been, and remains, a long-standing aim in cancer therapy. With the introduction of targeted approaches, including signal transduction therapies,[66] selected mAbs,[6,7,67] and several other sophisticated strategies, such as employment of cytotoxic chimeric proteins[68,69] and approaches based on an understanding of the proteasome,[70,71] the long-awaited aim of targeted therapies is beginning to look achievable. However, although some results are encouraging, these strategies promising efficacy with minimal toxicity have, with a small number of notable exceptions, so far brought minimal success.[66] For the authors' purposes here, targeted drugs have been divided into the natural or synthetic small molecules (ie, generally molecular weight <1 kDa) almost always of nonbiologic origin and the biologicals, in particular mAbs and recombinant fusion proteins, for example, denileukin diftitox[68] and aflibercept.[69]

Table 6
Handling procedures after severe reactions to chemotherapy

Drug	Management After Reactions
Platinum compounds	Desensitization
Taxanes	Premedication with steroids and antihistamines
L-Asparaginase	Substitution with different preparation Premedication with steroids or antihistamines Desensitization
Procarbazine	Discontinue
Epipodophyllotoxins	Premedication with antihistamines Slow infusion rate
Anthracyclines	Slow infusion rate Desensitization
Mercaptopurine, azathioprine	Desensitization
Methotrexate	Premedication with steroids or antihistamines Desensitization
Cytarabine	Discontinue
Cyclophosphamide and ifosfamide	Discontinue

Small Chemotherapeutic Drugs

The first example of using an understanding of the signaling network to design and employ targeted drugs was the application of the estrogen receptor antagonist tamoxifen for the treatment of some estrogen-dependent breast cancers.[72] Signal transduction therapy involves the identification of signaling molecules, such as hormones, ATP, growth factors, neurotransmitters, cytokines, and chemokines, and their altered pathways and consequent cell responses like cell division, gene expression, metabolic changes, and apoptosis.[66] The principle of signal transduction therapy is summarized in **Fig. 1**; some examples of differently targeted chemotherapeutic antineoplastic drugs are set out in **Table 7**, which also shows the structures, cancer indications, and mechanisms of action of the selected drugs (see reviews[3,88]). Protein kinases in particular, either in receptor or nonreceptor form, have been used as targets for a new generation of antitumor drugs. For example, the oncogene BCR-ABL (fusion of the breakpoint cluster region [BCR] gene on chromosome 22 and the ABL tyrosine kinase gene on chromosome 9) mutation formed by the so-called Philadelphia translocation[89] is present in most patients with chronic myeloid leukemia (CML); its fusion protein Bcr-Abl, essential in the induction of leukemia, is expressed in high levels. CML cells are absolutely dependent (ie, show oncogene addiction) on Bcr-Abl kinase activity, a dependence exploited by the drug imatinib (Gleevec), which inhibits the enzyme and has been successful in the treatment of the leukemia.[89] Dasatinib (Sprycel) is another protein tyrosine kinase inhibitor that shows a broader spectrum of enzyme activity blocking Bcr-Abl, Src, and other tyrosine kinases.[89] Gefitinib (Iressa)

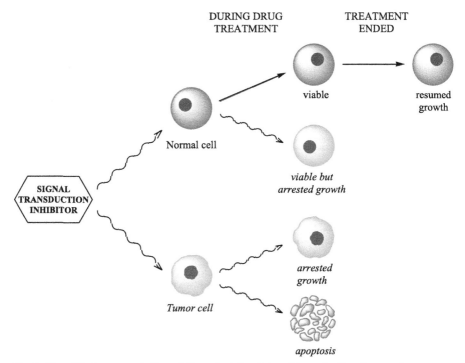

Fig. 1. Simplified representation of the principle of signal transduction therapy for cancers. (*Adapted from* Baldo BA, Pham NH. Adverse reactions to targeted and non-targeted chemotherapeutic drugs with emphasis on hypersensitivity responses and the invasive metastatic switch. Cancer Metastasis Rev 2013;32:737; with permission.)

Table 7
Detailed examples of differently targeted chemotherapeutic drugs[a] and their hypersensitivity/adverse reactions

Generic and Trade Name and Classification[b] on Basis of Mechanism	Structure	Cancer Indications	Mechanisms of Action[b]	Hypersensitivity[c]/Adverse[d] Reactions	References[e]
SIGNAL TRANSDUCTION INHIBITORS					
Nonreceptor tyrosine kinase inhibitors[f] Imatinib (Gleevec)		Ph+CML, Ph+ALL, GIST	Blocks Bcr-Abl tyrosine kinase from phosphorylating	*Systemic:* cytopenias, hypersens pneum, hepatotox, tls, CV, GI *Cutaneous:* pr, ppr, vasc, hyperpigm, agep, SJS, em	73,74
Receptor tyrosine kinase inhibitors[g] Erlotinib (Tarceva)		NSCL, pancreatic	EGFR inhibitor, binds ATP receptor site and interrupts signal cascade	*Systemic:* cytopenias, hepatotox, ild, renal and ocular disorders *Cutaneous:* ppr, pr, xerosis, hyperpigm, hfsr, digital fissures, paronychia	75
mTOR ser/threo kinase inhibitors[h] Everolimus (Afinitor)		Breast, RCC, PNET, SEGA	Binds protein FKBP12; this complex inhibits mTOR ultimately dephosphorylating S6K1 and causing apoptosis of cancer cells	*Systemic:* cytopenias, pneumonitis, renal failure, edema, oral ulcers, dyspnea, GI *Cutaneous:* acneiform rash, erythema, st, nail disorders, xerosis	76
Histone deacetylase inhibitors[i] Vorinostat (Zolinza)		CTCL	Accumulation of acetylated proteins including BCL6, p53, Hsp90l → growth arrest and apoptosis	*Systemic:* cytopenia, pulm embolism, thrombosis, GI *Cutaneous:* exfol dermatitis, pr, alopecia	77

(continued on next page)

Table 7
(continued)

Generic and Trade Name and Classification[b] on Basis of Mechanism	Structure	Cancer Indications	Mechanisms of Action[b]	Hypersensitivity[c]/Adverse[d] Reactions	References[e]
Target the PML-RARα oncoprotein[k] Tretinoin (Vesanoid)		APL	Downregulates S100A 10[l] and fibrinolytic activity	*Systemic*: retinoic acid syndrome, cls, retinoid toxicity, resp and ear disorders *Cutaneous*: pr, photosens, erythema, xeroderma	78
Bind retinoid receptors Bexarotene (Targretin)		CTCL	Activates retinoid X receptors changing gene expression, decreasing cell proliferation and producing tumor regression and apoptosis	*Systemic*: lipid abnormalities, pancreatitis, anemia, leuko, hypothyroidism, edema, infections *Cutaneous*: ppr, acne, keratitis, bullous rash, corneal lesions, photosens, xerosis, alopecia	79
PROTEASOME INHIBITORS[m]					
Bortezomib (Velcade)		MM, MCL, NHL	Inhibits proteasome by binding to chymotrypsin and caspase sites, may suppress degradation of proapoptotic factors	*Systemic*: cytopenias, hypotension, cardiac disorders, ARDS, tls, hepatic events, pneumonia, dyspnea *Cutaneous*: rash,[n] pr, erythema, U, facial edema, vasc, ten	80
HORMONAL EFFECTS					
Inhibitors of hormone synthesis Anastrozole[o] (Arimidex)		Breast	Binds aromatase preventing conversion of androgens → estrogens	*Systemic*: hot flushes, arthritis, arthralgia, dyspnea, osteoporosis, hypertension *Cutaneous*: rashes, pr, mpr, erythema nodosum, lupus, vasc, em, SJS	81

Drug	Indication	Mechanism	Side effects	Ref
GnRH[p] agonists Goserelin (Zoladex)	Prostate, breast	Synth analogue of GnRH, binds GnRH receptor → increase in Gn and reduction in hormone levels	*Systemic:* hot flushes, anemia, didf, osteoporosis, anaphylaxis, vaginitis. *Cutaneous:* rash, itch, rpcs, acne, seborrhea, alopecia	82
Hormone receptor antagonists Tamoxifen[q] (Nolvadex)	Breast (estrogen receptor positive and postmenopausal women)	Antagonist of estrogen receptor inhibiting breast cancer cells requiring estrogen, antiangiogenic effect	*Systemic:* hot flushes, vaginal discharge, endometriosis, interstit pneumonia, thrombosis, vision reduction. *Cutaneous:* U, angio, vasc,[r] pr vulvae, em, bullous pemphigoid, SJS	83
Antiandrogens Bicalutamide (Casodex)	Prostate, assessed for ovarian and metastatic breast cancer	Binds androgen receptor preventing its activation and accelerates degradation of receptor	*Systemic:* hot flushes, thrombo, interstit pneumonia, gynecomastia. *Cutaneous:* U, angio, pr, alopecia	84

TARGETED ANTIFOLATE DRUGS

Drug	Indication	Mechanism	Side effects	Ref
Pralatrexate (Folotyn)	PTCL	Folate analogue antimetabolite accumulates in cancer cells, which overexpress RFC-1 and interferes with DNA synth → cell death	*Systemic:* thrombo, febrile neutro, anemia, mucositis, fetal harm, pyrexia, tls. *Cutaneous:* rash, pr, exfoliation, ulceration, ten	85

(continued on next page)

Table 7
(continued)

Generic and Trade Name and Classification[b] on Basis of Mechanism	Structure	Cancer Indications	Mechanisms of Action[b]	Hypersensitivity[c]/Adverse[d] Reactions	References[e]
TARGETED CYTOTOXIC CHIMERIC PROTEINS					
Denileukin diftitox (Ontak)	Diphtheria toxin–IL-2 fusion protein	CTCL	Modified diphtheria toxin released causing ADP-ribosyltransferase-mediated inhibition of protein synthesis and death	*Systemic:* infusion reaction, cls, pyrexia, vision disturbances, periph edema, dyspnea, cough, GI *Cutaneous:* pr, ten	68,86
Ziv-aflibercept (Zaltrap)	Fusion protein of IgG1 Fc and VEGFR1 and VEGFR2 ligand-binding domains	MCRC	Acts as soluble decoy VEGF receptor and angiogenesis inhibitor	*Systemic:* leuko, neutro, thrombo, GI perforation, hemorrhage, hypertension, proteinuria, venous thromboembolism *Cutaneous:* acral erythema, hyperpigm, st, compromised wound healing	69,87

Abbreviations: agep, acute generalized exanthematous pustulosis; ALL, acute lymphoblastic leukemia; angio, angioedema; APL, acute promyelocytic leukemia; ARDS, acute (adult) respiratory distress syndrome; BCL6, B cell lymphoma 6 protein; cls, capillary leak syndrome; CML, chronic myelogenous leukemia; CTCL, cutaneous T-cell lymphoma; CV, cardiovascular disorders; didf, drug-induced disease flare (tumor-flare effect); EGFR, epidermal growth factor receptor; em, erythema multiforme; exfol, exfoliative; GI, gastrointestinal adverse events; GIST, gastrointestinal stromal tumor; Gn, gonadotropin; GnRH, gonadotropin-releasing hormone; hepatotox, hepatotoxicity; hfsr, hand-foot skin reaction; Hsp90, heat shock protein 90; hyperpigm, hyperpigmentation; hypersens, hypersensitivity; ild, interstitial lung disease; interstit, interstitial; leuko, leukopenia; MCL, mantle cell lymphoma; MCRC, metastatic colorectal cancer; MM, multiple myeloma; mpr, maculopapular rash; mTOR, mechanistic (or mammalian) target of rapamycin; neutro, neutrocytopenia; NHL, non-Hodgkin lymphoma; NSCL, non–small cell lung cancer; p53, tumor protein 53; periph, peripheral; Ph+, Philadelphia chromosome positive; photosens, photosensitization; PML-RARα, promyelocytic leukemia retinoic acid receptor α oncogene fusion protein; PNET, pancreatic neuroendocrine tumor; pneum, pneumonitis; ppr, papulopustular rash; pr, pruritus; PTCL, peripheral T cell lymphoma; pulm, pulmonary; RCC, renal cell carcinoma; RFC-1, reduced folate carrier type 1; rpcs, relapsing polychondritis cutaneous symptoms; SEGA, subependymal giant cell astrocytoma; ser/threo, serine/threonine; SJS, Stevens-Johnson syndrome; st, stomatitis; synth, synthesis; ten, toxic epidermal necrolysis; tls, tumor lysis syndrome; thrombo, thrombocytopenia; U, urticaria; vasc, vasculitis; VEGFR, vascular endothelial growth factor receptor.

a MAbs not included (see **Table 8**).

b Some drugs exert their actions by more than one mechanism and might, therefore, be classified into more than one category. The classification shown is deemed to be the most appropriate one.

c Reactions known, or suspected, of having an immunologic basis.

d Reactions, such as weakness, fatigue, headache, and so forth, and gastrointestinal (GI) symptoms like nausea, vomiting, diarrhea, constipation, appetite reduction, dyspepsia, and so forth, are not recorded here because they are common to so many of the drugs. Where such reactions are important, they are referred to collectively as GI.

e For additional references for all drugs listed here see.[3]

f Other frequently used registered drugs in this group include bosutinib, crizotinib, dasatinib, nilotinib, and ponatinib.

g Other frequently used registered drugs in this group include axitinib, gefitinib, lapatinib, pazopanib, regorafenib, sorafenib, sunitinib, and vandetanib.

h Temsirolimus and rapamycin are also in this group.

i Romidepsin is also in this group.

j BCL6 protein is a zinc finger transcription factor, a sequence-specific repressor of transcription. p53 (tumor protein 53), is a tumor suppressor protein that regulates the cell cycle. Hsp90, heat shock protein 90, is a molecular chaperone, assisting protein folding and stabilizing some proteins in tumor growth.

k Arsenic trioxide, also used for acute promyelocytic leukemia, also binds to PML-RARα.

l A plasminogen receptor.

m Carfilzomib is also used as a proteasome inhibitor for multiple myeloma.

n Incidence is 8% to 18%.

o An aromatase inhibitor. Other registered aromatase inhibitors include exemestane and letrozole.

p Other analogues include leuprolide.

q A selective estrogen receptor modulator.

r Nineteen percent of patients experience skin reactions.

and erlotinib (Tarceva) target the epidermal growth factor receptor (EGFR; also known as ErB1 and HER1), a member of the ErbB family of receptors. Other receptor tyrosine kinase inhibitors are used to target growth factor receptors, including vascular endothelial growth factor receptors (VEGFRs) and platelet-derived growth factor receptors (PDGFRs). Lapatinib (Tykerb) inhibits ErbB1 and ErbB2 (human epidermal growth factor receptor 2 [HER2]); sorafenib (Nexavar) inhibits VEGFR and PDGFR; sunitinib (Sutent) inhibits VEGFR and PDGFR; and pazopanib (Votrient) targets several tyrosine kinases, including VEGFRs, PDGFRs, and fibroblast growth factor receptor 2 (FGFR2). Increased understanding of the proteasome and its role in protein degradation via the ubiquitin-proteasome pathway has led on to the development of proteasome inhibitor drugs. These drugs, such as bortezomib (Velcade), seem to bind to chymotrypsin and caspase catalytic sites in the proteasome core where degradation of proapoptotic factors leads to death of multiple myeloma and mantle lymphoma cells.[6,70,71] Other signal transduction strategies are represented in **Table 7**.

mAbs

Table 8 lists the 15 mAbs currently approved for cancer therapy together with the specific target and approved indications for each mAb. These mAbs are directed to a limited number of targets: 4 to the B lymphocyte antigen CD20; 3 to EGFR2 (HER2, ErbB2); 2 to EGFR; and one each against CD30, CD52, VEGF, epithelial cell adhesion molecule (EpCAM), cytotoxic T lymphocyte–associated protein 4 (CTLA4), and tumor necrosis factor ligand superfamily member 11 (TNFSF-11 or receptor activator of nuclear factor κ-B ligand [CD254] best known as RANKL).[6,7]

Adverse Events

The small chemotherapeutic targeted drugs and targeted chimeric proteins (see **Table 7**) and mAbs (see **Table 8**) are considered separately.

Small chemotherapeutic drugs and cytotoxic chimeric proteins

Although it is true to say that targeted therapies generally produce less collateral damage to patients than nontargeted chemotherapies, for example, less nausea, vomiting, asthenia, diarrhea, and cytotoxic effects, the former still induce a wide range of adverse effects, only a few of which are true hypersensitivities.[3,106] **Table 7** details the systemic and cutaneous reactions of a representative drug from each of the 6 different categories of signal transduction inhibitors; the proteasome inhibitors; 4 different categories of drugs affecting sex hormones; the targeted antifolate drugs; and targeted cytotoxic chimeric proteins. **Table 9**, assembled from recorded adverse and hypersensitivity reactions of the large number of different non-mAb targeted agents currently being administered, summarizes the major hematologic, respiratory, cardiovascular, gastrointestinal, dermatologic, and other adverse events. Cytopenias occur less often and are less severe than the reactions induced by, for example, nontargeted alkylating and antimetabolite drugs but several reactions more or less unique to the targeted therapies are seen, including a lengthened QT interval, decreased left ventricular ejection fraction (LVEF), and a hand-foot skin reaction[107] (a distinct entity from hand-foot syndrome or acral erythema induced by nontargeted drugs, such as capecitabine, docetaxel, oxaliplatin, and methotrexate[6]). Cardiac toxicities are being increasingly recognized with targeted therapies.[108] Asymptomatic and symptomatic cardiac events were reported in 1.6% and 0.2%, respectively, of 3689 patients treated with the HER2 inhibitor lapatinib, and the multikinase angiogenesis inhibitors sunitinib and sorafenib have been associated with heart failure and hypertension, LVEF decrease, and a 6-fold higher chance of hypertension, respectively.[108] Mucocutaneous reactions to

Table 8
Hypersensitivity/adverse reactions of registered mAbs used for cancer therapy[a]

Monoclonal Antibody[a] Generic[b] and Trade Names	Target[c]	Approved Indications	Hypersensitivity[d]/Adverse[e] Reactions	References[f]
Catumaxomab[g] (Removab)	EpCAM[h]/CD3[i]	Malignant ascites	*Systemic:* cytopenias, CRS, SIRS, hepatotoxicity, abdominal disorders, pyrexia, infections, immunogenicity, dyspnea *Cutaneous:* rash, erythema, allergic dermatitis, hyperhidrosis, pruritus	90
Ibritumomab tiuxetan[j] (Zevalin)	CD20[k]	Non-Hodgkin lymphoma	*Systemic:* IR, severe cytopenia, infections, immunogenicity, secondary malignancies *Cutaneous:* exfoliative dermatitis, bullous dermatitis, EM, SJS, TEN	91
Tositumomab-[131]I[l] (Bexxar)	CD20	Non-Hodgkin lymphoma	*Systemic:* severe cytopenias, IR, hypothyroidism, infection, immunization, secondary malignancies, fetal harm, anaphylaxis *Cutaneous:* rash, pruritus, sweating, exfoliative dermatitis	92
Rituximab (MabThera, Rituxan)	CD20	Non-Hodgkin lymphoma	*Systemic:* IR, TLS, renal toxicity, pulmonary events,[m] cardiac events, bowel obstruction and perforation, neutropenias, infections, PML, RA, SS, HBR, anaphylaxis *Cutaneous:* paraneoplastic pemphigus, lichenoid dermatitis, vesiculobullous dermatitis, SJS, TEN	7,93,94
Ofatumumab (Arzerra)	CD20	Chronic lymphocytic leukemia	*Systemic:* cytopenias, IR, infections, pneumonia, intestinal obstruction, HBR, pyrexia, dyspnea, cough, diarrhea, fatigue, PML *Cutaneous:* rash, urticaria, hyperhidrosis	95
Brentuximab vedotin[n] (Adcetris)	CD30[o]	Anaplastic large cell lymphoma, Hodgkin lymphoma	*Systemic:* cytopenias, IR, TLS, immunogenicity, fetal harm, PML, anaphylaxis, PN *Cutaneous:* rash, pruritus, SJS, alopecia	96
Cetuximab (Erbitux)	EGFR[p]	Colorectal, head and neck cancers	*Systemic:* IR, pulmonary events,[m] cardiopulmonary arrest, electrolyte imbalance, infection, GI, anaphylaxis	93,97

(continued on next page)

Table 8 *(continued)*

Monoclonal Antibody[a] Generic[b] and Trade Names	Target[c]	Approved Indications	Hypersensitivity[d]/Adverse[e] Reactions	References[f]
Panitumumab[q] (Vectibix)	EGFR	Colorectal cancer	*Systemic:* IR, pulmonary events,[r] pulmonary embolism, electrolyte depletion, GI, fatigue *Cutaneous[s]:* rash, dermatitis acneiform, erythema, exfoliation, paronychia, skin fissures, photosensitivity, xerosis, pruritus *Cutaneous:* acneiform rash, nail changes, xeroderma, paronychial inflammation, pruritus	93,98
Bevacizumab (Avastin)	VEGF[t]	Colorectal, lung, kidney, brain cancers	*Systemic:* IR, pulmonary events,[m] GI perforation, hemorrhage, wound healing, non-GI fistula, arterial thromboembolic events, hypertension, necrotizing fasciitis, proteinuria, reversible posterior leukoencephalopathy *Cutaneous:* exfoliative dermatitis, alopecia	99
Pertuzumab (Perjeta)	HER2[u]	Metastatic breast cancer	*Systemic:* IR, cytopenias, hypersensitivity/anaphylaxis, LVD, embryo-fetal toxicity, GI, PN *Cutaneous:* rash, paronychia, pruritus, alopecia	100
Trastuzumab (Herceptin)	HER2	Breast cancer	*Systemic:* IR, neutropenia,[v] anemia, pulmonary events,[m] embryo-fetal toxicity, cardiomyopathy,[w] LVD, GI, anaphylaxis/angioedema *Cutaneous:* rash, nail disorders, pruritus	93,101
Trastuzumab emtansine[x] (Kadcyla)	HER2	Advanced metastatic breast cancer	*Systemic:* hepatotoxicity, pulmonary events, thrombocytopenia, fetal harm, LVD, neurotoxicity, hypersensitivity/IR *Cutaneous:* rash, pruritus	102
Alemtuzumab[y] (Campath-1H)	CD52[z]	Chronic lymphocytic leukemia	*Systemic:* IR, cytopenias, pulmonary events,[m] infections,[aa] immunogenicity, cardiac events *Cutaneous:* rash, urticaria, erythema, pruritus	103
Denosumab (Prolia, Xgeva)	RANKL[ab]	Bone metastases, giant cell tumor of the bone	*Systemic:* hypocalcemia, embryo-fetal toxicity, ONJ & osteomyelitis, dyspnea, fatigue/asthenia *Cutaneous:* rash, pruritus, dermatitis, eczema	104
Ipilimumab (Yervoy)	CTLA-4[ac]	Metastatic melanoma	*Systemic:* IMR, diarrhea, fatigue *Cutaneous:* rash, pruritus, dermatitis	105

Abbreviations: CRS, cytokine release syndrome; CTLA-4, cytotoxic T lymphocyte–associated protein 4; EM, erythema multiforme; EpCAM, epithelial cell adhesion molecule; GI, gastrointestinal symptoms (eg nausea, diarrhea, vomiting, constipation, and so forth); HBR, hepatitis B reactivation; IMR, immune-mediated reactions caused by T-cell activation and proliferation (enterocolitis, hepatitis, dermatitis, neuropathies, endocrinopathies); IR, infusion reactions; LVD, left ventricular dysfunction; ONJ, osteonecrosis of the jaw; PML, progressive multifocal leukoencephalopathy; PN, peripheral neuropathy; RA, rheumatoid arthritis; RANKL, receptor activator of nuclear factor kappa-B ligand (CD254); SIRS, systemic inflammatory response syndrome; SS, serum sickness-like reactions, Stevens-Johnson syndrome; TEN, toxic epidermal necrolysis; TLS, tumor lysis syndrome.

[a] Approved by the Food and Drug Administration and/or European Medicines Agency.

[b] Nomenclature: mAbs of murine origin are given the suffix *omab*; chimeric antibodies in which the V region is spliced into human C region is given the *ximab* stem; humanized antibodies with murine hypervariable region spliced into human antibody have the *zumab* stem; and antibodies with complete human sequence are given the *umab* stem.

[c] Specificity of mAb.

[d] Reactions known or suspected of having an immunologic basis.

[e] Other adverse reactions with no clearly established, or yet to be demonstrated, immune mechanism (nausea, cough, diarrhea, fatigue, sweating, and so forth).

[f] For additional references for all mAbs listed here see.[7]

[g] Registered by the European Medicines Agency, Health Canada, and Ministry of Health, Israel but not the Food and Drug Administration. Catumaxomab is a bispecific mouse–rat hybrid (given the suffix *axomab*) recognizing both the epithelial cell adhesion molecule and CD3.

[h] EpCAM, epithelial cell adhesion molecule. Expressed on epithelial and epithelial-derived neoplasms.

[i] CD3 is part of the T cell receptor (TCR) complex on T lymphocytes.

[j] With Yttrium-90 or Indium-111. Tiuxetan is a chelator.

[k] Expressed on B lymphocytes where it aids optimum B cell response to T-independent antigens.

[l] Kills B cells with [131]I.

[m] See **Table 9.**

[n] Conjugated to cytotoxic monomethyl auristatin E (MMAE).

[o] CD30 is a cell membrane protein of the tumor necrosis receptor family. Expressed on activated T and B lymphocytes.

[p] EGFR, epidermal growth factor receptor (HER1, ErbB-1).

[q] Not indicated for use in combination with chemotherapy because of the increased toxicity.

[r] See **Table 9.** It should be discontinued in patients developing interstitial lung disease, pneumonitis, and lung infiltrates.

[s] The most common drug-induced reactions following this mAb are skin toxicities.

[t] VEGF, vascular endothelial growth factor.

[u] HER2, human epidermal growth factor receptor 2. Also known as Neu, ErbB2, CD340, or p185.

[v] Highest risk with myelosuppressive therapy.

[w] Greatest risk (left ventricular dysfunction) when administered with anthracyclines.

[x] Called Ado-trastuzumab emtansine in the United States to distinguish from trastuzumab. Trastuzumab linked to the cytotoxin mertansine (deacetyl mercaptomaytansine [DM1]), a tubulin inhibitor.

[y] Withdrawn from the United States and Europe in 2012 to be relaunched for multiple sclerosis (MS).

[z] CD52 is present on the surface of mature lymphocytes and associated with some lymphomas.

[aa] In particular *Pneumocystis jiroveci,* cytomegalovirus (CMV), Epstein-Barr virus (EBV), and herpes virus.

[ab] RANKL, receptor activator of nuclear factor kappa-B ligand (CD254), a member of the tumor necrosis factor cytokine family.

[ac] CTLA-4, cytotoxic T-lymphocyte antigen 4 (CD152). Binds CD80/CD86 on antigen-presenting cells.

Table 9
Summary of major adverse effects of targeted anticancer chemotherapies

Targeted Therapy	Hematologic	Respiratory	Cardiovascular	GI	Dermatologic	Other
Multikinase Abl inhibitors[a]	Neutropenia; thrombocytopenia	Pneumonitis/pulm edema/alveolar damage; pulm hypertension	↓LVEF[b]/congest heart failure; QT prolongation	Mucositis/stomatitis; diarrhea/colitis	Rash[c]	Hypoglycemia; ↑transaminase; hyperlipasemia; hyperphosphatemia
EGFR inhibitors[d]	—	Pneumonitis/pulm edema/alveolar damage	—	Mucositis/stomatitis; diarrhea/colitis	Rash[c], HFSR[e]	Ocular - corneal abnormalities; conjunctivitis
Angiogenesis inhibitors[f]	Neutropenia; thrombocytopenia	Pneumonitis/pulm edema/alveolar damage	↓LVEF/congest heart failure; QT prolongation; hypertension; thromboembolic events	Mucositis/stomatitis; diarrhea/colitis	Rash; HFSR[e]	Hypothyroidism; hypoglycemia; ↑transaminase; hyperlipasemia; hypophosphatemia; hypomagnesemia
HER2 inhibitors[g]	—	Pneumonitis/pulm edema/alveolar damage	↓LVEF/congest heart failure	Mucositis/stomatitis; diarrhea/colitis	Rash	↑transaminase
mTOR inhibitors[h]	Neutropenia; thrombocytopenia	Pneumonitis/pulm edema/alveolar damage	—	Mucositis/stomatitis	Rash	↑transaminase; hyperglycemia; hypophosphatemia; hypercholesterolemia; hypertriglyceridemia

HDAC inhibitors[i]	Neutropenia; thrombocytopenia	—	QT prolongation	—	Rash	—
RXR agonists[j]	Neutropenia	—	—	—	Rash	↑transaminase; hypothyroidism; hypercholesterolemia; hypertriglyceridemia; hypoglycemia
Proteasome inhibitors[k]	Thrombocytopenia	—	Pneumonitis/pulm edema/alveolar damage; pulm hypertension	—	Rash	Neuropathy; pyrexia; infections (herpes zoster); ↑transaminase

For targeted drugs with hormonal effects and targeted antifolate drugs see.[3]

Abbreviations: Congest, congestive; GI, gastrointestinal; HDAC inhibitors, histone deacetylase inhibitors; HFSR, hand-foot skin reaction; LVEF, left ventricular ejection fraction; mTOR, mammalian target of rapamycin; pulm, pulmonary; RXR, retinoid X receptor.

[a] For example, imatinib, nilotinib, dasatinib, and ponatinib.
[b] LVEF, left ventricular ejection fraction.
[c] Papulopustular rash, sometimes with pruritus, the most common dermatologic event.
[d] For example, erlotinib, gefitinib, vandetanib, cetuximab, and panitumumab.
[e] HFSR, hand-foot skin reaction, not to be confused with hand-foot syndrome or acral erythema.
[f] Sunitinib, sorafenib, axitinib, ponatinib, and pazopanib; also includes ligand binders, (eg, aflibercept, bevacizumab).
[g] For example, lapatinib, pertuzumab, and trastuzumab.
[h] For example, everolimus and temsirolims.
[i] Histone deacetylase inhibitors (eg, romidepsin, vorinostat).
[j] Retinoid X receptor agonists (eg, bexarotene).
[k] For example, bortezomib and carfilzomib.

Data from Baldo BA, Pham NH. Adverse reactions to targeted and non-targeted chemotherapeutic drugs with emphasis on hypersensitivity responses and the invasive metastatic switch. Cancer Metastasis Rev 2013;32:723–61; and Dy GK, Adjei AA. Understanding, recognizing, and managing toxicities of targeted anticancer therapies. CA Cancer J Clin 2013;63:249–79.

EGFR inhibitors, particularly a papulopustular rash, pruritus, xerosis, pigmentary changes, fissures on fingers and toes, alopecia, trichomegaly of the eye lashes, paronychia, stomatitis, and mucositis occur fairly commonly.[109]

Although systemic and cutaneous responses to denileukin diftitox[86] are relatively few, with most reactions being infusion related (incidence ~70%) and vascular leak syndrome (27%), aflibercept has been implicated in causing hypertension and thromboembolic events. Other side effects with the drug, namely, mucositis/stomatitis, diarrhea, neutropenia, thrombocytopenia, and elevated transaminase levels, occur more often in combination therapy (eg, with 5-fluoruracil or FOLFIRI [FOL, folinic acid; F, fluoruracil; IRI, ironotecan]) than with chemotherapy alone.[87,106] One fatal case of toxic epidermal necrolysis (TEN) occurred following the administration of denileukin diftitox.[110]

Hypersensitivity is a loosely used term sometimes incorrectly employed to describe responses that have no immune basis or component, whereas other reactions where the term would be appropriate have been overlooked.[3] There are far fewer reports of each of the 4 types of hypersensitivities classified according to Coombs and Gell[111] for targeted than for nontargeted chemotherapeutic drugs, but this may be, in part, a reflection of the so-far inadequate study of many targeted drug-induced responses and because of their more recent introduction. Specific examples of reactions shown in **Box 4** summarize the current general view of the 4 different hypersensitivity responses seen to the small, targeted drugs.

mAbs

MAbs are also better tolerated than conventional antineoplastic drugs; but again, reactions to the agents are quite diverse, ranging from mild gastrointestinal symptoms and transient rash to anaphylaxis, severe cardiac and pulmonary toxicities, cytopenias, and life-threatening toxidermias (see **Table 8**).[6,7,93,106] Several reactions to mAbs are immune mediated (see later discussion); some may or may not have an immune component (eg, some infusion reactions/cytokine release syndrome [CRS] and systemic inflammatory response syndrome [SIRS]), whereas heart and some pulmonary, kidney, hepatic, and neurologic toxicities seem to be caused by nonimmune mechanisms (**Box 5**).[7,41,93]

Even with the development of humanized and fully human mAbs, the possibility of generating anti-idiotype antibodies remains[7]; although type I anaphylactic reactions

---

Box 4
Hypersensitivity reactions to targeted chemotherapeutic drugs (for additional references see[3])

- Type I IgE antibody-mediated reactions seen more often with tamoxifen, aromatase inhibitors exemestane and letrozole, gonadotropin-releasing hormone agonists goserelin and leuprolide, the mTOR inhibitor everolimus, and tyrosine kinase inhibitor bosutinib

- Type II hypersensitivities represented in few reports of autoimmune hypothyroidism and immune thrombocytopenia to tyrosine kinase inhibitors, especially sunitinib[112,113]

- Type III hypersensitivities also infrequently described: chiefly drug-induced vasculitis to tamoxifen and aromatase inhibitors (eg, anastrozole) and erlotinib (implicated in at least 14 cases)

- Type IV hypersensitivities reported to imatinib (drug reaction with eosinophilia and systemic symptoms [DRESS]); imatinib and exemestane (acute generalized exanthematous pustulosis); imatinib, exemestane, and letrozole (erythema multiforme); tamoxifen (erythema multiforme and Stevens-Johnson syndrome [SJS]); imatinib and vandetanib (SJS); imatinib letrozole, pralatrexate, and bortezomib (TEN); erlotinib, sorafenib, and bexarotene (bullous eruptions)

> **Box 5**
> **Nonimmune-mediated adverse events to mAbs used for cancer therapy**
>
> - Mechanisms of mAb-induced thrombocytopenia, neutropenia, hemolytic anemia, and vasculitis are often not investigated. Some may be immune mediated (see **Box 6**).
>
> - MAb-induced lung diseases, drug-induced lung disease (DILD): The mechanisms are generally not known; therefore, classification on the basis of pathogenesis is difficult (see **Box 7**).
>
> - Cardiac events occur with at least 5 mAbs: trastuzumab ($\downarrow$LVEF, cardiomyopathy); pertuzumab ($\downarrow$LVEF); bevacizumab ($\downarrow$LVEF, hypertension, thromboembolic events, $\uparrow$ heart failure)[106,108]; rituximab (cardiac arrhythmias); cetuximab (cardiopulmonary arrest in patients exposed to radiation therapy).
>
> - Tumor lysis syndrome is well known after brentuximab vedotin and rituximab.
>
> - Progressive multifocal leukoencephalopathy is occasionally seen after brentuximab, ofatumumab, and especially rituximab.
>
> - Papulopustular (acneiform) eruptions occur to EGFR-targeted mAbs (eg, cetuximab and panitumumab).
>
> *Data from* Baldo BA. Adverse events to monoclonal antibodies used for cancer therapy. Focus on hypersensitivity responses. Oncoimmunology 2013;2(10):e26333. http://dx.doi.org/10.4161/onci.26333; and Hansel TT, Kropshofer H, Singer T, et al. The safety and side effects of monoclonal antibodies. Nat Rev Drug Discov 2010;9;325–38.

might be expected, these responses to therapeutic mAbs are relatively uncommon. Other adverse reactions to mAbs, such as urticaria, serum sickness, SJS, TEN, and autoimmune diseases (eg, ipilimumab-induced autoimmune enterocolitis),[114] are clear examples of an immune-mediated reaction. However, some cytopenias, pulmonary and liver toxicities, infections, some other systemic responses, and cutaneous reactions are often difficult to categorize and may (eg, infusion reactions/CRS and SIRS) or may not (eg, tumor lysis syndrome [TLS], some cytopenias and pulmonary reactions, heart, embryo-fetal and neurologic toxicities) have an immune component.[3,7] **Box 6** summarizes known hypersensitivities to the mAbs currently administered as cancer therapies; but it is clear that mechanisms of many reactions induced by

> **Box 6**
> **Hypersensitivity reactions to mAbs used for cancer therapy**
>
> - Type I: There is a low incidence of reactions. Chimeric molecules, catumaxomab, ibritumomab, tositumomab, cetuximab, rituximab, and brentuximab carry warnings. Anaphylaxis is reported for cetuximab, rituximab, brentuximab, ibritumomab, trastuzumab, pertuzumab, and tositumomab.
>
> - Type II: There is little or no good evidence for immune thrombocytopenia. Rituximab-induced late-onset neutropenia may be immune mediated. Autoimmune hemolytic anemia is induced by rituximab and alemtuzumab.
>
> - Type III: Cellular and humoral processes may be involved in some cases of mAb-induced vasculitis. Chimeric mAbs can induce serum sickness (eg, rituximab).
>
> - Type IV: Rare reactions seem to be confined to ibritumomab, brentuximab, and especially rituximab (SJS, TEN, lichenoid dermatitis, vesiculobullous dermatitis, and paraneoplastic pemphigus). Dermatitis is induced by catumaxomab, bevacizumab, denosumab, ipilimumab, panitumumab, and tositumomab; they may be type IV reactions, but the mechanisms are not established.
>
> *Data from* Refs.[6,7,93,106]

individual mAbs remain inadequately investigated, and the list of mAb-induced hypersensitivities is likely to be extended. **Box 7** lists the mAbs implicated in pulmonary adverse events. Rituximab is the agent most commonly involved causing, in particular, bronchiolitis obliterans organizing pneumonia (BOOP), followed by interstitial pneumonitis, acute respiratory distress syndrome (ARDS), and hypersensitivity pneumonitis.

Diagnosis

Diagnostic procedures for hypersensitivities to targeted chemotherapeutic agents are generally not well developed, widely applied, or validated. For type I and IV reactions, few (if any) convincing skin test studies with sufficient numbers of patients seem to have been carried out.[3,6,7] Some immunoassays to aid the diagnosis of immune thrombocytopenia by detecting platelet-reactive serum IgE antibodies are available in only a few laboratories but, in general, the tests are not standardized, do not detect the drug-dependent antibodies, often present technical difficulties, and can produce false-positive results. The time delay in obtaining results in an urgent situation is also a major drawback. Some recommendations for testing for immune thrombocytopenia have been published.[115] Although neutrophil antigens involved in immune neutropenia have been identified, immunoassays to aid the diagnosis of immune-mediated neutropenia and agranulocytosis are not widely available. The monoclonal antibody immobilization of granulocyte antigens assay (MAIGA) seems to be the most specific test; but again, technical difficulties, autoantibodies, and drug-dependent antibodies can be a problem.[116] Diagnosis of drug-induced vasculitis, liver injury, lung disease, and some delayed cutaneous reactions all present difficulties because of a lack of specific tests, suitable laboratory markers, and/or convincing experimental models (see review[3] for discussion and references).

Premedication and Desensitization

Corticosteroids, often dexamethasone, and antihistamines, such as diphenhydramine and cimetidine/ranitidine/famotidine, are generally given in premedication protocols

---

Box 7
Pulmonary adverse events caused by mAbs

- *-ximabs*
  - Cetuximab: interstitial pneumonitis
  - Rituximab: ARDS, BOOP, bronchospasm, diffuse alveolar hemorrhage, hypersensitivity pneumonitis
- *-zumabs*
  - Alemtuzumab: bronchospasm, diffuse alveolar hemorrhage, pulmonary infections
  - Bevacizumab: anaphylaxis/bronchospasm, pulmonary hemorrhage from tumor site
  - Trastuzumab: ARDS, BOOP, dyspnea, interstitial pneumonitis, pleural effusions, pulmonary infiltrates/pulmonary fibrosis/pulmonary edema
- *-umabs*
  - Panitumumab: interstitial lung disease, lung infiltrates, pneumonitis, pulmonary fibrosis

Data from Baldo BA. Adverse events to monoclonal antibodies used for cancer therapy. Focus on hypersensitivity responses. Oncoimmunology 2013;2(10):e26333. http://dx.doi.org/10.4161/onci.26333.

often 12 and 6 hours before infusions of drugs. The corticosteroid is sometimes given for several days before infusion.[6]

As already emphasized,[117] desensitization has become a cornerstone in the management of hypersensitivity reactions to chemotherapeutic drugs and mAbs. By comparison with the nontargeted drugs, there are, as yet, fewer published studies on desensitization for the targeted chemotherapeutic drugs. Desensitization to the multikinase inhibitor sunitinib was accomplished following premedication with prednisone and promethazine and 10 escalating dosage steps beginning with a dose of 0.05 mg.[118] Most procedures have been undertaken with imatinib. Starting with a dose of 0.005 mg and building to a total of 400 mg, desensitizations were achieved with gradual dose escalations over 10 weeks in one case and over 5 days in another.[119] Success has also been reported using a 4-hour outpatient oral protocol beginning with 10 ng of imatinib and proceeding with increasing doses every 10 minutes.[120]

More data are available for mAbs. Successful desensitization to cetuximab commenced with premedication with prednisolone 12 hours and 1 hour before and diphenhydramine 30 minutes before commencement. From a starting dose of 0.001 mg cetuximab, doses were doubled every 15 minutes before a final dose of 325 mg at step 20, giving a cumulative dose of 844 mg. Any reactions were managed with diphenhydramine, a 30-minute waiting period, and dose and infusion reductions.[121] In another protocol, a 5-step procedure was used beginning with 5.07 mg and ending with 694.0 mg for a total of 769.9 mg.[122] In a rapid desensitization protocol for rituximab, patients first received premedication with H1 and H2 antihistamines and sometimes acetaminophen and/or corticosteroids before undergoing a 12-step procedure in which the dose was increased every 15 minutes from an initial dose of 0.022 mg. At step 12, the dose of 1020.5 mg represented approximately half of the total desensitization time taken and 92% of the total dose given. Most reactions that occurred were seen at this stage and responded to antihistamine treatment and an infusion pause.[27] Note that a negative skin test did not override a strong clinical history of a hypersensitivity reaction in determining whether or not to desensitize.[122] Unlike other hypersensitivity reactions to mAbs, particularly rituximab, reactions to trastuzumab are usually seen after multiple exposures.[123] Here again, a 12-step protocol has been used, with 92.3% being administered at the final step.[27,123] In a recently published rapid desensitization procedure for antineoplastic agents, including rituximab,[32] starting doses were 80% higher than the previously used successful 12-step procedures. It should be remembered, however, that higher starting doses are generally accompanied by higher potential risks.

FUTURE CONSIDERATIONS

The realization that antiangiogenic therapy, initially effective by inhibiting vascularization and tumor growth, may lead on to the reverse effect of enhanced tumor growth, invasiveness, and distal metastasis highlights the need to understand how tumor resistance develops.[124] This resistance of tumors has consequences for the appearance of some changed patterns of drug-induced adverse effects as new drugs are sought to inhibit hypoxia signaling. Combination therapies (using, for example, cytotoxic topoisomerase, mTOR, histone deacetylase (HDAC), and proteasome inhibitors) are being increasingly used to overcome the resistance.[3] Other possible new therapies that will each bring their own spectrum of adverse reactions include the introduction of further soluble decoy receptors for growth factors; drugs that inhibit VEGF, angiopoietins, placental growth factor, hypoxia-inducible factor-1alfa (HIF-1α), c-Met, E-cadherin, and matrix degrading enzymes; targeting of angiopoietin-Tie2 signaling; and the study of inhibitors of vascular integrin for antiangiogenic therapy.[3] Lastly, the terminology used to define hypersensitivity needs to be standardized so that investigators in oncology, immunology, and allergy can work from a common definition to distinguish true hypersensitivities from other adverse reactions. Misuse of the term *hypersensitivity* is particularly apparent in cancer chemotherapy; the fact that allergists and clinical immunologists are often so little involved in the diagnosis and management of adverse reactions is to the detriment of patients, the disciplines of oncology and allergology, the interpretation of observed reactions, and perhaps even the integrity of some of the data from clinical trials.[3]

REFERENCES

1. Weiss RB, Baker JR Jr. Hypersensitivity reaction from antineoplastic agents. Cancer Metastasis Rev 1987;6(3):413–32.
2. Pagani M. The complex clinical picture of presumably allergic side effects to cytostatic drugs: symptoms, pathomechanism, reexposure, and desensitization. Med Clin North Am 2010;94(4):835–52.
3. Baldo BA, Pham NH. Adverse reactions to targeted and non-targeted chemotherapeutic drugs with emphasis on hypersensitivity responses and the invasive metastatic switch. Cancer Metastasis Rev 2013;32:723–61.
4. Ardavanis A, Tryfonopoulos D, Yiotis I, et al. Non-allergic nature of docetaxel-induced acute hypersensitivity reactions. Anticancer Drugs 2004;15(6):581–5.
5. National Cancer Institute NCI drug dictionary. Available at: www.cancer.gov/drugdictionary. Accessed September 30, 2013.
6. Baldo BA, Pham NH. Ch. 11 Biologics; Ch. 13 Drugs used for chemotherapy. In: Drug allergy: clinical aspects, diagnosis, mechanisms, structure-activity relationships. New York: Springer; 2013. p. 369–85, 399–418.
7. Baldo BA. Adverse events to monoclonal antibodies used for cancer therapy. Focus on hypersensitivity responses. Oncoimmunology 2013;2(10):e26333. http://dx.doi.org/10.4161/onci.26333.
8. Syrigou E, Syrigos K, Saif MW. Hypersensitivity reactions to oxaliplatin and other antineoplastic agents. Curr Allergy Asthma Rep 2008;8:56–62.
9. Zanotti KM, Markman M. Prevention and management of antineoplastic-induced hypersensitivity reactions. Drug Saf 2001;24:767–79.
10. Shepherd GM. Hypersensitivity reactions to chemotherapeutic drugs. Clin Rev Allergy Immunol 2003;24:253–62.
11. Gadducci A, Tana R, Teti G, et al. Analysis of the pattern of hypersensitivity reactions in patients receiving carboplatin retreatment for recurrent ovarian cancer. Int J Gynecol Cancer 2008;18:615–20.
12. Weiss RB. Hypersensitivity reactions. Semin Oncol 1992;19:458–77.
13. Grosen E, Siitari E, Larrison E, et al. Paclitaxel hypersensitivity reactions related to bee-sting allergy. Lancet 2000;355:288–9.
14. Markman M, Zanotti K, Kulp B, et al. Relationship between a history of systemic allergic reactions and risk of subsequent carboplatin hypersensitivity. Gynecol Oncol 2003;89:514–6.
15. Sendo T, Sakai N, Itoh Y, et al. Incidence and risk factors for paclitaxel hypersensitivity during ovarian cancer chemotherapy. Cancer Chemother Pharmacol 2005;56:91–6.
16. Schwartz JR, Bandera C, Bradley A, et al. Does the platinum-free interval predict the incidence or severity of hypersensitivity reactions to carboplatin? The experience from Women and Infants' Hospital. Gynecol Oncol 2007;105:81–3.

17. Mori Y, Nishimura T, Kitano T, et al. Oxaliplatin-free interval as a risk factor for hypersensitivity reaction among colorectal cancer patients treated with FOLFOX. Oncology 2010;79:136–43.

18. Joly F, Ray-Coquard I, Fabbro M, et al. Decreased hypersensitivity reactions with carboplatin-pegylated liposomal doxorubicin compared to carboplatin-paclitaxel combination: analysis from the GCIG CALYPSO relapsing ovarian cancer trial. Gynecol Oncol 2011;122(2):226–32.

19. Syrigou E, Dannos I, Kotteas E, et al. Hypersensitivity reactions to docetaxel: retrospective evaluation and development of a desensitization protocol. Int Arch Allergy Immunol 2011;156(3):320–4.

20. Piovano E, Pivetta E, Modaffari P, et al. A search for predictive factors for hypersensitivity reactions to paclitaxel and platinum salts in chemotherapy for gynecologic pelvic neoplasms. Gynecol Obstet Invest 2012;74(1):21–7.

21. Lee C, Gianos M, Klausermeyer WB. Diagnosis and management of hypersensitivity reactions related to common cancer chemotherapy agents. Ann Allergy Asthma Immunol 2009;102:179–87.

22. Demoly P, Bousquet J. Drug allergy diagnosis work up. Allergy 2002;57(Suppl 72):37–40.

23. Wang H, Diepgen TL. Is atopy a protective or a risk for cancer? A review of epidemiological studies. Allergy 2005;60:1098–111.

24. Herrero T, Tomero P, Infante S, et al. Diagnosis and management of hypersensitivity reactions caused by oxaliplatin. J Investig Allergol Clin Immunol 2006; 16:327–30.

25. Leguy-Seguin V, Jolimoy G, Coudert B, et al. Diagnosis and predictive value of skin testing in platinum salts hypersensitivity. J Allergy Clin Immunol 2007;119:726–30.

26. Pagani M, Bonadonna P, Senna GE, et al. Standardization of skin test for diagnosis and prevention of hypersensitivity reactions to oxaliplatin. Int Arch Allergy Immunol 2008;145:54–7.

27. Castells MC, Tennant NM, Sloane DE, et al. Hypersensitivity reactions to chemotherapy: outcomes and safety of rapid desensitization in 413 cases. J Allergy Clin Immunol 2008;122(3):574–80.

28. Garufi C, Cristaudo A, Vanni B, et al. Skin testing and hypersensitivity reactions to oxaliplatin. Ann Oncol 2003;14:497–502.

29. Meyer L, Zuberbier T, Worm M, et al. Hypersensitivity reactions to oxaliplatin: cross-reactivity to carboplatin and the introduction of a desensitization schedule. J Clin Oncol 2002;20:1146–7.

30. Goldberg A, Altaras MM, Mekori YA, et al. Anaphylaxis to cisplatin: diagnosis and value of pretreatment in prevention of recurrent allergic reactions. Ann Allergy 1994;73:271–2.

31. Lee CW, Matulonis UA, Castells MC. Rapid inpatient/outpatient desensitization for chemotherapy hypersensitivity: standard protocol effective in 55 patients for 255 courses. Gynecol Oncol 2005;99(2):393–9.

32. Madrigal-Burgaleta R, Berges-Gimeno MP, Angel-Pereira D, et al. Hypersensitivity and desensitization to antineoplastic agents: outcomes of 189 procedures with a new short protocol and novel diagnostic tools assessment. Allergy 2013; 68(7):853–61.

33. Pagani M, Venemalm L, Bonadonna P, et al. An experimental biological test to diagnose hypersensitivity reactions to carboplatin: new horizons for an old problem. Jpn J Clin Oncol 2012;42:347–50.

34. Weiss RB, Donehower RC, Wiernik PH, et al. Hypersensitivity reactions from. Taxol J Clin Oncol 1990;8(7):1263–8.

35. Popescu NA, Sheehan MG, Kouides PA, et al. Allergic reactions to cyclophosphamide: delayed clinical expression associated with positive immediate skin tests to drug metabolites in five patients. J Allergy Clin Immunol 1996;97:26–33.

36. Rosas-Vargas MA, Casas-Becerra B, Velázquez-Armenta Y, et al. Cyclophosphamide hypersensitivity in a leukemic child. Ther Drug Monit 2005;27:263–4.

37. Khan A, Hill JM. Atopic hypersensitivity to L-asparaginase: resistance to immunosuppression. Int Arch Allergy Appl Immunol 1971;40:463–9.

38. Giguere JK, Douglas DM, Lupton GP, et al. Procarbazine hypersensitivity manifested as a fixed drug eruption. Med Pediatr Oncol 1988;16:378–80.

39. de Souza P, Friedlander M, Wilde C, et al. Hypersensitivity reactions to etoposide. Am J Clin Oncol 1994;17:387–9.

40. Brockow K, Garvey LH, Aberer W, et al. Skin test concentrations for systemically administered drugs – an ENDA/EAACI Drug Allergy Interested Group position paper. Allergy 2013;68:702–12.

41. National Cancer Institute. Common Terminology Criteria for Adverse Events v4.03 (CTCAE). 2009. Available at: http://ctep.cancer.gov. Accessed October 30, 2013.

42. Dizon DS, Sabbatini PJ, Aghahanian C. Analysis of patients with epithelial ovarian cancer of fallopian tube carcinoma retreated with cisplatin after the development of a carboplatin allergy. Gynecol Oncol 2002;84:378–82.

43. Elligers KT, Davies M, Sanchis D, et al. Rechallenge with cisplatin in a patient with pancreatic cancer who developed a hypersensitivity reaction to oxaliplatin. Is skin test useful in this setting? JOP 2008;9:197–202.

44. Enrique E, Malek T, Castello JV, et al. Usefulness of skin testing with platinum salts to demonstrate lack of cross-reactivity between carboplatin and cisplatin. Ann Allergy Asthma Immunol 2008;100:86.

45. Lokich J, Anderson N. Paclitaxel hypersensitivity reactions: a role for docetaxel substitution. Ann Oncol 1998;9:573–4.

46. Moon C, Verschraegen CF, Bevers M, et al. Use of docetaxel (Taxotere) in patients with paclitaxel (Taxol) hypersensitivity. Anticancer Drugs 2000;11:565–8.

47. Dizon DS, Schwartz J, Rojan A, et al. Cross-sensitivity between paclitaxel and docetaxel in a women's cancer program. Gynecol Oncol 2006;100:149–51.

48. Sanchez-Munoz A, Jimenez B, Garcia-Tapiador A, et al. Cross-sensitivity between taxanes in patients with breast cancer. Clin Transl Oncol 2011;13:904–6.

49. Hak LJ, Relling MV, Cheng C, et al. Asparaginase pharmacodynamics differ by formulation among children with newly diagnosed acute lymphoblastic leukemia. Leukemia 2004;18:1072–7.

50. Silverman L, Gelber RD, Dalton VK, et al. Improved outcome for children with acute lymphoblastic leukemia: results of Dana-Farber consortium protocol 91-01. Blood 2001;97:1211–8.

51. Soyer OU, Aytac S, Tuncer A, et al. Alternative algorithm for L-asparaginase allergy in children with acute lymphoblastic leukemia. J Allergy Clin Immunol 2009;123:895–8.

52. Kintzel PE. Prophylaxis for paclitaxel hypersensitivity reactions. Ann Pharmacother 2001;35:1114–7.

53. Berger MJ, Dunlea LJ, Rettig AE, et al. Feasibility of stopping paclitaxel premedication after two doses in patients not experiencing previous infusion hypersensitivity reaction. Support Care Cancer 2012;20:1991–7.

54. Olson JK, Sood AK, Sorosky JI, et al. Taxol hypersensitivity: rapid retreatment is safe and cost effective. Gynecol Oncol 1998;68:25–8.
55. Markman M, Kennedy A, Webster K, et al. Paclitaxel-associated hypersensitivity reactions: experience of the gynaecologic oncology program of the Cleveland Clinic Cancer Center. J Clin Oncol 2000;18:102–5.
56. Stock W, Douer D, De Angelo DJ, et al. Prevention and management of asparaginase/pegasparaginase-associated toxicities in adults and older adolescents: recommendations of an expert panel. Leuk Lymphoma 2011;52:2237–53.
57. Brandi G, Pantaleo MA, Galli C, et al. Hypersensitivity reactions related to oxaliplatin (OHP). Br J Cancer 2003;89:477–81.
58. Maindrault-Goebel F, Andrè T, Turnigard C, et al. Allergic-type reactions to oxaliplatin: retrospective analysis of 42 patients. Eur J Cancer 2005;41:2262–7.
59. Polyzos A, Tsavaris N, Kosmos C, et al. Hypersensitivity reactions to oxaliplatin: cross-reactivity to carboplatin and the introduction of a desensitization schedule. Oncology 2001;61:129–33.
60. Markman M, Zanotti K, Peterson G, et al. Expanded experience with an intradermal skin test to predict for the presence or absence of carboplatin hypersensitivity. J Clin Oncol 2003;21:4611–4.
61. Pagani M, Bonadonna P. Skin test protocol for the prevention of hypersensitivity reactions to oxaliplatin. Anticancer Res 2014;34:537–40.
62. Limsuwan T, Castells MC. Outcomes and safety of rapid desensitization for chemotherapy hypersensitivity. Expert Opin Drug Saf 2010;9(1):39–53.
63. Scherer K, Brockow K, Aberer W, et al. Desensitization in delayed drug hypersensitivity reactions: an EAACI position paper of the Drug Allergy Interesting Group. Allergy 2013;68:844–52.
64. Cernadas JR, Brockow K, Romano A. General considerations on rapid desensitization for drug hypersensitivity – a consensus statement. Allergy 2010;65:1357–66.
65. Patil SU, Long AA, Ling M, et al. A protocol for risk stratification of patients with carboplatin-induced hypersensitivity reactions. J Allergy Clin Immunol 2012;129:443–7.
66. Levitski A, Klein S. Signal transduction therapy of cancer. Mol Aspects Med 2010;31(4):287–329.
67. Scott AM, Wolchok JD, Old LJ. Antibody therapy of cancer. Nat Rev Cancer 2012;12:278–87.
68. Turturro F. Denileukin diftitox: a biotherapeutic paradigm shift in the treatment of lymphoid- derived disorders. Expert Rev Anticancer Ther 2007;7(1):11–7.
69. Lockhart AC, Rothenberg ML, Dupont J, et al. Phase I study of intravenous vascular endothelial growth factor trap, aflibercept, in patients with advanced solid tumors. J Clin Oncol 2010;28(2):207–14.
70. Kisselev AF, van der Linden WA, Overkleeft HS. Proteasome inhibitors: an expanding army attacking a unique target. Chem Biol 2012;19(1):99–115.
71. Moreau P, Richardson PG, Cavo M, et al. Proteasome inhibitors in multiple myeloma: ten years later. Blood 2012;120:947–59.
72. Ward HW. Anti-oestrogen therapy for breast cancer: a trial of tamoxifen at two dose levels. Br Med J 1973;1(5844):13–4.
73. Gleevec. FDA: full prescribing information. Adverse reactions. Available at: http://www.accessdata.fda.gov/drugsatfda_docs/label/2012/021588s035lbl.pdf. Accessed October 1, 2013.
74. Kantarjian H, Sawyers C, Hochhaus A, et al. Hematologic and cytogenetic responses to imatinib mesylate in chronic myelogenous leukemia. N Engl J Med 2002;346(9):645–52.

75. Tarceva. FDA: full prescribing information. Adverse reactions. Available at: http://www.accessdata.fda.gov/drugsatfda_docs/label/2010/021743s14s16lbl.pdf. Accessed October 1, 2013.

76. Afinitor. FDA: full prescribing information. Adverse reactions. Available at: http://www.accessdata.fda.gov/drugsatfda_docs/label/2012/022334s016lbl.pdf. Accessed October 1, 2013.

77. Zolinza. FDA: full prescribing information. Adverse reactions. Available at: http://www.accessdata.fda.gov/drugsatfda_docs/label/2011/021991s002lbl.pdf. Accessed October 1, 2013.

78. Vesanoid. FDA: full prescribing information. Adverse reactions. Available at: http://www.accessdata.fda.gov/drugsatfda_docs/label/2004/20438s004lbl.pdf. Accessed October 1, 2013.

79. Targretin. FDA: full prescribing information. Adverse reactions. Available at: http://www.accessdata.fda.gov/drugsatfda_docs/label/2011/021055s006lbl.pdf. Accessed October 1, 2013.

80. Velcade. FDA: full prescribing information. Adverse reactions. Available at: http://www.accessdata.fda.gov/drugsatfda_docs/label/2012/021602s027lbl.pdf. Accessed October 1, 2013.

81. Arimidex. FDA: full prescribing information. Adverse reactions. Available at: http://www.accessdata.fda.gov/drugsatfda_docs/label/2011/020541s026lbl.pdf. Accessed October 1, 2013.

82. Zoladex. FDA: full prescribing information. Adverse reactions. Available at: http://www.accessdata.fda.gov/drugsatfda_docs/label/2011/019726s054,020578s032lbl.pdf. Accessed October 1, 2013.

83. Nolvadex. FDA: full prescribing information. Adverse reactions. Available at: http://www.accessdata.fda.gov/drugsatfda_docs/label/2005/17970s053lbl.pdf. Accessed October 1, 2013.

84. Casodex. FDA: full prescribing information. Adverse reactions. Available at: http://www.accessdata.fda.gov/drugsatfda_docs/label/2009/020498s019s021lbl.pdf. Accessed October 1, 2013.

85. Folotyn. FDA: full prescribing information. Adverse reactions. Available at: http://www.accessdata.fda.gov/drugsatfda_docs/label/2011/022468s003s004s005lbl.pdf. Accessed October 1, 2013.

86. Ontak. FDA: full prescribing information. Adverse reactions. Available at: http://www.accessdata.fda.gov/drugsatfda_docs/label/2008/103767s5094lbl.pdf. Accessed October 2, 2013.

87. Zaltrap. FDA: full prescribing information. Adverse reactions. Available at: http://www.accessdata.fda.gov/drugsatfda_docs/label/2012/125418s000lbl.pdf. Accessed October 2, 2013.

88. Thurston DE. Chemistry and pharmacology of anticancer drugs. Boca Raton (FL): CRC Press; 2007. p. 95–150.

89. Druker BJ. Translation of the Philadelphia chromosome into therapy for CML. Blood 2009;112:4808–17.

90. European Medicines Agency evaluation of medicines for human use. Assessment report for Removab. Proc. no. EMEA/H/C/000972, 2009. Available at: http://www.ema.europa.eu/docs/en_GB/document_library/EPAR_-_Public_assessment_report/human/000972/WC500051808.pdf. Accessed October 2, 2013.

91. Zevalin. FDA: full prescribing information. Adverse reactions. Available at: http://www.accessdata.fda.gov/drugsatfda_docs/label/2009/125019s0156.pdf. Accessed October 2, 2013.

92. Bexxar. FDA: full prescribing information. Adverse reactions. Available at: http://www.accessdata.fda.gov/drugsatfda_docs/label/2012/125011s102lbl.pdf. Accessed October 2, 2013.

93. Hansel TT, Kropshofer H, Singer T, et al. The safety and side effects of monoclonal antibodies. Nat Rev Drug Discov 2010;9:325–38.

94. Rituxan. FDA: Full prescribing information. Adverse reactions. Available at: http://www.accessdata.fda.gov/drugsatfda_docs/label/2012/103705s5367s5388lbl.pdf. Accessed October 2, 2013.

95. Arzerra. FDA: full prescribing information. Adverse reactions. Available at: http://www.accessdata.fda.gov/drugsatfda_docs/label/2009/125326lbl.pdf. Accessed October 2, 2013.

96. Adcetris. FDA: full prescribing information. Adverse reactions. Available at: http://www.accessdata.fda.gov/drugsatfda_docs/label/2012/125388s0005lbl.pdf. Accessed October 2, 2013.

97. Erbitux. FDA: full prescribing information. Adverse reactions. Available at: http://www.accessdata.fda.gov/drugsatfda_docs/label/2009/125084s168lbl.pdf. Accessed October 2, 2013.

98. Vectibix. FDA: full prescribing information. Adverse reactions. Available at: http://www.accessdata.fda.gov/drugsatfda_docs/label/2009/125147s080lbl.pdf. Accessed October 2, 2013.

99. Avastin. FDA: full prescribing information. Adverse reactions. Available at: http://www.accessdata.fda.gov/drugsatfda_docs/label/2012/125085s0238lbl.pdf. Accessed October 2, 2013.

100. Perjeta. FDA: full prescribing information. Adverse reactions. Available at: http://www.accessdata.fda.gov/drugsatfda_docs/label/2012/125409lbl.pdf. Accessed October 2, 2013.

101. Herceptin. FDA: full prescribing information. Adverse reactions. Available at: http://www.accessdata.fda.gov/drugsatfda_docs/label/2010/103792s5256lbl.pdf. Accessed October 2, 2013.

102. Kadcyla. FDA: full prescribing information. Adverse reactions. Available at: http://www.accessdata.fda.gov/drugsatfda_docs/label/2013/125427lbl.pdf. Accessed October 2, 2013.

103. Campath-1H. FDA: full prescribing information. Adverse reactions. Available at: http://www.accessdata.fda.gov/drugsatfda_docs/label/2007/103948s5070lbl.pdf. Accessed October 2, 2013.

104. Xgeva. FDA: full prescribing information. Adverse reactions. Available at: http://www.accessdata.fda.gov/drugsatfda_docs/label/2013/125320s094lbl.pdf. Accessed October 2, 2013.

105. Yervoy. FDA: full prescribing information. Adverse reactions. Available at: http://www.accessdata.fda.gov/drugsatfda_docs/label/2011/125377s0000lbl.pdf. Accessed October 2, 2013.

106. Dy GK, Adjei AA. Understanding, recognizing, and managing toxicities of targeted anticancer therapies. CA Cancer J Clin 2013;63:249–79.

107. Degan A, Alter M, Schenck F, et al. The hand-foot-syndrome associated with medical tumor therapy - classification and management. J Dtsch Dermatol Ges 2010;8(9):652–61.

108. Criscitiello C, Metzger-Filho O, Saini KS, et al. Targeted therapies in breast cancer: are heart and vessels also being targeted? Breast Cancer Res 2012;14:209.

109. Balagula Y, Lacouture ME, Cotliar JA. Dermatologic toxicities of targeted anticancer therapies. J Support Oncol 2010;8(4):149–61.

110. Polder K, Wang C, Duvic M, et al. Toxic epidermal necrolysis associated with denileukin diftitox (DAB389IL-2) administration in a patient with follicular large cell lymphoma. Leuk Lymphoma 2005;46(12):1807–11.
111. Coombs RR, Gell PG. Classification of allergic reactions responsible for clinical hypersensitivity and disease. In: Gell PG, Coombs RR, Lachmann PJ, editors. Clinical aspects of immunology. Oxford (United Kingdom): Blackwells; 1975. p. 761–81.
112. Ansari Z, George MK. Drug-induced immune-mediated thrombocytopenia secondary to sunitinib in a patient with metastatic renal cell carcinoma: a case report. J Med Case Rep 2013;7:54.
113. Barak AF, Bonstein L, Lauterbach R, et al. Tyrosine kinase inhibitors induced immune thrombocytopenia in chronic myeloid leukemia? Hematol Rep 2011;3:e29, 95–6.
114. Weber J. Review: anti-CTLA-4 antibody ipilimumab: case studies of clinical response and immune-related adverse events. Oncologist 2007;12:864–72.
115. Arnold DM, Santoso S, Greinacher A, on behalf of the Platelet Immunology Scientific Subcommittee of the ISTH. Recommendations for the implementation of platelet autoantibody testing in clinical trials of immune thrombocytopenia. J Thromb Haemost 2012;10(4):695–7.
116. Salama A, Schütz B, Kiefel V, et al. Immune-mediated agranulocytosis related to drugs and their metabolites: mode of sensitization and heterogeneity of antibodies. Br J Haematol 1989;72(2):127–32.
117. Giavina-Bianchi P, Caiado J, Picard M, et al. Rapid desensitization to chemotherapy and monoclonal antibodies is effective and safe. Allergy 2013;68: 1482–3.
118. Bar-Sela G, Kedem E, Hadad S, et al. Successful desensitization protocol for hypersensitivity reaction caused by sunitinib in a patient with a gastrointestinal stromal tumor. Jpn J Clin Oncol 2010;40(2):163–5.
119. Chou V, McClelland S, Resnick DJ, et al. Successful desensitization of an adult with type I hypersensitivity to imatinib. Internet J Asthma Allergy Immunol 2005; 4(2). http://dx.doi.org/10.5580/1a78.
120. Nelson RP Jr, Cornetta K, Ward KE, et al. Desensitization to imatinib in patients with leukemia. Ann Allergy Asthma Immunol 2006;97(2):216–22.
121. Jerath MR, Kwan M, Kannarkar M, et al. A desensitization protocol for the mAb cetuximab. J Allergy Clin Immunol 2009;123:260–2.
122. Hong DI, Bankova L, Cahill KN, et al. Allergy to monoclonal antibodies: cutting-edge desensitization methods for cutting-edge therapies. Expert Rev Clin Immunol 2012;8(1):43–52.
123. Brennan PJ, Rodriguez-Bouza T, Hsu FI, et al. Hypersensitivity reactions to mAbs: 105 desensitizations in 23 patients, from evaluation to treatment. J Allergy Clin Immunol 2009;124:1259–66.
124. Pàez-Ribes M, Allen E, Hudock J, et al. Antiangiogenic therapy elicits malignant progression of tumors to increased local invasion and distant metastasis. Cancer Cell 2009;15(3):220–31.

Vaccine Allergy

Jean-Christoph Caubet, MD[a],*, Claude Ponvert, MD, PhD[b]

KEYWORDS

- Vaccine allergy • Vaccine components • Toxoids • Hypersensitivity • Egg • Gelatin
- Children

KEY POINTS

- Overdiagnosis of vaccine allergy is common and is considered a major public health problem.
- Usually, no allergy test is required in patients developing local reactions after vaccine administration as they are not associated with a higher rate of systemic reactions.
- In patients with a history suggestive of an immediate IgE-mediated hypersensitivity, a complete allergic work is mandatory to confirm or exclude an allergy.
- Egg allergic patients can received safely the influenza vaccine with some precautions and skin test to the influenza vaccine is no longer recommended before.
- In almost all cases, the vaccines can be administered using adapted protocols, even if the allergy tests are positive.

INTRODUCTION

Adverse events after vaccine administration are commonly reported in the general population and constitute a common problem in clinical practice. The most frequent reactions after immunization are local reactions and nonimmediate skin eruptions (ie, delayed urticaria or maculopapular or nonspecific skin rashes), particularly after injection of vaccines containing toxoids[1–5] and hepatitis B virus (HBV) vaccine.[6–9] The literature data strongly suggest that most of these clinical manifestations do not result from a hypersensitivity reaction but, instead, from a nonspecific inflammation as reflected by the usual tolerance of booster doses.[10,11] In the study by Gold and colleagues,[11] only 10% of children reporting generalized allergic reactions developed a reaction on reexposure but most of these reactions were not suggestive of a hypersensitivity reaction. A correct management of these reactions is an essential

Disclosure: None.
[a] Department of Pediatrics, University Hospitals of Geneva and Medical School, University of Geneva, Geneva, Switzerland; [b] Pulmonology & Allergology Service, Department of Pediatrics, Sick Children's Hospital, Paris, France
* Corresponding author. Département de Pédiatrie, Hôpitaux Universitaires de Genève, 6 rue Willy-Donzé, Genève 14 CH-1211, Switzerland.
E-mail address: Jean-Christoph.Caubet@hucge.ch

Immunol Allergy Clin N Am 34 (2014) 597–613
http://dx.doi.org/10.1016/j.iac.2014.04.004   immunology.theclinics.com
0889-8561/14/$ – see front matter © 2014 Elsevier Inc. All rights reserved.

component of health care because they are clearly associated with a decreased vaccination rate in the general population. Indeed, most of these patients are falsely labeled as allergic, with a major impact on health, both individual and public. In addition, the economic impact is very important.

True allergic reactions to vaccines are rare but their identification is important because they can be life-threatening. Rarely, the vaccine itself is responsible for immediate hypersensitivity reactions, especially vaccines containing toxoids[2,12–14] and pneumococcal antigens.[15,16] In addition to microbial components, residual components of the culture medium, as well as preservatives, stabilizers, and adjuvants added to vaccines, may elicit hypersensitivity reactions in susceptible individuals. Particularly, gelatin used as a stabilizer in many vaccines has been incriminated in allergic reactions to vaccine.[17–22] Several recent studies led to a major change in paradigm. They showed that most patients with egg allergy, even those with severe egg allergy, can safely receive influenza vaccine under certain conditions.[23,24] Finally, local and generalized nonimmediate reactions can result from hypersensitivity to the excipient,[25–27] adjuvant,[28–31] stabilizer,[19,32–34] and microbial component itself.[35]

This article discusses the different types of allergic reactions after immunization based on the timing (immediate vs nonimmediate) and the extent of the reaction (local vs systemic). The different vaccine components potentially responsible for an allergic reaction are discussed, as well as the management of patients with a history of reaction to a specific vaccine and those with a history of allergy to one of the vaccine components.

LOCAL REACTIONS TO VACCINES

Local reactions are the most frequent adverse event after immunization and have an important impact in clinical practice. Indeed, these reactions are often associated with major discomfort, particularly pain, and patients are often falsely labeled as allergic.

Different Types of Local Reactions and Pathomechanisms

Based on the clinical aspect and the timing of reaction, different types of local reactions can be distinguished:

- Mild local reactions are the most frequent type of local reaction after vaccine administration and are benign. These mild local reactions result from a nonspecific inflammation due to the injection itself as well as injection of foreign material.
- Large local reactions are less common and are characterized by pain, swelling, and redness at the injection site, usually occurring within 24 to 72 hours after vaccine administration and regressing typically in 2 to 3 days.[36–42] Important local inflammatory reactions are particularly encountered after injection of vaccines containing toxoids but can occur after administration of other vaccines, particularly HBV, pneumococcal, and *Hemophilus influenzae* vaccines.[6–8,43,44] These reactions may represent an Arthus reaction (ie, important local inflammatory reaction) in patients with preexisting IgG antibodies from earlier immunizations.[3,45,46] Of note, although receiving multiple doses of vaccine has been identified as a risk factor, shorter interval between the doses was not associated with higher rates of Arthus reactions.[47,48] Nevertheless, these typical large local reactions can occur at the first vaccine injection or during booster doses made with batches of vaccines containing high concentrations of toxoids or aluminium hydroxide, independent of the concentrations of serum antibodies to tetanus, diphtheria, or *Bordetella pertussis*.[41,42] The relationship between the content of toxoids or aluminium hydroxide in the vaccine and the frequency of local

inflammatory reactions is inconstant. A recent study showed that the frequency of large local reactions to Diphtheria-Tetanus (DT) vaccines was significantly increased in mice preimmunized with combined vaccines containing vaccine acellular pertussis; however, the pathomechanisms explaining this adjuvant effect is far from clear.[49] Based on these data, it is likely that most of these accelerated large local reactions result from a nonspecific inflammation induced by a variety of factors, including a high content of aluminium hydroxide and/or substances of microbial origin. In most cases, boosters injected sequentially with monovalent vaccines containing limited number of vaccine antigens are well tolerated.[11,13,50]

- Extensive limb swelling is less common but may be impressive for the patients. It looks like a benign edema (ie, swelling and mild redness) and is usually painless. It probably results from extravasation mechanisms still poorly understood.[51–53] By definition, these reactions extend at least to the elbow or knee.

- Subcutaneous nodules have been described in up to 19% of patients receiving vaccines containing aluminium hydroxide.[28,54–58] Although these lesions usually regress spontaneously within a few weeks, few cases of persistent nodules have been reported.[54,56–58] Patch tests with aluminium salts are often negative. Most of these reactions result from a nonspecific foreign body inflammation as demonstrated by a significant positive correlation between the concentration of aluminium hydroxide and the frequency and size of nodules.[58,59] However, Bergfors and colleagues[57] found that most subjects who developed persistent nodules had positive patch tests to aluminium.[60] Finally, the positivity of delayed-reading intradermal tests to tetanus toxoid suggested a nonimmediate hypersensitivity to toxoids in children developing sterile abscesses.[35] However, a relatively high number of positive responses in skin tests to toxoids were also observed in control subjects.[45,61–63]

- Local eczema lesions have been mainly reported in adults immunized with vaccines containing aluminium hydroxide,[29–31] thimerosal,[26,64] and formaldehyde.[27] A nonimmediate hypersensitivity has been suggested by positive patch tests to these components.[28–30,64–66] Of note, generalized eczema has also been reported after vaccine administration.[67,68]

- Nevi associated with hypertrichosis are rarely reported after administration of various vaccines (eg, bacille Calmette-Guérin [BCG], tetanus, and smallpox), as well as after allergenic extracts used for desensitization.[69–71] The causal components responsible for the reaction, as well as the exact pathomechanisms of such reaction, remain unknown.

Diagnosis and Management of Local Reactions After Vaccine Administration

Management of patients with history of local reaction after vaccine injection is described in **Fig. 1**. Usually, no allergy test is required in patients developing local reactions after vaccine administration because they are not associated with a higher rate of systemic reactions on reexposure. However, measurements of serum vaccine-specific antibodies (IgM or IgG) are indicated in patients with suspicion of Arthus reaction.[24] Indeed, levels of antibodies associated with protection from vaccine-preventable disease has been proposed.[24] If patients reach the established level associated with protection from disease, consideration can be given to withholding additional doses, although the induced immunity might be lower than if all doses were injected.[24] From another point of view, positive late responses to intradermal tests have been reported in adult subjects who developed an Arthus reaction after receiving a booster dose of DT vaccine[45] but these results were not found in

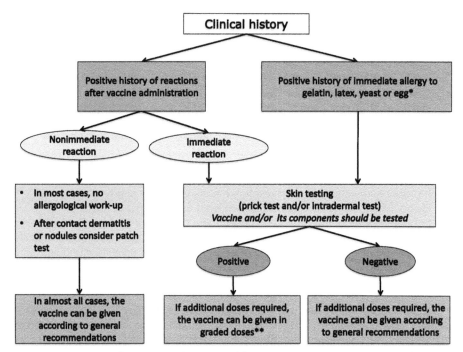

Fig. 1. Management of patients with suspected hypersensitivity to a vaccine and of patients with known allergy to a vaccine component. * for egg allergic patients, see text; ** Ref[110] (*Form* Caubet JC, Rudzeviciene O, Gomes E, et al. Managing a child with a possible allergy to vaccine. Pediatr Allergy Immunol 2013 http://dx.doi.org/10.1111/pai.12132. [Epub ahead of print]; with permission.)

children.[13] In patients reporting important local inflammatory reactions after injection of combined vaccines, sequential injections of single or limited numbers of vaccinating agents, every few days, preferably intramuscularly, are usually well tolerated.[72,73]

In patients developing eczema or persistent nodules after vaccine administration, patch tests may be useful to demonstrate a delayed hypersensitivity to preservatives or adjuvants and to guide the physician to avoid vaccine and other products containing these incriminated components. However, a positive patch test is not accurate for the purpose of assessing a patient's ability to tolerate a vaccine and is not a contraindication to administer the vaccine following a risk-benefit analysis.[74]

Prevention

The risks of developing a local reaction after immunization are not well defined. However, decreasing the frequency of local reactions would clearly improve the vaccination rate in the general population. Recently, it was demonstrated that reactogenicity is reduced by using a correct needle length because a longer needle is associated with a lower rate of local reactions.[72,73] Similarly, the site of injection may influence the development of local reactions. Injection in the thigh in children less than 3 years is associated with fewer local reactions, which supports current recommendations.[75] On the other hand, patients with known sensitization to one of the vaccine components should receive a vaccine free of this component, if available. All these preventive measures will help improve the vaccination cover of the population.

SYSTEMIC REACTIONS TO VACCINES

Systemic reactions are far less common, with an estimated incidence between one and three reactions per million vaccine doses.[76,77] However, identification of these reactions is of major importance because they carry the risk of life-threatening anaphylaxis if the patient is exposed again.

Different Types of Systemic Reactions and Pathomechanisms

Different types of systemic reactions can be discerned, mostly based on the clinical characteristics and the timing of the reaction:

- Delayed urticaria and/or angioedema, or maculopapular or other nonspecific rashes, occurring a few hours after vaccine administration, are relatively common. The pathomechanisms of these reactions is not fully understood; however, a nonspecific activation of the immune system as well as a nonspecific degranulation of mastocytes has been proposed.[65]
- Immediate reactions usually occur within 1 hour after immunization and manifest as various combinations of IgE-mediated symptoms, mainly urticaria and/or angioedema, rhinitis, or wheezing and/or hypotension.
- Rarely, other serious reactions have been linked with some vaccines, including Guillain-Barré syndrome with swine flu influenza vaccine, transient rash with measles vaccine, and encephalopathy with *B pertussis* vaccine. These reactions are not discussed in this article.[24]

Patients with a History of Systemic Reaction to Vaccine

The main cause of consultation with an allergist regarding vaccine allergy is an adverse event following vaccine administration,[78] including systemic immediate or nonimmediate hypersensitivity reactions.

Systemic reactions due to hypersensitivity to microbial components

Rarely, hypersensitivity to a microbial component itself has been incriminated in patients who develop systemic allergic reactions after immunization. Although the most well known example is hypersensitivity to tetanus and diphtheria toxoids, specific hypersensitivity to other microbial components, such as pneumococcal or *B pertussis* antigens, has been described, mostly in single-case reports.

Hypersensitivity to toxoids Delayed urticaria and/or angioedema, as well as nonspecific skin rashes, have been reported in 5% to 13% of patients receiving vaccines containing toxoids.[3,5] Several studies, including skin tests (both immediate- and delayed-reading) and measurement of specific antibodies (IgE, IgM, IgG), suggest that most of these generalized reactions result from a nonspecific activation of the immune system by a significant amount of microbial substances and will not relapse on reexposure to the same vaccine.[11–13]

Although rare, real anaphylactic reactions to vaccines containing toxoids have been reported. Since the introduction of highly purified toxoids, the incidence of those reactions has decreased, ranging from 0 to 1 per 10,000.[79–85] Ponvert and colleagues[13] reported four subjects with positive skin tests to toxoids (one to diphtheria and three to tetanus toxoids) among six children with a history of severe anaphylactic reactions to vaccines containing toxoids. In addition, an immediate hypersensitivity to tetanus and diphtheria toxoids has been suggested by positive skin tests and/or specific IgE in six patients who developed an immediate urticaria. These results confirmed results from other investigators based on single-case reports.[2,3,13,14,79,86] However, Jacobs and colleagues[3] reported on 95 adults with history of anaphylactoid reactions occurring within 2 hours after immunization. Only one subject had a positive immediate skin test to tetanus toxoid and tolerated the challenge without reaction. These discrepancies are probably explained by differences in subject selection, based on positive clinical history. On the other hand, false-positive specific IgE to these toxoids have been reported in many patients tolerating injections of vaccines containing tetanus toxoids (higher levels found in atopic subjects).[86–89]

Hypersensitivity to _B pertussis_ antigen Urticaria and/or angioedema, as well as anaphylactic reactions after immunization, have been attributed to specific hypersensitivity to _B pertussis_ antigen.[90,91] However, most of these studies did not include an allergic workup. Up to 65% of children immunized with _B pertussis_ vaccines produce specific IgE to the microbial antigen, particularly atopic children immunized with acellular vaccines.[91–94] The concentrations of specific IgE to _B pertussis_ are positively correlated with IgG responses and primarily reflect the immunogenicity of _B pertussis_ antigens, instead of the allergenicity. In fact, no correlation has been demonstrated between IgE levels and the number of adverse reactions to vaccines, with the exception of inflammatory local reactions.[91] In animal experiments, the antigens of _B pertussis_ have been shown to be potent adjuvants for IgE responses to unrelated antigens.[95,96] However, in humans, simultaneous administration of _B pertussis_ vaccine and DT vaccine tends to inhibit IgE responses to toxoids.[88] The frequency of allergic reactions has been shown to be similar in subjects vaccinated with DT and DT combined with _B pertussis_ (DTaP).

Hypersensitivity to pneumococcal antigens Except relatively frequent mild-to-moderate local reactions, pneumococcal vaccines are generally well tolerated. In the literature, most case reports of anaphylactic reactions to pneumococcal vaccine do not include an allergic workup.[43] However, immediate responses to skin tests and specific IgE were positive in two children reporting a severe anaphylactic reaction after injection of a pneumococcal vaccine.[15,16] Of note, skin tests and specific IgE were negative with the vaccine solvent (phenol) and the vaccine itself in 10 and 9 controls, respectively. Only one negative control (unvaccinated) had a positive skin test to the vaccine, suggesting a sensitization to _Streptococcus_, either through portage or unknown infection. These results support the good diagnostic value of these tests in patients with positive history of allergic reaction to pneumococcal vaccines.

Systemic reactions due to hypersensitivity to other vaccine components
In addition to microbial components, residual components of the culture medium, as well as preservatives, stabilizers, and adjuvants added to vaccines, may be responsible for allergic reactions to vaccines.

Gelatin and egg Gelatin and egg are among the most frequently incriminated components in hypersensitivity to vaccine. Although reactions to vaccine administration can be the revealing factor of an allergy to these components, the clinician is more often confronted with patients with a known allergy to these components who need to receive a vaccine containing these (see later discussion).

Yeast HBV and human papilloma virus (HPV) vaccines may contain traces of yeast proteins derived from cell cultures,[97] with a potential risk of allergic reactions in patients sensitized to yeast. However, anaphylactic reactions to these vaccines are rare and after-marketing surveillance data suggest that recombinant yeast-derived HBV and HPV vaccines pose minimal risk of allergic reaction in yeast-sensitized individuals.[98,99] Sensitization to *Saccharomyces cerevisiae*, shown by positive skin tests and specific IgE, has been found in a patient with a history of allergy to hepatitis B vaccine.[100] Although the diagnostic value of these tests is not well defined, international guidelines recommend performing skin tests with yeasts in the rare patients reporting reactions to yeast-containing vaccines.[24]

Dextran Dextran hypersensitivity is rare and has been mainly implicated in allergic reactions to particular brands of measles-mumps-rubella (MMR) vaccine and BCG, both no longer available on the market.[101–103] However, dextran is found sporadically in other vaccines, such as some rotavirus vaccines. These allergic reactions were related to the presence of IgG antibodies to dextran and the mechanism was hypothesized to be complement activation and anaphylatoxin release.[101–103] In newborns, these antibodies are believed to derive from a placental transfer from the mother. In older children and adults, the origin of these antibodies remains obscure and may result from a previous sensitization by sugars expressed on infectious microorganisms or saprophytes. These could explain the presence of specific antibodies (IgM or IgG) to dextran found in 70% to 80% of the patients in the general population.[104] Nonimmediate reactions to dextran are rarely reported in the literature.[65]

Preservatives and adjuvants Preservatives are added to a large variety of vaccines and can be responsible for allergic reactions. Although thimerosal is one of the most effective preservatives, it has been used less often during the last few years because of its mercury content.[105] On the other hand, phenoxyethanol and formaldehyde have been increasingly used. As shown by several single-case reports, these preservatives might trigger allergic, mainly nonimmediate, reactions (contact dermatitis and generalized maculopapular rash).[27,67,106,107] Some vaccines require an adjuvant, such as aluminium, to become immunogenic. In addition to local reactions discussed above, patients sensitized to aluminium can rarely develop generalized contact dermatitis after vaccine administration.[29]

Antibiotics MMR, polio, and influenza vaccines are likely to contain small amounts of antibiotics, including neomycin, gentamicin, polymyxin B, and streptomycin. These are used to avoid contamination of the culture with bacteria or fungus. Although not confirmed by a complete allergic workup, an antibiotic allergy has been incriminated as a potential cause of nonimmediate reactions, such as contact dermatitis, and of immediate reactions (more rare) to a vaccine.[108,109] The rare patients with a confirmed immediate allergy to these antibiotics should avoid a vaccine containing them,[97] whereas most patients who develop a nonimmediate reaction can receive the vaccine with a low risk of mild reaction outweighed by the benefit of the vaccination.[97,109]

General management of patients with a history of systemic reaction to vaccine

Systematic approaches have been proposed for the management of patients with a suspicion of vaccine allergy (see **Fig. 1**). Although essential, the clinical history is not sufficient and a complete allergic workup is required in all patients with a suspicion of vaccine allergy, even if no further dose of the suspected vaccine is needed because of the potential for cross-reaction with common components in other vaccines or foods.[24,74] Allergy tests will be adapted, depending whether an immediate or a nonimmediate reaction is suspected. In patients with a suspicion of immediate hypersensitivity, the workup should include immediate-reading skin tests (prick tests full dose, or 1/10 in case of severe anaphylactic reaction) as well as intradermal tests (1/100) and/or specific IgE to the vaccine itself and the related vaccines (i.e. DTaP, DT, T and Polio vaccine in suspected allergy to DTaP-Polio vaccine), but also to the potential single components that may have cause the reaction (egg, gelatin, yeast, formalde-hyde and latex). In the decision to administer a vaccine, the ratio between risk and therapeutic benefit should be assessed. The physician should determine whether subsequent doses of the suspected vaccine, or other vaccines with similar components, are required. Measurement of vaccines antibodies to determine whether they are at protective levels can help determine whether booster injection can be withheld. The discussion should always involve the primary care physician, the allergist, and the patient and/or family. If the allergic workup confirms a hypersensitivity to one of the vaccine components, the vaccine can still be administered following the protocol proposed by the American Academy of Pediatrics.[110] Of note, monovalent vaccine should be preferred.[111] Regarding patient reporting generalized nonimmediate reaction, the diagnostic value of skin tests, particularly delayed-reading intradermal tests, remains highly uncertain.

Patients with History of Allergy to Vaccine Components

The other circumstance that often brings a patients to the allergist regarding vaccine allergy is that a patient needs a vaccine but has a positive history of allergy to one or several vaccine components.[78]

Patients allergic to eggs

Owing to manufacturing process, MMR vaccines, as well as influenza, yellow fever, and tick-borne encephalitis vaccines, may contain various amounts of ovalbumin and are, therefore, associated with a potential risk of anaphylactic reactions in patients who are allergic to egg.[112–116] Since the 1990s, the production methods of MMR and influenza vaccines have been modified. MMR vaccines are prepared on fibroblasts from chicken embryo and, therefore, contain no to trace ovalbumin (0–1 ng/mL). Several studies have confirmed the safety of this vaccine in patients allergic to egg.[115,117] In consequence, skin tests are not required and these patients can receive full-dose MMR regardless of the nature and severity of their allergy.[24,65,97]

The administration of influenza vaccine in patients allergic to egg has been a major concern for a long time. However, a major change of paradigm recently occurred.[118–127] Several studies have assessed the safety of influenza vaccine in these patients, including patients with severe egg allergy. More than 4800 subjects have been evaluated, including nearly 600 subjects with severe egg allergy.[23,24] Although some subjects developed mild cutaneous reaction (ie, generalized urticaria), no anaphylactic reaction has been reported in these studies. Also, it has been shown that skin tests with influenza vaccines may provide false-positive responses and that the risk of reaction was similar in subjects with positive skin tests compared with subjects who tested negative.[118,119,124] Based on these data, the current consensus indicates that skin testing to influenza vaccine is useless in egg allergic patients.[23,24] Recently, the ovalbumin content of currently used influenza vaccines was evaluated in several studies and three categories can be distinguished:

- Influenza vaccine obtained by genetic engineering do not contain ovalbumin, so they can be administered safely in patients allergic to egg.
- Influenza vaccines produced on chicken egg embryo contain very small amounts of ovalbumin (less than 1 μg/0.5 mL), even if the manufacturers often mention higher content. These vaccines can be administered full dose with some precaution (in the primary care office for patients with mild egg allergy [urticaria] and in the allergist office for patients with more severe egg allergy).[23,24] However, some investigators recommend administering the vaccine in two doses in patients with more severe egg allergy (1/10, then 9/10 30 minutes later).[65,111] In this case, if the

patient reacts to the first dose, the risk-benefit ratio should be evaluated. If the vaccine is absolutely required, it can be administered in graded dose.[110]

- Other influenza vaccines containing significant amounts of ovalbumin (>1.2 μg/mL) are potentially associated with a risk of reaction in patients allergic to egg[128,129]; therefore, administration of these vaccines in these patients should be avoided.

Regarding other vaccines containing egg proteins, such as yellow fever vaccines, unfortunately only a few studies have assessed their safety in patients allergic to egg. Skin tests to the vaccine before administration are recommended.[24] A recent study proposed a desensitization protocol in patients with positive skin tests.[130] However, a safe administration of influenza vaccine with an ovalbumin content much higher than yellow fever vaccine has been recently reported in patients allergic to egg.[131] Further studies are needed to evaluate the safety of yellow fever vaccine in these patients, particularly to determine the usefulness of skin tests and the optimal protocol to administer the vaccine (comparison of graded dose with full dose administration).

Patients allergic to gelatin

Anaphylactic reactions have been reported in patients without egg allergy after injection of vaccines containing gelatin used as a stabilizer, including MMR, Japanese encephalitis, and chickenpox vaccines.[17–22,132,133] Recently, gelatin hypersensitivity has been incriminated in a child allergic to egg who developed an anaphylactic reaction after receiving an influenza vaccine.[134] In these patients, the diagnosis of allergy to gelatin was based on positive skin test and/or specific IgE to gelatin. A history more or less suggestive of food allergy to gelatin was subsequently found in several of these patients. On the other hand, a study showed that food allergy to gelatin developed secondarily to vaccine administration in 20% to 25% of subjects.[20,21] Of note, a negative history of reaction to gelatin on ingestion should not exclude a hypersensitivity to gelatin.[20,135] Since gelatin was removed from several vaccines and hydrolyzed gelatin was used in others, anaphylactic reactions to vaccines have decreased significantly.[136–138] In patients with suspicion of hypersensitivity to gelatin, the first step is to confirm the allergy by a complete allergic workup, including skin tests and/or specific IgE to gelatin. In patients with a confirmed gelatin allergy, a gelatin-free vaccine should be preferred. If unavailable, the risk-benefit ratio to administer the vaccine should be discussed. If the vaccine is required, a skin test with the vaccine itself should be performed before vaccine administration. Patients with negative skin tests can receive the vaccine full dose, whereas patients with positive skin tests should receive the vaccine following the protocol proposed by the American Academy of Pediatrics.[110]

Of note, nonimmediate urticaria and/or angioedema, as well as nonspecific rashes have also been reported after injection of vaccine containing gelatin.[32] Some of these reactions may result from a nonimmediate hypersensitivity to gelatin, as suggested by high levels of serum specific IgG gelatin found in many of those subjects.[33] Another study showed that most subjects reporting nonimmediate reactions to vaccines containing gelatin had positive delayed-reading responses to an intradermal test and/or lymphocyte transformation test (LTT), supporting the hypothesis that these reactions may also result from an hypersensitivity to gelatin.[34] However, other studies have shown that LTT gelatin were positive in many subjects tolerating vaccine containing gelatin.[139]

Patients allergic to milk

DT vaccines are prepared on milk proteins and may contain nanoscale quantities of milk proteins. A recent case series incriminated casein in allergic reaction to DT vaccines in subjects with severe milk allergy and high levels of specific IgE to cow's milk.[140] Similarly, allergy to cow's milk has been incriminated in an allergic reaction to Sabin vaccine.[141] However, these data must be confirmed by further study.

Patients allergic to antibiotics
To the authors' knowledge, there is no case report of immediate allergic reactions to vaccine attributed to antibiotic. However, regarding the rare patient with a confirmed immediate allergic reaction to antibiotics added to vaccine (ie, neomycin, gentamicin, polymyxin B, and streptomycin), it is recommended to avoid vaccines containing them. If the vaccine is really needed, skin tests with the vaccine itself and the antibiotics (if validated) are recommended. If the skin tests are negative, the vaccine can be administered full dose. If antibiotic hypersensitivity is confirmed (skin or provocation tests) or highly likely, based on clinical history, a graded protocol should be used to administer the vaccine.

General management of patients with an allergy to vaccine components
In patients with a suspected allergy to vaccine components, the first step is to confirm this allergy by skin tests, specific IgE measurement, and/or a provocation test, which is considered the gold standard. If an allergy is confirmed, skin tests with the vaccine itself are recommended. If negative, the vaccine can be administered full dose, whereas if the skin test is positive, the vaccine should be administered in graded dose following the protocol proposed by the American Academy of Pediatrics.[110] The decision to administer the vaccine should be based on risk-benefit assessment and should be discussed between the primary care physician, the allergist, and the patient and/or family. Usually, measurements of vaccine antibodies to determine if the patient already reaches the protective antibodies levels are needed before making this decision. As mentioned above, patients with egg allergy can be managed differently. Skin tests with the vaccine itself and graded-dose administration are no longer recommended.[23,24,111] However, the vaccine should be administered with some precautions (ie, in the primary care office in patients with mild egg allergy and in the allergist office or in the hospital in patients with severe egg allergy). Of note, skin test to the influenza vaccine is still recommended in patients who reacted after influenza vaccine administration.

SUMMARY

Overdiagnosis of vaccine allergy is common and is considered a major public health problem. The diagnosis of allergy to vaccine is complex and is often retained owing to fear of severe anaphylactic reactions. However, most patients labeled as allergic to a vaccine tolerate a subsequent injection of the vaccine without clinical reaction. This is particularly the case in patients who develop local reactions or delayed benign skin rashes. Regarding patients with a history suggestive of an immediate IgE-mediated hypersensitivity, a complete workup is mandatory. It should be primarily based on skin tests and/or specific IgE measurements. In almost all cases, the vaccines can be administered using adapted protocols, even if the allergy tests are positive. However, some vaccine administrations carry a relatively high risk of severe anaphylactic reactions and should always be performed by well-trained physicians and emergency equipment must be readily available.

REFERENCES

1. Bernstein DI, Smith VE, Schiff GM, et al. Comparison of acellular pertussis vaccine with whole cell vaccine as a booster in children 15 to 18 months and 4 to 6 years of age. Pediatr Infect Dis J 1993;12:131–5.

2. Carey AB, Meltzer EO. Diagnosis and "desensitization" in tetanus vaccine hypersensitivity. Ann Allergy 1992;69:336–8.
3. Jacobs RL, Lowe RS, Lanier BQ. Adverse reactions to tetanus toxoid. JAMA 1982;247:40–2.
4. Long SS, Deforest A, Smith DG, et al. Longitudinal study of adverse reactions following diphtheria-tetanus-pertussis vaccine in infancy. Pediatrics 1990;85: 294–302.
5. Mortimer EA, Sorensen RU. Urticaria following administration of diphtheria-tetanus toxoids-pertussis vaccine. Pediatr Infect Dis J 1987;6:876–7.
6. Andre FE. Overview of a 5-year clinical experience with a yeast-derived hepatitis B vaccine. Vaccine 1990;8(Suppl):S74–8 [discussion: S79–80].
7. Dienstag JL, Werner BG, Polk BF, et al. Hepatitis B vaccine in health care personnel: safety, immunogenicity, and indicators of efficacy. Ann Intern Med 1984;101:34–40.
8. McMahon BJ, Helminiak C, Wainwright RB, et al. Frequency of adverse reactions to hepatitis B vaccine in 43,618 persons. Am J Med 1992;92:254–6.
9. Szmuness W, Stevens CE, Harley EJ, et al. Hepatitis B vaccine: demonstration of efficacy in a controlled clinical trial in a high-risk population in the United States. N Engl J Med 1980;303:833–41.
10. Andrews RM, Kempe AE, Sinn KK, et al. Vaccinating children with a history of serious reactions after vaccination or of egg allergy. Med J Aust 1998;168: 491–4.
11. Gold M, Goodwin H, Botham S, et al. Re-vaccination of 421 children with a past history of an adverse vaccine reaction in a special immunisation service. Arch Dis Child 2000;83:128–31.
12. Piletta PA, Pasche-Koo F, Saurat JH, et al. Immediate local reaction to tetanus toxoid booster. Allergy 1997;52:676–7.
13. Ponvert CS, Scheinmann P, Karila C, et al. Une étude de 30 cas fondée sur les tests cutanés à lecture immédiate, semi-retardée et retardée, sur les dosages des anticorps spécifiques et sur les injections de rappel. Revue française d'allergologie et d'immunologie clinique 2001;41:701–11.
14. Skov PS, Pelck I, Ebbesen F, et al. Hypersensitivity to the diphtheria component in the Di-Te-Pol vaccine. A type I allergic reaction demonstrated by basophil histamine release. Pediatr Allergy Immunol 1997;8:156–8.
15. Ponvert C, Ardelean-Jaby D, Colin-Gorski AM, et al. Anaphylaxis to the 23-valent pneumococcal vaccine in child: a case-control study based on immediate responses in skin tests and specific IgE determination. Vaccine 2001;19: 4588–91.
16. Ponvert C, Scheinmann P, de Blic J. Anaphylaxis to the 23-valent pneumococcal vaccine: a second explored case by means of immediate-reading skin tests with pneumococcal vaccines. Vaccine 2010;28:8256–7.
17. Sakaguchi M, Yamanaka T, Ikeda K, et al. IgE-mediated systemic reactions to gelatin included in the varicella vaccine. J Allergy Clin Immunol 1997;99: 263–4.
18. Kelso JM, Jones RT, Yunginger JW. Anaphylaxis to measles, mumps, and rubella vaccine mediated by IgE to gelatin. J Allergy Clin Immunol 1993;91: 867–72.
19. Kumagai T, Yamanaka T, Wataya Y, et al. Gelatin-specific humoral and cellular immune responses in children with immediate- and nonimmediate-type reactions to live measles, mumps, rubella, and varicella vaccines. J Allergy Clin Immunol 1997;100:130–4.

20. Sakaguchi M, Nakayama T, Inouye S. Food allergy to gelatin in children with systemic immediate-type reactions, including anaphylaxis, to vaccines. J Allergy Clin Immunol 1996;98:1058–61.
21. Sakaguchi M, Yoshida M, Kuroda W, et al. Systemic immediate-type reactions to gelatin included in Japanese encephalitis vaccines. Vaccine 1997;15:121–2.
22. Singer S, Johnson CE, Mohr R, et al. Urticaria following varicella vaccine associated with gelatin allergy. Vaccine 1999;17:327–9.
23. Kelso JM, Greenhawt MJ, Li JT. Update on influenza vaccination of egg allergic patients. Ann Allergy Asthma Immunol 2013;111:301–2.
24. Kelso JM, Greenhawt MJ, Li JT, et al. Adverse reactions to vaccines practice parameter 2012 update. J Allergy Clin Immunol 2012;130:25–43.
25. Noel I, Galloway A, Ive FA. Hypersensitivity to thiomersal in hepatitis B vaccine. Lancet 1991;338:705.
26. Rietschel RL, Adams RM. Reactions to thimerosal in hepatitis B vaccines. Dermatol Clin 1990;8:161–4.
27. Ring J. Exacerbation of eczema by formalin-containing hepatitis B vaccine in formaldehyde-allergic patient. Lancet 1986;2:522–3.
28. Bohler-Sommeregger K, Lindemayr H. Contact sensitivity to aluminium. Contact Derm 1986;15:278–81.
29. Cox NH, Moss C, Forsyth A. Allergy to non-toxoid constituents of vaccines and implications for patch testing. Contact Dermatitis 1988;18:143–6.
30. Cox NH, Moss C, Forsyth A. Cutaneous reactions to aluminium in vaccines: an avoidable problem. Lancet 1988;2:43.
31. Fisher AA. Reactions to aluminium and its salts. Cutis 1984;33:154, 159.
32. Sakaguchi M, Miyazawa H, Inouye S. Sensitization to gelatin in children with systemic non-immediate-type reactions to varicella vaccines. Ann Allergy Asthma Immunol 2000;84:341–4.
33. Sakaguchi M, Miyazawa H, Inouye S. Specific IgE and IgG to gelatin in children with systemic cutaneous reactions to Japanese encephalitis vaccines. Allergy 2001;56:536–9.
34. Taniguchi K, Fujisawa T, Ihara T, et al. Gelatin-induced T-cell activation in children with nonanaphylactic-type reactions to vaccines containing gelatin. J Allergy Clin Immunol 1998;102:1028–32.
35. Church JA, Richards W. Recurrent abscess formation following DTP immunizations: association with hypersensitivity to tetanus toxoid. Pediatrics 1985;75:899–900.
36. Pichichero ME, Casey JR. Acellular pertussis vaccines for adolescents. Pediatr Infect Dis J 2005;24:S117–26.
37. Pichichero ME, Deloria MA, Rennels MB, et al. A safety and immunogenicity comparison of 12 acellular pertussis vaccines and one whole-cell pertussis vaccine given as a fourth dose in 15- to 20-month-old children. Pediatrics 1997;100:772–88.
38. Halperin SA, Eastwood BJ, Barreto L, et al. Adverse reactions and antibody response to four doses of acellular or whole cell pertussis vaccine combined with diphtheria and tetanus toxoids in the first 19 months of life. Vaccine 1996;14:767–72.
39. Liese JG, Stojanov S, Berut F, et al. Large scale safety study of a liquid hexavalent vaccine (D-T-acP-IPV-PRP–T-HBs) administered at 2, 4, 6 and 12-14 months of age. Vaccine 2001;20:448–54.
40. Pichichero ME, Edwards KM, Anderson EL, et al. Safety and immunogenicity of six acellular pertussis vaccines and one whole-cell pertussis vaccine given as a fifth dose in four- to six-year-old children. Pediatrics 2000;105:e11.

41. Rennels MB, Deloria MA, Pichichero ME, et al. Lack of consistent relationship between quantity of aluminum in diphtheria-tetanus-acellular pertussis vaccines and rates of extensive swelling reactions. Vaccine 2002;20(Suppl 3):S44–7.

42. Rennels MB, Deloria MA, Pichichero ME, et al. Extensive swelling after booster doses of acellular pertussis-tetanus-diphtheria vaccines. Pediatrics 2000;105: e12.

43. Nichol KL, MacDonald R, Hauge M. Side effects associated with pneumococcal vaccination. Am J Infect Control 1997;25:223–8.

44. Broder KR, Cortese MM, Iskander JK, et al. Preventing tetanus, diphtheria, and pertussis among adolescents: use of tetanus toxoid, reduced diphtheria toxoid and acellular pertussis vaccines recommendations of the Advisory Committee on Immunization Practices (ACIP). MMWR Recomm Rep 2006;55:1–34.

45. Facktor MA, Bernstein RA, Fireman P. Hypersensitivity to tetanus toxoid. J Allergy Clin Immunol 1973;52:1–12.

46. Siegrist CA. Mechanisms underlying adverse reactions to vaccines. J Comp Pathol 2007;137(Suppl 1):S46–50.

47. Talbot EA, Brown KH, Kirkland KB, et al. The safety of immunizing with tetanus-diphtheria-acellular pertussis vaccine (Tdap) less than 2 years following previous tetanus vaccination: experience during a mass vaccination campaign of healthcare personnel during a respiratory illness outbreak. Vaccine 2010;28: 8001–7.

48. Beytout J, Launay O, Guiso N, et al. Safety of Tdap-IPV given one month after Td-IPV booster in healthy young adults: a placebo-controlled trial. Hum Vaccin 2009;5:315–21.

49. Yamamoto A, Nagata N, Ochiai M, et al. Enhanced sensitisation of mice with diphtheria tetanus acellular pertussis vaccine to local swelling reaction to the booster immunisation. Vaccine 2002;20:3088–94.

50. Ponvert C. Allergic and pseudo-allergic reactions to vaccines. Immuno-analyse & Biologie spécialisée 2006;21:99–104.

51. Schmitt HJ, Beutel K, Schuind A, et al. Reactogenicity and immunogenicity of a booster dose of a combined diphtheria, tetanus, and tricomponent acellular pertussis vaccine at fourteen to twenty-eight months of age. J Pediatr 1997; 130:616–23.

52. Marshall HS, Gold MS, Gent R, et al. Ultrasound examination of extensive limb swelling reactions after diphtheria-tetanus-acellular pertussis or reduced-antigen content diphtheria-tetanus-acellular pertussis immunization in preschool-aged children. Pediatrics 2006;118:1501–9.

53. Halperin SA, Scheifele D, Barreto L, et al. Comparison of a fifth dose of a five-component acellular or a whole cell pertussis vaccine in children four to six years of age. Pediatr Infect Dis J 1999;18:772–9.

54. Bordet AL, Michenet P, Cohen C, et al. Post-vaccination granuloma due to aluminium hydroxide. Ann Pathol 2001;21:149–52 [in French].

55. Castelain PY, Castelain M, Vervloet D, et al. Sensitization to aluminium by aluminium-precipitated dust and pollen extracts. Contact Dermatitis 1988;19: 58–60.

56. Nagore E, Martinez-Escribano JA, Tato A, et al. Subcutaneous nodules following treatment with aluminium-containing allergen extracts. Eur J Dermatol 2001;11: 138–40.

57. Bergfors E, Trollfors B, Inerot A. Unexpectedly high incidence of persistent itching nodules and delayed hypersensitivity to aluminium in children after the use of adsorbed vaccines from a single manufacturer. Vaccine 2003;22:64–9.

58. Slater DN, Underwood JC, Durrant TE, et al. Aluminium hydroxide granulomas: light and electron microscopic studies and X-ray microanalysis. Br J Dermatol 1982;107:103–8.

59. Pineau A, Durand C, Guillard O, et al. Role of aluminium in skin reactions after diphtheria-tetanus-pertussis-poliomyelitis vaccination: an experimental study in rabbits. Toxicology 1992;73:117–25.

60. Bergfors E, Bjorkelund C, Trollfors B. Nineteen cases of persistent pruritic nodules and contact allergy to aluminium after injection of commonly used aluminium-adsorbed vaccines. Eur J Pediatr 2005;164:691–7.

61. Delafuente JC, Eisenberg JD, Hoelzer DR, et al. Tetanus toxoid as an antigen for delayed cutaneous hypersensitivity. JAMA 1983;249:3209–11.

62. Johnson C, Walls RS, Ruwoldt A. Delayed hypersensitivity to tetanus toxoid in man: in vivo and in vitro studies. Pathology 1983;15:369–72.

63. Fairshter RD, Thornton DB, Gottschalk HR, et al. In vivo and in vitro cell-mediated immunity to tetanus toxoid in adults. J Allergy Clin Immunol 1980; 66:452–7.

64. Osawa J, Kitamura K, Ikezawa Z, et al. A probable role for vaccines containing thimerosal in thimerosal hypersensitivity. Contact Dermatitis 1991;24:178–82.

65. Barbaud A, Deschildre A, Waton J, et al. Hypersensitivity and vaccines: an update. Eur J Dermatol 2013;23(2):135–41.

66. Aberer W. Vaccination despite thimerosal sensitivity. Contact Dermatitis 1991; 24:6–10.

67. Vogt T, Landthaler M, Stolz W. Generalized eczema in an 18-month-old boy due to phenoxyethanol in DPT vaccine. Contact Dermatitis 1998;38:50–1.

68. Ghadially R, Ramsay CA. Gentamicin: systemic exposure to a contact allergen. J Am Acad Dermatol 1988;19:428–30.

69. Kumar LR, Goyal BG. Pigmented hairy scar following smallpox vaccination. Indian J Pediatr 1968;35:283–4.

70. Pembroke AC, Marten RH. Unusual cutaneous reactions following diphtheria and tetanus immunization. Clin Exp Dermatol 1979;4:345–8.

71. Ozkan H, Dundar NO, Ozkan S, et al. Hypertrichosis following measles immunization. Pediatr Dermatol 2001;18:457–8.

72. Diggle L, Deeks J. Effect of needle length on incidence of local reactions to routine immunisation in infants aged 4 months: randomised controlled trial. BMJ 2000;321:931–3.

73. Diggle L, Deeks JJ, Pollard AJ. Effect of needle size on immunogenicity and reactogenicity of vaccines in infants: randomised controlled trial. BMJ 2006;333: 571.

74. Caubet JC, Rudzeviciene O, Gomes E, et al. Managing a child with possible allergy to vaccine. Pediatr Allergy Immunol 2013. [Epub ahead of print].

75. Jackson LA, Peterson D, Nelson JC, et al. Vaccination site and risk of local reactions in children 1 through 6 years of age. Pediatrics 2013;131:283–9.

76. Zent O, Arras-Reiter C, Broeker M, et al. Immediate allergic reactions after vaccinations–a post-marketing surveillance review. Eur J Pediatr 2002;161: 21–5.

77. Bohlke K, Davis RL, Marcy SM, et al. Risk of anaphylaxis after vaccination of children and adolescents. Pediatrics 2003;112:815–20.

78. Kelso JM. Allergic reactions after immunization. Ann Allergy Asthma Immunol 2013;110:397–401.

79. Brindle MJ, Twyman DG. Allergic reactions to tetanus toxoid. A report of four cases. Br Med J 1962;1:1116–7.

80. Cody CL, Baraff LJ, Cherry JD, et al. Nature and rates of adverse reactions associated with DTP and DT immunizations in infants and children. Pediatrics 1981;68:650–60.
81. Pollock TM, Morris J. A 7-year survey of disorders attributed to vaccination in North West Thames region. Lancet 1983;1:753–7.
82. Smith RE, Wolnisty C. Allergic reactions to tetanus, diphtheria, influenza and poliomyelitis immunization. Ann Allergy 1962;20:809–13.
83. Leung AK. Anaphylaxis to DPT vaccine. J R Soc Med 1985;78:175.
84. Ovens H. Anaphylaxis due to vaccination in the office. CMAJ 1986;134:369–70.
85. Zaloga GP, Chernow B. Life-threatening anaphylactic reaction to tetanus toxoid. Ann Allergy 1982;49:107–8.
86. Lewis K, Jordan SC, Cherry JD, et al. Petechiae and urticaria after DTP vaccination: detection of circulating immune complexes containing vaccine-specific antigens. J Pediatr 1986;109:1009–12.
87. Dannemann A, van Ree R, Kulig M, et al. Specific IgE and IgG4 immune responses to tetanus and diphtheria toxoid in atopic and nonatopic children during the first two years of life. Int Arch Allergy Immunol 1996;111:262–7.
88. Aalberse RC, van Ree R, Danneman A, et al. IgE antibodies to tetanus toxoid in relation to atopy. Int Arch Allergy Immunol 1995;107:169–71.
89. Nagel J, Svec D, Waters T, et al. IgE synthesis in man. I. Development of specific IgE antibodies after immunization with tetanus-diphtheria (Td) toxoids. J Immunol 1977;118:334–41.
90. Deloria MA, Blackwelder WC, Decker MD, et al. Association of reactions after consecutive acellular or whole-cell pertussis vaccine immunizations. Pediatrics 1995;96:592–4.
91. Decker MD, Edwards KM, Steinhoff MC, et al. Comparison of 13 acellular pertussis vaccines: adverse reactions. Pediatrics 1995;96:557–66.
92. Edelman K, Malmstrom K, He Q, et al. Local reactions and IgE antibodies to pertussis toxin after acellular diphtheria-tetanus-pertussis immunization. Eur J Pediatr 1999;158:989–94.
93. Hedenskog S, Bjorksten B, Blennow M, et al. Immunoglobulin E response to pertussis toxin in whooping cough and after immunization with a whole-cell and an acellular pertussis vaccine. Int Arch Allergy Appl Immunol 1989;89:156–61.
94. Nilsson L, Gruber C, Granstrom M, et al. Pertussis IgE and atopic disease. Allergy 1998;53:1195–201.
95. Kosecka U, Berin MC, Perdue MH. Pertussis adjuvant prolongs intestinal hypersensitivity. Int Arch Allergy Immunol 1999;119:205–11.
96. Ishizaka K. Cellular events in the IgE antibody response. Adv Immunol 1976;23:1–75.
97. Fritsche PJ, Helbling A, Ballmer-Weber BK. Vaccine hypersensitivity—update and overview. Swiss Med Wkly 2010;140:238–46.
98. DiMiceli L, Pool V, Kelso JM, et al. Vaccination of yeast sensitive individuals: review of safety data in the US vaccine adverse event reporting system (VAERS). Vaccine 2006;24:703–7.
99. Halsey NA. The human papillomavirus vaccine and risk of anaphylaxis. CMAJ 2008;179:509–10.
100. Brightman CA, Scadding GK, Dumbreck LA, et al. Yeast-derived hepatitis B vaccine and yeast sensitivity. Lancet 1989;1:903.
101. Zanoni G, Puccetti A, Dolcino M, et al. Dextran-specific IgG response in hypersensitivity reactions to measles-mumps-rubella vaccine. J Allergy Clin Immunol 2008;122:1233–5.

102. Ponnighaus JM, Fine PE, Moreno C. Hypersensitivity to dextran in BCG vaccine. Lancet 1991;337:1039.
103. Rudin C, Gunthard J, Halter C, et al. Anaphylactoid reaction to BCG vaccine containing high molecular weight dextran. Eur J Pediatr 1995;154:941–2.
104. Hedin G, Richter W, Ring J. Dextran-induced anaphylactoid reactions in man. Role of dextran-reactive antibodies. Int Arch Allergy Appl Immunol 1976;52:145–59.
105. Bigham M, Copes R. Thiomersal in vaccines: balancing the risk of adverse effects with the risk of vaccine-preventable disease. Drug Saf 2005;28:89–101.
106. Sasseville D. Hypersensitivity to preservatives. Dermatol Ther 2004;17:251–63.
107. Fabry H. Formaldehyde sensitivity. Two interesting cases. Contact Derm Newsletter 1968;3:51.
108. Kwittken PL, Rosen S, Sweinberg SK. MMR vaccine and neomycin allergy. Am J Dis Child 1993;147:128–9.
109. Rietschel RL, Bernier R. Neomycin sensitivity and the MMR vaccine. JAMA 1981;245:571.
110. Wood RA, Berger M, Dreskin SC, et al. An algorithm for treatment of patients with hypersensitivity reactions after vaccines. Pediatrics 2008;122:e771–7.
111. Ponvert C, Bloch-Morot E. Allergic and non-allergic hypersensitivity to vaccines. Revue française d'allergologie 2013;53:9–17.
112. Aukrust L, Almeland TL, Refsum D, et al. Severe hypersensitivity or intolerance reactions to measles vaccine in six children. Clinical and immunological studies. Allergy 1980;35:581–7.
113. Baxter DN. Measles immunization in children with a history of egg allergy. Vaccine 1996;14:131–4.
114. Beck SA, Williams LW, Shirrell MA, et al. Egg hypersensitivity and measles-mumps-rubella vaccine administration. Pediatrics 1991;88:913–7.
115. Fasano MB, Wood RA, Cooke SK, et al. Egg hypersensitivity and adverse reactions to measles, mumps, and rubella vaccine. J Pediatr 1992;120:878–81.
116. Herman JJ, Radin R, Schneiderman R. Allergic reactions to measles (rubeola) vaccine in patients hypersensitive to egg protein. J Pediatr 1983;102:196–9.
117. O'Brien TC, Maloney CJ, Tauraso NM. Quantitation of residual host protein in chicken embryo-derived vaccines by radial immunodiffusion. Appl Microbiol 1971;21:780–2.
118. James JM, Zeiger RS, Lester MR, et al. Safe administration of influenza vaccine to patients with egg allergy. J Pediatr 1998;133:624–8.
119. Gagnon R, Primeau MN, Des Roches A, et al. Safe vaccination of patients with egg allergy with an adjuvanted pandemic H1N1 vaccine. J Allergy Clin Immunol 2010;126:317–23.
120. Greenhawt MJ, Chernin AS, Howe L, et al. The safety of the H1N1 influenza A vaccine in egg allergic individuals. Ann Allergy Asthma Immunol 2010;105:387–93.
121. Owens G, MacGinnitie A. Higher-ovalbumin-content influenza vaccines are well tolerated in children with egg allergy. J Allergy Clin Immunol 2011;127:264–5.
122. Howe LE, Conlon AS, Greenhawt MJ, et al. Safe administration of seasonal influenza vaccine to children with egg allergy of all severities. Ann Allergy Asthma Immunol 2011;106:446–7.
123. Webb L, Petersen M, Boden S, et al. Single-dose influenza vaccination of patients with egg allergy in a multicenter study. J Allergy Clin Immunol 2011;128:218–9.
124. Chung EY, Huang L, Schneider L. Safety of influenza vaccine administration in egg-allergic patients. Pediatrics 2010;125:e1024–30.

125. Fung I, Spergel JM. Administration of influenza vaccine to pediatric patients with egg-induced anaphylaxis. J Allergy Clin Immunol 2012;129:1157–9.

126. Des Roches A, Paradis L, Gagnon R, et al. Egg-allergic patients can be safely vaccinated against influenza. J Allergy Clin Immunol 2012;130:1213–6.e1.

127. Greenhawt MJ, Spergel JM, Rank MA, et al. Safe administration of the seasonal trivalent influenza vaccine to children with severe egg allergy. Ann Allergy Asthma Immunol 2012;109:426–30.

128. Li JT, Rank MA, Squillace DL, et al. Ovalbumin content of influenza vaccines. J Allergy Clin Immunol 2010;125:1412–3 [author reply: 1413–4].

129. Waibel KH, Gomez R. Ovalbumin content in 2009 to 2010 seasonal and H1N1 monovalent influenza vaccines. J Allergy Clin Immunol 2010;125:749–51, 751.e1.

130. Rutkowski K, Ewan PW, Nasser SM. Administration of yellow fever vaccine in patients with egg allergy. Int Arch Allergy Immunol 2013;161:274–8.

131. Kelso JM. Administration of influenza vaccines to patients with egg allergy: update for the 2010–2011 season. J Allergy Clin Immunol 2010;126:1302–4.

132. Sakaguchi M, Inouye S. IgE sensitization to gelatin: the probable role of gelatin-containing diphtheria-tetanus-acellular pertussis (DTaP) vaccines. Vaccine 2000;18:2055–8.

133. Sakaguchi M, Yoshida T, Asahi T, et al. Development of IgE antibody to gelatin in children with systemic immediate-type reactions to vaccines. J Allergy Clin Immunol 1997;99:720–1.

134. Albin S N-WA. A Patient with gelatin allergy and anaphylaxis to the influenza vaccine. Abstract P104. The American College of Allergy, Asthma & Immunology 2013.

135. Nakayama T, Aizawa C, Kuno-Sakai H. A clinical analysis of gelatin allergy and determination of its causal relationship to the previous administration of gelatin-containing acellular pertussis vaccine combined with diphtheria and tetanus toxoids. J Allergy Clin Immunol 1999;103:321–5.

136. Nakayama T, Onoda K. Vaccine adverse events reported in post-marketing study of the Kitasato Institute from 1994 to 2004. Vaccine 2007;25:570–6.

137. Kumagai T, Nakayama T, Kamada M, et al. The lymphoproliferative response to enzymatically digested gelatin in subjects with gelatin hypersensitivity. Clin Exp Allergy 2000;30:1430–5.

138. Nakayama T, Aizawa C. Change in gelatin content of vaccines associated with reduction in reports of allergic reactions. J Allergy Clin Immunol 2000;106:591–2.

139. Kumagai T, Ozaki T, Kamada M, et al. Gelatin-containing diphtheria-tetanus-pertussis (DTP) vaccine causes sensitization to gelatin in the recipients. Vaccine 2000;18:1555–61.

140. Kattan JD, Konstantinou GN, Cox AL, et al. Anaphylaxis to diphtheria, tetanus, and pertussis vaccines among children with cow's milk allergy. J Allergy Clin Immunol 2011;128:215–8.

141. Parisi CA, Smaldini PL, Gervasoni ME, et al. Hypersensitivity reactions to the Sabin vaccine in children with cow's milk allergy. Clin Exp Allergy 2013;43:249–54.

Hypersensitivity Reactions to Biologic Agents

Alessandra Vultaggio, MD, PhD[a], Mariana C. Castells, MD, PhD[b],*

KEYWORDS

- Antidrug antibodies • Biologic agents • Drug allergy • Hypersensitivity reactions
- Immunogenicity

KEY POINTS

- Biologic agents (BAs) are important therapeutic tools, but their use may be limited by adverse drug reactions.
- Procedures for management of BA-induced reactions, including preventive, diagnostic work-up and desensitization, are becoming available in the clinical setting.
- The knowledge of such procedures for management of BA-induced reactions may be useful to increase the safety profile of current and forthcoming BAs.

INTRODUCTION

Many BAs have become available as new therapeutic tools, including monoclonal antibody (mAb), cytokines, and fusion proteins. Since their approval, BA therapy had a positive impact on the long-term outcomes, such as disability and mortality, associated with both inflammatory chronic diseases and cancers; thus, in a short period of time, they have entered the mainstream of their treatment.[1,2] There is a large amount of research and development being undertaken to create BAs for many serious diseases, such as rheumatoid arthritis, multiple sclerosis, bowel inflammatory diseases, and different types of cancers.[3] These medications each have their unique profile in terms of efficacy, tolerability, and adverse effects; they are not deprived in toxicity, which can impair quality of life and may occasionally be life-threatening or, more frequently, lead to the interruption of treatment.[4]

DEFINITIONS

Generally, adverse events (AEs) are defined as any untoward medical occurrences associated with the use of a drug in humans, whether or not considered drug related,

The authors have nothing to disclose.
[a] Immunoallergology Unit, Department of Biomedicine, Azienda Ospedaliero-Universitaria Careggi, Viale Morgagni 85, Florence 50134, Italy; [b] Drug Hypersensitivity and Desensitization Center, Mastocytosis Center, Brigham and Women's Hospital, Harvard Medical School, Boston, MA, USA
* Corresponding author.
E-mail address: mcastells@partners.org

whereas any AE caused by an injected drug is defined as an infusion reaction. The term, *allergic hypersensitivity reactions (HRs)*, refers to antibody- or cellular-mediated infusion reactions. Infusion reactions may be divided into local and systemic reactions.[5] Local infusion reactions, which are induced by subcutaneous BAs, are referred to as injection site reactions (ISRs). Lastly, acute infusion reactions occur during or within 1 hour after infusion or within a few minutes after subcutaneous injection, whereas delayed reactions occur from 1 hour to 14 days after.[6,7]

CLINICAL PRESENTATION: SYMPTOMS AND MANAGEMENT

The clinical manifestations of both acute and delayed reactions vary considerably, ranging from mild to severe and life threatening; thus, important clinical consequences, such as drop-out therapy or fatal cases, may occur.

Acute Infusion Reactions

Acute reactions include mainly cutaneous symptoms, such as itching, urticaria, and flushing, but sometimes anaphylaxis may occur characterized by respiratory distress, laryngeal edema, and bronchospasm, accompanied by gastrointestinal and cardiovascular involvement. In some cases, patients may display fever, skills, or myalgia.[7] The severity of the reaction should be determined to better define the clinical management of such infusion. Mild to moderate events may be managed by reducing the infusion rate (after a temporary interruption) and administering H_1 antihistamines and corticosteroids for symptom control. In cases of severe reactions, the infusion must be stopped and rescue treatment promptly administered, such as epinephrine, liquids, oxygen supply, H_1 antihistamines, and high doses of intravenous steroids, according to the clinical features of the reaction.[8]

Acute infusion reactions may occur at the first dose or during the course of treatment, thus suggesting different underlying pathogenic mechanisms. Matucci and colleagues[9] have recently analyzed the clinical characteristics of infliximab-induced immediate infusion reactions: severe events were 1 in 3 reactions; a majority of reactions occurred within 15 minutes after the beginning of the infusion; and cutaneous and respiratory symptoms were the most frequent clinical features.

Delayed Infusion Reactions

Delayed reactions usually occur within the first 2 weeks after the administration of a BA. They usually present with arthralgia, myalgia, exanthems, fever, urticaria, and itching.[10] The clinical presentation of delayed reactions may be consistent with a classic serum sickness characterized by the production of antibody to foreign immunoglobulin with formation of antigen-antibody complexes. Patchy lung infiltrates and skin necrotizing vasculitis may be present, sustained by inflammatory infiltrates involving small blood vessels and complement deposition at immunofluorescence staining. In addition, there can be lymphadenopathy, splenomegaly, gastrointestinal symptoms (nausea, vomiting, abdominal pain, and melena), and extremity weakness.[11] It has been reported that approximately 2.5% of patients receiving infliximab infusion develop serum sickness–like reactions,[12] but other chimeric molecules used to treat various conditions, such as abciximab for acute coronary syndromes, trastuzumab for breast cancer, rituximab for lymphoma, omalizumab for asthma, and natalizumab for multiple sclerosis, have been associated to these reactions.[12–15] Some delayed reactions associated with mAb infusions may be characterized by a prevalent hematologic involvement, such as hemolytic anemia and immune thrombocytopenia.[16,17] The course of delayed reactions is usually self-limiting, but severe acute respiratory distress syndrome and fatal outcomes have been observed.[18] Patients displaying serum sickness disease must be treated with steroids and for those most severely affected, plasma exchange may be used; serum sickness is a well-recognized indication of this therapeutic modality. On the other hand, premedication plays no established and secure role in exanthems or serum sickness and is often without effect.

Systemic Skin Reactions

During therapy with BAs, such as rituximab and anti–TNF-α agonists, disseminated skin reactions have been reported, including exanthems (maculopapular, eczematous, lichenoid, and granulomatous) and erythema multiforme.[19] A lymphocyte infiltration at the dermoepidermal junction has been reported in the case of infliximab-related generalized erythemato-squamous exanthema in patients treated for rheumatoid arthritis with infliximab, occurring 2 to 4 weeks after the treatment was introduced.[20] In cases of these dermatoses, clinicians may discontinue infliximab or try to continue it in conjunction with corticosteroid application or switch to a different TNF-α antagonist. Some severe systemic events, such as Stevens-Johnson syndrome after rituximab and a case of toxic epidermal necrolysis (TEN) associated with cetuximab, have been described.[21,22] Among disseminated skin reactions related to the use of BAs, the development of psoriasiform eruption during TNF-α antagonists can be included.[23] In addition, acneiform exanthems and folliculitides during treatment with antagonists of epidermal growth factor receptor, such as cetuximab, or tyrosine kinase inhibitors, such as erlotinib, may be present.[24]

Injection Site Reactions

Regarding subcutaneously administered BAs, even if they can also induce systemic reactions, the most common adverse events are represented by ISRs, characterized by erythema, swelling, itching, or infiltrated plaques.[10] ISRs may occur within a few minutes (immediate reactions) or later (delayed reactions). Patients treated with subcutaneous TNF-α blockers, such as etanercept and adalimumab, may develop ISRs around the sites of injection, mainly reported in the first 2 months of inception of therapy, usually occurring 1 to 2 days after the last injection, and resolving within a few days. It has been observed that some patients treated with anti-TNF blockers develop recall ISRs that are reactions at sites were the BA was previously injected after the last injection.[25] ISRs are usually mild and disappear when the treatment is continued, uncommonly leading to the drug interruption. The use of local corticosteroids is usually sufficient in the management of ISRs along with a follow-up of the lesions to assess their severity and the compliance of patients to the treatment.

PATHOGENIC MECHANISMS OF ACUTE REACTIONS

Regarding the pathogenesis of immediate systemic HRs, they are a complex picture, not fully clarified. Non–antibody- and antibody-mediated reactions can, however, be distinguished.[26]

Among non–antibody-mediated reactions, complement-mediated events can be presumed but not clearly demonstrated as yet, whereas cytokine release syndrome (CRS) is identified as the most defined type, usually occurring at first dose of treatment. Antibody-mediated adverse reactions (HRs) usually occur during an ongoing treatment and are unpredictable despite preventive measures, and both IgE and non IgE antibodies can be involved.[26]

The CRS is sustained by a massive release of cytokine from different immune cells (monocytes, macrophages, cytotoxic T cells, and NK cells). Both in vivo and in vitro studies indicate that TNF-α, interferon-γ, and interleukin 6 are the main actors of CRS.[27] The postulated mechanism is related to the interaction of the mAb with the Fcγ receptors of immune cells, leading to their activation and/or lysis and subsequent cytokine release.[28] CRS can be clinically heterogeneous, ranging from a flulike syndrome to a multiorgan failure due to a cytokine storm, but sometimes these reactions raise concern for immediate hypersensitivity, being clinically indistinguishable from an anaphylaxis. Some clinical manifestations of CRS and hypersensitivity may overlap, such as rash, fever, hypotension, dyspnea, and tachycardia.

In contrast to delayed systemic infusion reactions or ISRs, for which the role of antibody formation is still unclear, acute systemic reactions to biologicals are deeply related to the development of antidrug antibodies (ADAs). The authors' findings, obtained in infliximab-treated patients, indicate that the development of ADAs is definitely correlated with clinical outcome, in terms of infusion reactions.[9] The authors' data confirm results previously published on a Crohn diseases patient treated with infliximab.[29] Patients who develop antibodies to biologicals are more likely to show immediate infusion-related reactions. Concerning antibody-dependent mechanisms, even if ADAs mainly are of IgG class, in particular IgG1 subclass, different ADA isotypes may be involved: IgE and non-IgE (**Fig. 1**). It is important to underline that IgE- and IgG-mediated reactions may be clinically indistinguishable. Svenson and coworkers[30] have clearly shown that IgG toward infliximab correlates with immediate infusion reactions. In mice models, the role of allergen-specific IgG in induction of anaphylaxis has been shown, whereas their role in humans is controversial. In the authors' opinion, adverse effects of biologicals may be an interesting model to confirm the role of this alternative pathway of anaphylaxis in humans. In mice, the IgG pathway of anaphylaxis requires a high amount of antigen and of IgG antibody; thus, human anaphylaxis induced by therapeutic mABs, after repeated infusion of high amount of the protein, may be the most likely candidates for human IgG-mediated anaphylaxis.[31] IgG ADAs can directly activate circulating basophils, through the binding of Fcγ receptors, and indirectly they can activate tissue mast cells through activation of the complement cascade and release of anaphylatoxins.

An IgE-mediated mechanism has been described for several BAs in reactive patients, through the use of skin testing, in vitro assay for the detection of IgE, or both.[32–35] Vultaggio and colleagues[36] first identified the presence of serum infliximab-specific IgE in some reactive patients. To date, among 30 reactive patients, they have identified 23 subjects as ADA positive, and 6 of them had a positive result in a *carotid artery plaque* (CAP) analysis for infliximab-specific IgE.[9] In addition, IgE-mediated reactions seem more severe than non–IgE-mediated events. The same investigators have been able to detect circulating rituximab-specific IgE antibodies in an autoimmune patient treated with rituximab who experienced 2 infusion-related reactions.[37] By using a non–isotype-specific assay for the screening, they found rituximab-specific ADA, and by using an ImmunoCAP platform (ThermoFisher, Uppsala, Sweden), they defined the presence of IgE ADAs, closely time-related to the reactions. These findings confirmed data obtained in vivo (positive results of skin testing) in rituximab-reactive patients obtained by Brennan and coworkers.[38] In addition, these results confirm that a specific BA may trigger infusion reaction via different mechanisms according to the patient and the situation. A majority of acute infusion reactions to rituximab occur during the first exposure and are usually induced by CRS.

The development of ADAs usually results from repeated exposure to BAs and is associated with reactions occurring after initial doses. In particular, immunogenicity-related infusion reactions for infliximab occur within the first 10 infusions and IgE-mediated events occur early on, within the first 5 administrations.[9,39,40] In addition,

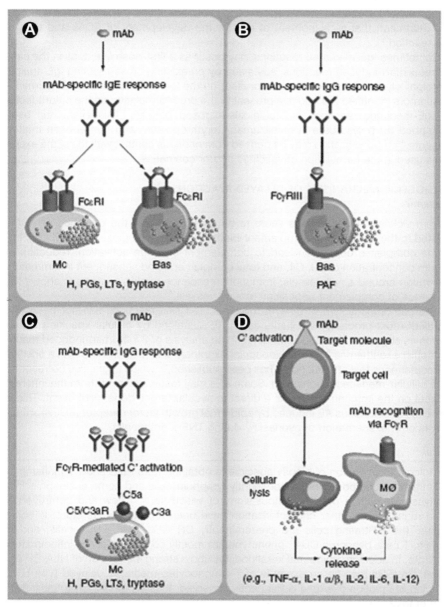

Fig. 1. Antibody (IgE and non-IgE) and non–antibody-mediated mechanisms of reactions to BAs. (*A*) Cross-linking of FcεRI induced by specific IgE antibodies on mast cells and basophils. (*B*) Activation of basophils trough FcγRIII by IgG antibodies. (*C*) Complement activation by drug-antibodies immunocomplexes and subsequent activation of mast cells by anaphylotoxins. (*D*) mAb-induced cytokine release. H, histamine; LTs, leukotrienes; Mc, mast cells; PAF, platelet activation factor; PGs, prostaglandins. (*From* Maggi E, Vultaggio A, Matucci A. Acute infusion reactions induced by monoclonal antibody therapy. Expert Rev Clin Immunol 2011;7:57; with permission.)

a majority of IgE-related events occur at re-exposure after a period of interruption of the treatment, that is, a moment of risk for the development of ADAs and then of the reaction.[9]

Sometimes IgE-mediated reactions may occur as a first-dose event, as in the case of cetuximab-induced reactions, sustained by preexisting cross-reacting IgE against "foreign" glycan structures that are present on the therapeutic antibody.[41] Some investigators identified the additive present in the drug formulation as the culprit factor of IgE-mediated reactions in biologicals-exposed patients. This event has been described for polysorbate in omalizumab-, erythropoietin- and darbepoetin-treated patients.[42,43] Sensitization may be derived from previous contact with the same excipients used in the formulation of vaccines and/or cosmetics.

PATHOGENIC MECHANISMS OF DELAYED REACTIONS
Systemic

Serum sickness–like reactions seem to be associated with the presence of ADAs, related to the formation of complement-binding immune complexes (type III HR). Immune complexes deposition lead to complement cascade activation; reduction of serum concentration of C3, C4, and total complement; and subsequent inflammatory infiltration around small vessels. Immunofluorescence of skin specimens shows the presence of complement deposition around vessels.[11]

The pathomechanism of delayed disseminated skin reactions has not been well studied; most probably, it constitutes an AE sustained by cellular-specific mechanisms as suggested by results obtained in an analysis of 2 infliximab-induced maculopapular exanthemas.[44] A maculopapular exanthem due to abciximab with a positive intracutaneous test after 48 hours has been published,[45] which might also correspond to a cellular-mediated mechanism. Some AEs may result, however, from the inherent effects on the immune system as a direct molecular target–dependent event. This is the case of cutaneous AE induced by epidermal growth factor receptor (EGFR) antagonists or of exacerbation of psoriasis[21] during TNF-α antagonist.

Local

Histologic examination of biopsy specimens obtained from ISRs show an inflammatory infiltrate composed of predominantly lymphoid cells and some eosinophils in a perivascular cuffing pattern without signs of vasculitis.[46,47] Few and controversial data regarding a further characterization have been reported in literature; in some cases, the infiltrating cells are predominantly $DR^+CD3^+CD4^-CD8^+$ cells, and in others, T cells bearing a $CD4^+$ phenotype are mostly composed of the inflammatory infiltrate. In addition, epidermal keratinocytes show strong expression of HLA-DR antigen. So ISRs may be an example of T-lymphocytes–mediated delayed-type HRs. Waning of reaction overtime is frequently observed, thus suggesting eventual induction of tolerance.

VALUE OF SKIN TESTING FOR ACUTE REACTIONS

Skin tests are usually done and are of great importance in the diagnosis of drug allergy because they potentially reproduce IgE-mediated reactions or T-cell–mediated events. In vivo tests, however, are not currently standardized and approved for BAs; in this field of drug allergy, up to now, exact diagnostic tools to identify potentially reactive patients have not been defined.

Even if data in literature about skin testing for BAs are limited, during the last few years positive skin testing has been reported in patients with immediate HR caused by BAs,[32–34,38] such as rituximab, anti-TNF agents, and trastuzumab. More importantly, few studies involving small case series reported results of skin testing confirmed by in vitro tests, such as RAST or ImmunoCAP.[35,36] Regarding in vivo tests for BAs, there is insufficient evidence to recommend appropriate drug concentration as well as the timing to perform it. Some data on nonirritant concentrations for anti-TNF agents and other BAs are reported in literature (**Table 1**).

The utility of skin testing in 23 patients who have experienced infliximab-related reactions has been recently evaluated.[9] The investigators showed that it was essential to perform intradermal test in immediately reactive patients, because the prick test is usually negative. Seven of them (30.4%) had a positive result at an immediate-reading intradermal test and 6 of them displayed ImmunoCAP, positivity thus showing a great correlation between serologic IgE positivity and in vivo results. Considering that immediate intradermal tests for BAs had a specificity of approximately 100% in that small case series, they seem to be a useful method for the diagnosis of immediate type I HRs to BAs; however, they show a sensitivity of 30%, similar to the performance characteristics of in vitro IgE detection for BAs. The overall lack of sensitivity of IgE assay (in vivo and in vitro) could be explained by non–IgE-mediated hypersensitivity to BAs, as discussed previously.

It is an obvious factor that for skin testing the time between the reaction and the evaluation (**Fig. 2**) is a crucial point, due to temporary unresponsiveness of the skin mast cells after massive activation during the reaction. In addition, IgE specific for BAs displays a rapid decrease over time and, accordingly, Matucci and co-workers[9] reported that none of the patients had positivity when studied 8 months after the first analysis, suggesting that the allergological work-up of reactive patients should be performed early. The authors, however, do not have any negativization rate of skin testing for BAs. Concerning safety, there were also no unexpected adverse reactions to the in vivo procedures with BAs in patients experiencing severe reactions.

Easy clinical application, their safety, and high specificity may offer a new tool for the diagnosis of at least IgE-mediated HR. There is an urgent need, however, to establish, standardize, and share practical procedures in this field of drug allergy. These procedures could be used to design multicenter studies aimed at defining the diagnostic accuracy of skin testing for BAs in a prospective manner, which are lacking.

Table 1
Concentrations and dilutions for mAb skin testing

Biologic Agent	Concentration (mg/mL)	Dilutions	
		Prick Test	IDT (0.02 mL)
Infliximab[9,36,38]	10	1:100–1:1	1:1000–1:10
Adalimumab[48,68]	50	1:100–1:1	1:1000–1:10
Etanercept[34,48]	25	1:100–1:1	1:1000–1:10
Rituximab[37,38]	10	1:100–1:1	1:1000–1:10
Cetuximab[73]	5	1:100–1:1	1:1000–1:10
Trastuzumab[38]	21	1:100–1:1	1:1000–1:10
Natalizumab[35]	20	1:100–1:1	1:1000–1:10

Maxima and minima dilutions are reported for each BA based on literature data. For delayed reactions, reading at 24–48 h can be suggested.
For each test, positive (histamine) and negative controls (saline) must be used.
Abbreviation: IDT, intradermal test.

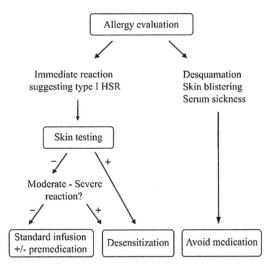

Fig. 2. Allergological evaluation of reactive patients to be submitted to desensitization procedure. (*From* Brennan PJ, Bouza TR, Hsu FI, et al. Hypersensitivity reactions to mAbs:105 desensitizations in 23 patients, from evaluation to treatment. J Allergy Clin Immunol 2009;124:1260; with permission.)

MANAGEMENT OF BA-INDUCED REACTIONS: PREVENTIVE MEASURES AND DIAGNOSIS

Considering the increased use of the biologic therapies in different pathologic conditions, the management of BA-induced reactions is becoming an unavoidable necessity in the clinical practice. The management of these reactions means defining their pathogenic mechanism as well as identifying patients at risk. If the authors deal with patients with previous reactions, the aim is to define the pathomechanism, whereas if the authors have patients with no previous reaction, it is to identify patients at risk and reduce the risk itself. The common clinical outcome is the prevention of further or first-time reactions.

Preventive Measures

Recognition of patients at risk

The identification of patients at risk is a key point in clinical practice. Taking a thorough history, in particular, including atopic status and any previous allergic reactions, is one of the most useful risk-assessment tools in allergy. Data show that there is no correlation between the atopic status and the incidence of HRs during therapy with TNF-α blocking agents; a similar prevalence of atopy and previous adverse drug reactions in reactive and unreactive patients also was seen.[39,48]

Excellent data have highlighted the associations between ADAs and adverse clinical outcomes; risk factors for immunogenicity represent risk factors for HRs. In particular, the presence of antibodies against anti–TNF mAbs confers a risk of development of HRs in all immune-mediated inflammatory diseases. The combined use of anti–TNF mAbs and disease-modifying antirheumatic drugs reduces the development of antibodies and subsequent risks; information on other BAs is fragmentary.[49] A higher incidence of infliximab reactions in rheumatoid arthritis patients than in patients suffering from seronegative ankylosing spondyloarthritis and vasculitis confirmed that the underlying disease itself can be an important factor in the context of developing an unwanted immune response toward the therapeutic agent.[39] Concordantly, a higher detection rate of antirituximab antibodies in systemic lupus erythematosus than in lymphoma patients suggests that chimeric antibodies may be more immunogenic in autoimmune disease because of the highly activated B-lymphocytes status.[50,51] The high expression of costimulatory molecules on dendritic cells in patients with immune-mediated diseases may accelerate the development of ADAs.[52] Some reports indicate an increased proportion of BA reactions in patients who have discontinued therapy.[53] Adults and children with Crohn disease experienced severe systemic reactions when a distant reinfusion interval was attempted.[54] Patients receiving regularly scheduled infliximab infusions have a decreased likelihood of forming ADAs. On the contrary, intermittent therapy may favor ADA formation and increase the likelihood of infusion reaction.[55]

It is likely that regular drug infusion may induce a high-dose tolerance through efficient peripheral mechanisms, which need the continuous antigen intake. Thus, the avoidance of long intervals between infusions represents a useful strategy to increase BA safety.

CRS seen during the treatment of tumors is largely dependent on the disease burden; for example, in patients treated with rituximab suffering from non-Hodgkin lymphoma, the severity of reactions is related to the numbers of $CD20^+$ circulating cells.

Premedication
Prophylactic medication with acetaminophen and/or H_1 antihistamines could prevent infusion reactions in HRs even though solid evidence is lacking and there are controversial data.[56] Premedication seems to be not protective in patients who have already developed ADAs[39]; pretreatment with acetaminophen plus H_1 antihistamines, however, is recommended as prophylaxis for CRS induced by mAbs used in cancer therapy. The incidence and severity of CRS may also be reduced by premedication with high-dose steroids given before the administration of the first dose of the BA.[57]

Choice of the infusion rate
Specific guidelines of use and administration, including flow of infusion, for each BA are usually provided, aimed at significantly reducing the risk of reaction. Many mild-to-moderate events can be successfully managed by reducing the rate of infusion, although, at least for infliximab-induced events, it seems to be useful in ADA-negative but not in ADA-positive patients.[36,39]

In addition, in contrast to type I HRs, CRS may be managed by short-term cessation of the mAbs infusion (fractionized dosing) and restarting the infusion at a slower rate. These reactions can also be minimized by cautious incremental increases in the rate of infusion and ensuring appropriate hydration and diuresis.

Diagnosis: In Vitro and In Vivo Tests

In vitro tests useful in the clinical setting for the evaluation of BA-induced reactions are focused on the detection of ADAs. Different methods can be used, but solid-phase or solution ELISA is the most frequently used, generally displaying sensitivity, accuracy, and reproducibility.[58] Even if these assays are relatively simple, shortcomings related to matrix effects and detection of low-affinity ADAs, are present, leading to false-positive or -negative results. Thus, the initial ADA screening assay, able to detect all ADA-positive samples, should be followed by a confirmatory assay for distinguishing between true and false-positive results. For example, false-positive results can be due to rheumatoid factors cross-linking with the capture antibody[59] as well as drug interference, and rapidly dissociating or low-affinity antibodies may lead to an under-estimation of the number of patients producing ADAs (false-negative results). Serum samples should be taken shortly before a new dose of drug, because in currently used assays, ADA detection is only possible if the production of ADAs exceeds the amount of drug present in a patient's serum due to the formation of ADA-drug complexes. In addition, sample pretreatment methods with acid, for dissociation of drug-antidrug complexes, may be used to improve free drug tolerance in ADA as-says.[60] The evaluation of drug levels in parallel with the ADA detection could be neces-sary to understand ADA assay's results.

Although ADAs are mostly represented by IgG class,[6] multiple isotypes (IgM, IgE, and IgG) and subclasses (IgG1–4) can be produced during humoral antidrug response. Thus, a multitier testing strategy for assessment of immunogenicity is recommended, including the isotype definition of confirmed positive samples. The identification of BA-specific IgE may be difficult because these antibodies are usually quantitatively lower than all other isotypes, and IgG ADAs can deeply interfere with the detection of the low amounts of IgE. The ImmunoCAP platform is characterized by a high and reproducible binding capacity, leading to its ability to identify ADAs independently of their affinity and in the presence of interfering IgG.

Among other tests, the measurement of serum tryptase, the classical mediator ac-counting for mast cells activation, is currently used, and high levels are consistent with a true anaphylactic reaction. Tryptase levels within normal range, however, do not exclude IgE-mediated anaphylaxis, as described in patients with acute systemic reac-tions to BAs.[36] In these cases, the attention has been focused on basophils that ex-press high-affinity FcεRI and, after stimulation, release mediators but not tryptase. The measurement of serum cytokine levels as well as complement fractions may be supposed in the in vitro evaluation of acute BA-induced reactions, but they are not routinely performed as yet.

Taking into account that patients developing ADAs are more likely to show acute re-actions, whereas definitive data on their role in the induction of delayed reactions are lacking, no clear indications about the usefulness of ADA detection in patients with delayed reactions to BAs are available. Finally, to date, the role of in vitro T-cell analysis remains to be defined in the clinical setting for both acute and delayed BA-induced reactions.

Besides the value of skin testing for acute reactions already reported, there are few data regarding in vivo allergological tests for delayed HRs.[61,62] They have been carried out largely in patients with interferon-induced reactions. Controversial data are re-ported, however, and conclusive results are lacking.

DESENSITIZATION
Risk, Safety, and Outcomes

There is an inherent risk to the administration of an mAb to which a patient has had an HR and the risk should be weighed against the benefit of using the medication when the offending agent is the best option and can improve the quality of life. Rapid drug desensitization (RDD) is a groundbreaking treatment option, allowing patients to receive their full target doses while protecting them against severe HRs and anaphy-laxis. RDD is contraindicated in patients whose reactions suggest Stevens-Johnson syndrome or TEN, drug reaction with eosinophilia and systemic symptoms, or acute generalized exanthematous pustulosis. RDD has not provided benefit for the treat-ment of serum sickness–like reactions or hemolytic anemia. RDD is a temporary phe-nomenon that inhibits mast cell activation and the release of mediators, such as histamine leukotrienes and prostaglandins, which are responsible for the symptoms of anaphylaxis. Whether RDD can induce long-term tolerance needs further study, and current outcomes indicate that patients have to be redesensitized at each medication exposure. RDD is a safe and effective treatment option to increase the life expectancy and quality of life for indicated patients with HRs to mAbs. RDD can address infusion reactions consistent with cytokine storms and type I HRs, including anaphylaxis. Skin testing is a useful tool to provide evidence of IgE mechanism and validate the indication of RDD, although most mAbs skin tests have not been validated in large series and their negative predictive value is unknown. Different protocols are available for RDD and large series of patients are required for their validation. Trained allergists, nurses, and pharmacists are required for successful RDD to mAbs.

Rituximab

Rituximab is a chimeric mAB against CD20 effective in lymphomas, leukemias, transplant rejection, and autoimmune and inflammatory disorders. Desensitization to rituximab was initially described as part of a case series of 413 RDDs in 98 patients by Castells and colleagues.[63] Three of the 98 patients had 7 successful RDDs to rituximab; 2 patients had initially presented with rash and severe pruritis during the infusion of rituximab; and a third patient had presented syncope, preventing the completion of the rituximab infusion. The RDD protocol included three 250-mL solutions with 10-fold increasing concentrations and 12 steps in which the dose was advanced every 15 minutes by increasing the rate and/or the concentration. Reactions during the desensitizations were mild and occurred during this last step.

The 3 patients were able to complete full treatment doses over 7 RDDs with no severe reactions. No patient experienced any reaction during RDD that was more severe than the initial presenting reaction. Brennan and colleagues[38] described a group of 14 additional patients who experienced HRs to rituximab as part of a review of 105 RDDs to mAbs in 23 patients who had reactions to mAbs. The protocol for infusions and treatment of reactions was identical to that described but adapted to dosing of mAbs (rituximab, infliximab, and trastuzumab). Eleven of 14 rituximab-sensitive patients developed a reaction on their first exposure and had no known prior exposure to any other mAB. Data on rituximab skin testing were collected, but the sensitivity and specificity have not been on a larger scale and a negative skin test did not preclude desensitization over a strong clinical history of HR. One patient in the study converted from a positive to a negative skin test and was able to tolerate a subsequent rituximab infusion without RDD. Consistent with the findings of Castells and colleagues,[63] a majority of reactions that occurred to rituximab RDD occurred during the last step (#12, comprising approximately 90% of the therapeutic dose) with a majority of reactions consisting of mild cutaneous symptoms (flushing and hives), and all reactions were less severe than the initial presenting HR.

Infliximab

Infliximab is a chimeric mouse-human IgG1 mAB that binds with high affinity and specificity to tumor necrosis factor α (TNF-α) and is used primarily in the treatment of inflammatory bowel disease and rheumatoid arthritis.

To address acute infusion reactions, slowing the infusion rate has been shown helpful as has the use of premedication with steroids, antihistamines, and acetaminophen, but severe infusion reactions are not prevented by these premedications. RDD protocols have been successfully applied to treat infliximab hypersensitivity. Puchner and colleagues[64] first reported successful desensitization for anaphylactic reactions in 2 patients who were desensitized to infliximab with an 11-step protocol with 2-fold increase at each step starting at 1/100,000 of the final dose. The dose was increased every 15 minutes and the infusion was completed in 4 hours. Cheifetz and colleagues,[65] in a retrospective analysis of 165 patients who received a total of 479 infusions of infliximab, described a slow infusion protocol starting at 10 mL/h for 15 minutes, then doubled every 15 minutes to 20, 40, 80, and 100 mL/h after which the patient was continued at 150 mL/h for 30 minutes. There were 26 acute reactions of which 15 (58%) were mild, 6 (23%) were moderate, and 5 (19%) were severe. All patients with mild or moderate reactions were able to continue infliximab. Of the 4 patients who had severe reactions, 2 were able to continue treatment with desensitization, 1 had a breakthrough severe reaction, and 1 withdrew from further treatments. In 2006, Duburque and colleagues[66] reported their experience with desensitization in 14 patients with Crohn disease who had developed severe infusion reactions despite prophylactic administration of hydrocortisone and for whom infliximab was considered the only therapeutic option. The investigators used an 11-step protocol in which the final target dose was 5 mg/kg with a total infusion time of 2 hours and 45 minutes. Of the 14 patients studied, all were able to receive at least 1 full infliximab treatment. Three patients had mild reactions, 1 patient had angioedema necessitating stoppage of the protocol, and 1 patient had a delayed reactions consisting of generalized arthralgias, myalgias, and fever and requiring treatment with corticosteroids. Brennan and colleagues[38] reported 6 patients who had immediate-type HRs to infliximab. Four patients (67%) had a positive intradermal skin test at either 0.1 or 1.0 mg/mL concentration and all patients undergoing RDD had reactions after several exposures to infliximab. The same protocol used for rituximab RDD was used successfully for infliximab desensitization, with a majority of reactions occurring during the last step and consisting of mainly cutaneous symptoms of flushing, pruritis, and/or hives. All patients were able to receive their full treatment dose and no delayed reactions were observed.

Other Monoclonal TNF-α Inhibitors

Although local reactions with hives, local swelling, and pruritus are the most common allergic reaction with the injectable TNF-α inhibitors, systemic reactions after adalimumab administration have also been reported. Skin testing has been used to document the IgE-mediated mechanism of reactions to both etanercept and adalimumab. Rodriguez-Jimenez and colleagues[67] performed a successful desensitization in a patient with plaque psoriasis who had poor responses to methotrexate and etanercept. Infliximab was also tried but discontinued secondary to a cardiac dysrhythmia associated with its use. Adalimumab was effective but induced generalized urticaria and rhinitis after 6 doses. The patient was skin test positive to full strength adalimumab (50 mg/mL) compared with 10 negative control patients. Adalimumab was given over 6 injections spaced 60 minutes apart starting with a 0.5-mg dose. Each subsequent injection was an approximate doubling of the prior step. By the end of the 6-hour desensitization, the patient had received a full dose of 44.25 mg. Bavbek and colleagues[34] recently reported a successful desensitization to etanercept in a patient with ankylosing spondylitis who became sensitized to both adalimumab and etanercept. The patient had developed local swelling, diffuse pruritus, and shortness of breath after his 26th adalimumab injection and was then switched to etanercept. He developed a local reaction followed by a disseminated urticarial rash after his 22nd etanercept injection. The patient was positive on intradermal skin test to 1/100 dilution of etanercept compared with 2 negative control patients. An attempt to prevent a reaction with antihistamines was unsuccessful secondary to a breakthrough disseminated urticarial rash. The patient was then desensitized after a 3-day protocol and received 6 injections on each day spaced by 30 to 90 minutes starting at 1/100 dilution of the final dose and doubling the dose with each step. The patient achieved the target dose and was subsequently maintained on etanercept twice weekly as a single injections with only small (<3 cm in diameter) local ISRs. The same investigators describe a 26-year-old woman with rheumatoid arthritis and severe generalized urticaria associated with adalimumab who had a positive skin test at 0.05 mg/mL and was desensitized successfully with 6 doubling doses reaching the target dose of 55 mg in 3, 5 hours.[68]

Cetuximab

Cetuximab is a human-murine chimerized IgG1 mAB that targets the extracellular ligand-binding domain of the EGFR. It was the first Food and Drug Administration–approved mAB directed against EGFR and is approved for metastatic colorectal cancer and squamous-cell carcinoma of the head and neck. It carries a black box warning of severe infusion reactions, which have been reported to occur in 3% of patients, with 90% of those reactions occurring during the first infusion with rare fatalities (<1:1000). These reactions occurred despite the use of prophylactic antihistamines, and the reactions that developed were consistent with a type I HR with bronchospasm, hypotension, and/or urticaria. Most reactions to cetuximab occur with the first infusion. An unusually high rate of severe infusion reactions in North Carolina and Tennessee prompted an investigation, which led to the discovery of a high prevalence of preformed anticetuximab IgE directed against galactose-α–1,3-galactose in patients who had first-time infusion reactions and who had tick bites prior to the infusion. Cetuximab is generated in a mouse cell line, SP2/0, which expresses α1,3-galactosyltransferase, which is present on the Fab' portion of the cetuximab heavy chain, which is shared by the tick.[41]

The first published desensitization to cetuximab was a case report describing a female patient with metastatic breast cancer and preexisting anti–cetuximab-specific IgE. A 5-solution, 20-step protocol was used and four 10-fold serial dilutions were used in succession, starting from most the most dilute (0.0002 mg/mL) to the final, most concentrated solution (2 mg/mL), and each step doubling the prior step's dose, starting with 0.001 mg. The patient presented several reactions during desensitization but was able to complete the infusion.[69]

The 12-step RDD protocol has been successfully used to desensitized more than 10 patients with type I hypersensitivity symptoms, and skin testing to cetuximab was found positive in these patients during first administrations.[70] There have even been reports of successful readministration of cetuximab after an HR during the first administration using a premedication regimen of H_1 and H_2 antihistamines, steroids, and a test dose; however, caution needs to be exercised in the interpretation of these case reports because the underlying mechanism for the initial reactions are not described.

Trastuzumab

Trastuzumab is a humanized mouse IgG1 mAB with selective affinity for the human epidermal growth factor 2 protein, HER2. Traztuzumab is approved for the treatment of HER2-overexpressing metastatic breast cancer. Rates of severe HR to trastuzumab range from 0.6% to 5% with the bulk of reports in the literature reporting mild-to-moderate infusion reactions characterized by fevers or chills in 40% of patients.[71] The current recommendation of the manufacturer is to permanently discontinue trastuzumab in those who develop anaphylaxis, angioedema, or acute respiratory distress syndrome. The first reports of desensitization to trastuzumab in 2002 were in 2 female patients with metastatic breast cancer: one who developed urticaria and palmar pruritus after her third infusion and severe flushing, vaginal itching, nausea, vomiting, rigors, and angioedema of the face, lips, and tongue at the fourth infusion. Positive intradermal skin testing (0.5 mg/mL) was consistent with type I hypersensitivity. The second patient developed diffuse pruritus after 10 months of therapy with trastuzumab and then had throat tightness in the first minute of her infusion. Skin testing on prick and intradermal was negative. Desensitization protocols first 5 steps involved dose escalation starting with a 5-μg/mL solution and the final 10 steps used a 1-mg/mL solution. Both patients experienced hypersensitivity symptoms, the first with angioedema of the tongue and urticaria and the second diffuse pruritus during the desensitization protocol.[72]

Brennan and colleagues[38] described 3 patients and, unlike rituximab, HRs to trastuzumab occurred after multiple exposures to trastuzumab. Skin testing was positive in the 3 patients; they underwent 29 successful RDDs. Melamed and Stahlman[72] reported the induction of tolerance by performing weekly subcutaneous immunotherapy with trastuzumab. Two patients who underwent a 15-step desensitization were continued on subcutaneous injections with trastuzumab. During the first week, patients received daily injections of 15 mg and increased the frequency to 3 injections over the second week. During weeks 3 to 10, 20-mg injections were given twice weekly followed by weekly 20-mg injections thereafter for as long as patients were on trastuzumab therapy. This protocol worked for 1 patient with postinfusion reactions of rigors, chills, and occasional hives for several months, who was able to continue on trastuzumab infusions for 3 years with no further allergic symptoms.

This approach suggests that the desensitized state can be maintained as long as continuous exposure to the agent is not limited by its toxicity but the risk of antibody formation may limit its therapeutic efficacy.

SUMMARY

BAs are important therapeutic tools, but their use may be limited by adverse drug reactions. Procedures for management of BA-induced reactions, including preventive diagnostic work-up and desensitization, are becoming available in the clinical setting. The knowledge of such procedures may be useful to increase the safety profile of current and coming BAs.

REFERENCES

1. Kotsovilis S, Andreakos E. Therapeutic human monoclonal antibodies in inflammatory diseases. Methods Mol Biol 2014;1060:37–59.
2. Li GN, Wang SP, Xue X, et al. Monoclonal antibody-related drug for cancer therapy. Drug Discov Ther 2013;7(5):178–84.
3. Buss NA, Henderson SJ, McFarlane M, et al. Monoclonal antibody therapeutics: history and future. Curr Opin Pharmacol 2012;12(5):615–22.
4. Borchers AT, Leibushor N, Cheema GS, et al. Immune mediated adverse effects of biological used in the treatment of rheumatic diseases. J Autoimmun 2011;37: 273–88.
5. Vultaggio A, Nencini F, Pratesi S, et al. Manifestations of anti-drug antibodies response: hypersensitivity and infusion reactions. J Int Cyt Res, in press.
6. Pichler WJ. Adverse side-effects to biologicals. Allergy 2006;61(8):912–20.
7. Maggi E, Vultaggio A, Matucci A. Acute infusion reactions induced by monoclonal antibody therapy. Expert Rev Clin Immunol 2011;7:55–63.

8. Lenz HJ. Management and preparedness for infusion and hypersensitivity reactions. Oncologist 2007;12:601–9.

9. Matucci A, Pratesi S, Petroni G, et al. Allergological in vitro and in vivo evaluation of patients with hypersensitivity reactions to infliximab. Clin Exp Allergy 2013; 43(6):659–64.

10. Scherer K, Spoerl D, Bircher AJ. Adverse drug reactions to biologics. J Dtsch Dermatol Ges 2010;8(6):411–26.

11. Proctor L, Renzulli B, Warren S, et al. Monoclonal antibody-stimulated serum sickness. Transfusion 2004;44:955.

12. Gamarra RM, McGraw SD, Drelichman VS, et al. Serum sickness-like reactions in patients receiving intravenous infliximab. J Emerg Med 2006;30(1):41–4.

13. D'Arcy CA, Mannik M. Serum sickness secondary to treatment with the murine-human chimeric antibody IDEC-C2B8 (rituximab). Arthritis Rheum 2001;44: 1717–8.

14. Pilette C, Coppens N, Houssiayu FA, et al. Severe serum sickness-like syndrome after omalizumab therapy for asthma. J Allergy Clin Immunol 2007;120(4):972–3.

15. Hellwing K, Schimrigk S, Fischer M, et al. Allergic and nonallergic delayed infusion reactions during natalizumab therapy. Arch Neurol 2008;65(5):656–8.

16. Cuker A, Coles AJ, Sullivan H, et al. A distinctive form of immune thrombocytopenia in a phase 2 study of alemtuzumab for the treatment of relapsing-remitting multiple sclerosis. Blood 2011;118(24):6299–305.

17. Berzuini A, Montanelli F, Prati D. Hemolytic anemia after eculizumab in paroxysmal nocturnal hemoglobinuria. N Engl J Med 2010;363(10):993–4.

18. Calogiuri G, Ventura MT, Mason L, et al. Hypersensitivity reactons to last generation chimeric, humanized and human recombinant monoclonal antibodies for therapeutic use. Curr Pharm Des 2008;14:2883–91.

19. Bremmer M, Deng A, Gaspari A. A mechanism-based classification of dermatologic reactions to biologic agents used in the treatment of cutaneous disease. Part 1. Dermatitis 2009;20:182–92.

20. Vergara G, Silvestre JF, Betlloch I, et al. Cutaneous drug eruption to infliximab: report of 4 cases with an interface dermatitis pattern. Arch Dermatol 2002;138: 1258–9.

21. Bremmer M, Deng A, Gaspari A. A mechanism-based classification of dermatologic reactions to biologic agents used in the treatment of cutaneous disease. Part 2. Dermatitis 2009;20:243–56.

22. Lin WL, Lin WC, Yang JY, et al. Fatal toxic epidermal necrolysis associated with cetuximab in a patient with colon cancer. J Clin Oncol 2008;26:2779–80.

23. Sfikakis PP, Iliopoulos A, Elezoglou A, et al. Psoriasis induced by anti-tumor necrosis factor therapy: a paradoxical adverse reactrion. Arthritis Rheum 2005; 52(8):2513–8.

24. Lenz HJ. Anti-EGFR mechanism of action: antitumor effect and underlying cause of adverse events. Oncology (Williston Park) 2006;20:5–13.

25. Murdaca G, Spanò F, Puppo F. Selective TNF-a inhibitor induced-injection site reactions. Expert Opin Drug Saf 2013;12(2):187–93.

26. Vultaggio A, Maggi E, Matucci A. Immediate adverse reactions to biologicals: from pathogenic mechanisms to prophylactic management. Curr Opin Allergy Clin Immunol 2011;11(3):262–8.

27. Wing M. Monoclonal antibody first dose cytokine release syndrome - mechanisms and prediction. J Immunotoxicology 2008;5:11–5.

28. Brennan FR, Morton Dill L, Spindeldreher S, et al. Safety and immunotoxicity assessment of immunomodulatory monoclonal antibodies. MAbs 2010;2(3):233–55.

29. Baert F, Noman M, Vermeire S, et al. Influence of immunogenicity on the long-term efficacy of infliximab in Crohn's disease. N Engl J Med 2003;348(7): 601–8.

30. Svenson M, Geborek P, Saxne T, et al. Monitoring patients treated with anti-TNF-α biopharmaceuticals: assessing serum infliximab and anti-infliximab antibodies. Rheumatology 2007;46:1828–34.

31. Finkelman FD. Anaphylaxis: lessons from mouse model. J Allergy Clin Immunol 2007;120:506–15.

32. Georgitis JW, Browning MC, Steiner D, et al. Anaphylaxis and desensitization to the murine monoclonal antibody used for renal graft rejection. Ann Allergy 1991; 66:343–7.

33. Stubenrauch K, Wessels U, Birnboeck H, et al. Subset analysis of patients experiencing clinical events of a potentially immunogenic nature in the pivotal clinical trials of tocilizumab for rheumatoid arthritis: evaluation of an anti-drug antibody ELISA using clinical adverse event-driven immunogenicity testing. Clin Ther 2010;32:1597–609.

34. Bavbek S, Aydın O, Ataman S, et al. Injection-site reaction to etanercept: role of skin test in the diagnosis of such reaction and successful desensitization. Allergy 2011;66(9):1256–7.

35. Munoz-Cano R, Carnes J, Sanchez-Lopez J, et al. Biological agents: new drugs, old problems. J Allergy Clin Immunol 2010;126:394–5.

36. Vultaggio A, Matucci A, Nencini F, et al. Anti-infliximab IgE and non IgE antibodies and induction of infusion-related severe anaphylactic reactions. Allergy 2010;65:657–61.

37. Vultaggio A, Matucci A, Nencini F, et al. Drug-specific th2 cells and ige antibodies in a patient with anaphylaxis to rituximab. Int Arch Allergy Immunol 2012;359:321–6.

38. Brennan PJ, Bouza TR, Hsu FI, et al. Hypersensitivity reactions to mAbs:105 desensitizations in 23 patients, from evalutaion to treatment. J Allergy Clin Immunol 2009;124:1259–66.

39. Vultaggio A, Matucci A, Parronchi P, et al. Safety and tolerability of infliximab therapy: suggestions and criticisms based on wide clinical experience. Int J Immunopathol Pharmacol 2008;21:367–74.

40. Lee TW, Singh R, Fedorak RN. A one-hour infusion of infliximab during maintenance therapy is safe and well tolerated: a prospective cohort study. Aliment Pharmacol Ther 2001;34:181–7.

41. Chung CH, Mirakhur B, Chan E, et al. Cetuximab-induced anaphylaxis and IgE specific for galactose-α-1,3-galactose. N Engl J Med 2008;358:1109–17.

42. Price KS, Hamilton RG. Anaphylactoid reactions in two patients after omalizumab administration after successful long-term therapy. Allergy Asthma Proc 2007;28:313–9.

43. Steele RH, Limaye S, Cleland B, et al. Hypersensitivity reactions to the polysorbate contained in recombinant erythropoietin and darbepoietin. Nephrology (Carlton) 2005;10:317–20.

44. Torres MJ, Chaves P, Blanca-Lopez N, et al. T-cell involvement in delayed type hypersensitivity reactions to infliximab. J Allergy Clin Immunol 2011;128(6): 1365–7.

45. Moneret-Vautrin DA, Morisset M, Vignaud JM, et al. T cell mediated allergy to abciximab. Allergy 2002;57:269–70.

46. Winfield H, Lain E, Horn T, et al. Eosinophilic cellulitis like reaction to subcutaneous etanercept injection. Arch Dermatol 2006;142(2):218–20.

47. Werth VP, Levinson AI. Etanercept-induced injection site reactions, mechanistic insights from clinical fidings and immunohistochemistry. Arch Dermatol 2001; 137:953–5.
48. Benucci M, Mandredi M, Saviola G, et al. Correlation between atopy and hypersensitivity reactions during therapy with three different TNF-alpha blocking agents in rheumatoid arthritis. Clin Exp Rheumatol 2009;27(2):333–6.
49. Maneiro JR, Salgado E, Gomez-Reino JJ. Immunogenicity of monoclonal antibodies against tumor necrosis factor used in chronic immune-mediated Inflammatory conditions: systematic review and meta-analysis. JAMA Intern Med 2013;173(15):1416–28.
50. Lee S, Ballow M. Monoclonal antibodies and fusion proteins and their complications: targeting B cells in autoimmune disease. J Allergy Clin Immunol 2010;125: 814–20.
51. Sehn LH, Donaldson J, Filewich A, et al. Rapid infusion rituximab in combination with corticosteroid-containing chemotherapy or as maintenance therapy is well tolerated and can safetly be delivered in the community setting. Blood 2007; 109:4171–3.
52. Anderson PJ. Tumor necrosis factor inhibitors: clinical implications of their different immunogenicity profiles. Semin Arthritis Rheum 2005;34(Suppl 1):19–22.
53. Du Pan SM, Dehler S, Ciurea A, et al, Swiss Clinical Quality Management Physicians. Comparison of drug retention rates and causes of drug discontinuation between anti-tumor necrosis factor agents in rheumatoid arthritis. Arthritis Rheum 2009;61:560–8.
54. Rutgeerts P, Feagan BG, Lichtenstein GR, et al. Comparison of scheduled and episodic treatment strategies of infliximab in Crohn's disease. Gastroenterology 2004;126:402–13.
55. Lecluse LL, Piskin G, Mekkes JR, et al. Review and expert opinion on prevention and treatment of infliximab-related infusion reactions. Br J Dermatol 2008;159: 527–36.
56. Murdaca G, Colombo BM, Cagnati P, et al. Update upon efficacy and safety of TNF-a inhibitors. Expert Opin Drug Saf 2012;11(1):1–5.
57. Vogel WH. Infusion reactions: diagnosis, assessment and management. Clin J Oncol Nurs 2010;14:E10–21.
58. Mire-Sluis AR, Barrett YC, Devanarayan V, et al. Reccomendations for the design and optimization of immunoassay used in the detection of host antibodies against biotechnology products. J Immunol Methods 2004;289:1–16.
59. Rispens T, de Vrieze H, de Groot E, et al. Antibodies to constant domains of therapeutic monoclonal antibodies: anti-hinge antibodies in immunogenicity testing. J Immunol Methods 2012;375(1–2):93–9.
60. Aarden L, Ruuls SR, Wolbink G. Immunogenicity of anti-tumor necrosis factor antibodies-toward improved methods of anti-antibody measurement. Curr Opin Immunol 2008;20(4):431–5.
61. Serarslan G, Okuyucu E, Melek I, et al. Widespread maculopapular rash due to intramuscular interferon beta-1a during the treatment of multiple sclerosis. Mult Scler 2008;14:259–61.
62. Poreaux C, Waton J, Cuny JF, et al. Evaluation d'une pratique de prise en charge des taxidermies dues a l'interferon: a propos de 15 cas. Ann Dermatol Venereol 2009;136:s317–8.
63. Castells MC, Tennant NM, Sloane DE, et al. Hypersensitivity reactions to chemotherapy: outcomes and safety of rapid desensitization in 413 cases. J Allergy Clin Immunol 2008;122(3):574–80.

64. Puchner TC, Kugathasan S, Kelly KJ, et al. Successful desensitization and therapeutic use of infliximab in adult and pediatric Crohn's disease patients with prior anaphylactic reaction. Inflamm Bowel Dis 2001;7(1):34–7.
65. Cheifetz A, Smedley M, Martin S, et al. The incidence and management of infusion reactions to infliximab: a large center experience. Am J Gastroenterol 2003; 98(6):1315–24.
66. Duburque C, Lelong J, Iacob R, et al. Successful induction of tolerance to infliximab in patients with Crohn's disease and prior severe infusion reactions. Aliment Pharmacol Ther 2006;24(5):851–8.
67. Rodriguez-Jimenez B, Dominguez-Ortega J, González-Herrada C, et al. Successful adalimumab desensitization after generalized urticaria and rhinitis. J Investig Allergol Clin Immunol 2009;19(3):246–7.
68. Bavbek S, Ataman S, Bankova L, et al. Injection site reaction to adalimumab: positive skin test and successful rapid desensitization. Allergol Immunopathol 2013;41(3):204–6.
69. Saif MW, Syrigos KI, Hotchkiss S, et al. Successful desensitization with cetuximab after an infusion reaction to panitumumab in patients with metastatic colorectal cancer. Cancer Chemother Pharmacol 2009;65(1):107–12.
70. Jerath MR, Kwan M, Kannarkat M, et al. A desensitization protocol for the mAb cetuximab. J Allergy Clin Immunol 2009;123:260–2.
71. Cook-Bruns N. Retrospective analysis of the safety of herceptin immunotherapy in metastatic breast cancer. Oncology 2001;61(Suppl 2):S58–66.
72. Melamad J, Stahlman J. Rapid desensitization and rush immunotherapy to trastuzumab. J Allergy Clin Immunol 2002;110:813–4.
73. Jacquener S, Moneret-Vautrin DA, Bihain B. Mammalian meat-induced anaphylaxis: clinical relevance of anti-galactose-a-1,3-galactose IgE confirmed by means of skin tests to cetuximab. J Allergy Clin Immunol 2009;124:603–5.

Hypersensitivity to Antiepileptic Drugs

Young-Min Ye, MD[a], Bernard Yu-Hor Thong, MBBS, FRCP(Edin)[b], Hae-Sim Park, MD, PhD[a],*

KEYWORDS

- Antiepileptic drugs • Drug hypersensitivity • Pharmacogenetics
- Severe cutaneous adverse reactions

KEY POINTS

- Antiepileptic drug allergy is a rare but potentially fatal adverse reaction, associated most commonly with phenytoin, carbamazepine, and lamotrigine.
- Antiepileptic drug allergy generally occurs on first exposure to the drug, with symptoms such as skin rash, fever, and internal organ involvement that develop within several weeks of drug exposure.
- Early diagnosis is essential because primary treatment starts with cessation of the implicated drug.
- Avoidance of other aromatic anticonvulsants (eg, phenytoin, carbamazepine, phenobarbital, primidone, oxcarbazepine, and lamotrigine) is recommended in patients who develop allergic reactions to any one of these agents due to a high degree of cross-reactivity among them.
- Pharmacogenetic testing for HLA allele B*1502 should be considered before commencing carbamazepine in Han Chinese, South Asian, and East Indian patients.

INTRODUCTION

Adverse reactions to antiepileptic drugs (AEDs) may lead to treatment failure, morbidity, and mortality from both epilepsy and the adverse drug reaction (ADR).[1,2] It may also impair the quality of life for epilepsy patients.[1] Most adverse reactions to AEDs are predictable, dose-dependent, and pharmacologic-associated type A ADRs, which are usually reversible after discontinuation of the offending drugs. However, type B ADRs occur unexpectedly in susceptible patients and are pathogenically unrelated to the mechanism of action of the drugs. Despite the relatively low

---

The authors have no conflict of interest to disclose.

[a] Department of Allergy and Clinical Immunology, Ajou University School of Medicine, 206 World cup-ro, Yeongtong-gu, Suwon 443-721, Republic of Korea; [b] Department of Rheumatology, Allergy and Immunology, Tan Tock Seng Hospital, 11 Jalan Tan Tock Seng, Singapore 308433, Singapore
* Corresponding author.
E-mail address: hspark@ajou.ac.kr

Immunol Allergy Clin N Am 34 (2014) 633–643
http://dx.doi.org/10.1016/j.iac.2014.04.005
0889-8561/14/$ – see front matter © 2014 Elsevier Inc. All rights reserved.

incidence, drug hypersensitivity reactions (DHRs) that are type B may result in potentially fatal outcomes.[3] As for antibiotics, conventional aromatic AEDs are a common cause of drug allergy (immunologic-mediated DHRs) in hospitalized and general populations.[4,5] AED DHRs present with a variety of different clinical manifestations ranging from skin rashes and mucosal involvement to systemic involvement (fever, hepatitis, lymphadenopathy, eosinophilia, and blood dyscrasias). Cutaneous eruptions are the more common manifestation. However, severe cutaneous adverse reactions (SCARs) are not rare in AED users.[2] These include Stevens-Johnson syndrome (SJS), toxic epidermal necrolysis (TEN), drug-induced hypersensitivity syndrome (DIHS), drug reaction with eosinophilia and systemic symptoms (DRESS), and acute generalized exanthematous pustulosis (AGEP). The pathogenesis of AED DHR has not been fully elucidated. Bioactivation, detoxification, covalent adduct formation, presentation to the immune system, and consequent formation of antibody and T-cell immune effectors have been suggested.[6] The incidence and severity of AED DHRs may be affected by various factors that include age, gender, genetics, and the drug itself.[2] Identifying susceptible individuals and risk factors, as well as close clinical monitoring during the latent period are key to the prevention of AED DHR. This article summarizes the epidemiology, pathogenic mechanisms, risk factors, clinical features, and management of allergic reactions to the aromatic AEDs carbamazepine (CBZ), phenytoin (PHT), and lamotrigine (LTG).

EPIDEMIOLOGY

The prevalence of DHRs to AEDs varies according to the populations enrolled, offending drugs, and study design. Skin rash is a common adverse reaction of AEDs and is a leading cause of withdrawal from some AED trials.[7]

A retrospective chart review reported that the average rate of AED-associated rash was 2.8%, resulting in a rate of AED discontinuation of 2.1%.[8] Most reports on ADRs to AEDs have shown higher rates of rash with CBZ (5%–17% of the patients taking CBZ), PHT (5%–7%), and LTG (5%–10%).[8] Severe mucocutaneous reactions with internal organ involvement such as DIHS-DRESS and SJS-TEN are estimated between 1 in 1000 and 1 in 10,000 exposures.[9] The incidence of AED DHRs in patients with head injuries increases to 1 in 100.[10]

SJS-TEN can lead to significant disability or mortality (ranging from 10% to 40%) despite the low incidence.[11] Aromatic AEDs (including CBZ, PHT, phenobarbital, and LTG) are also associated with these SCARs.[9] In addition, aromatic AEDs are significantly associated with IgE-mediated (immediate) type I and cell-mediated (nonimmediate or delayed) type IV DHRs, with a reported odds ratio of 2.15 and 6.06, respectively.[12]

Cross-sensitivity among aromatic AEDs (particularly high in female patients) is reported to be 30% to 58%.[8,13] Among various AEDs, PHT and CBZ were reported as the two drugs with the most frequent cross-reactivity.[13] In addition, cross-reactivity between CBZ and tricyclic antidepressant agents has also been reported based on their structural similarity with the tricyclic nucleus.[14]

RISK FACTORS
Genetic Factors

Genetic markers are useful to predict individuals susceptible to AED DHR (**Box 1**). HLA alleles represent a major determinant of AED DHR since 2004 when Chung and colleagues[15] first reported a strong association of HLA-B*1502 in Han Chinese patients with CBZ-induced SCARs. This strong association was further confirmed by other

Box 1			
Genetic factors associated with carbamazepine-induced DHRs			
	No. Positive for Target Genotype/ Total No.		
Ethnicity	**Case**	**Control**	**Odds Ratio (95% CI)**
HLA-B*1502			
Whites			
Alfirevic et al,[28] 2006	0/2	0/43	NA
Lonjou et al,[29] 2008	4/12	1/1290	644.50 (64.69–6431.36)
Han-Chinese			
Hung et al,[16] 2006	59/60	6/144	1357.00 (159.84–11,520.40)
Shi et al,[19] 2012	13/18	12/93	17.55 (5.31–58.06)
Wu et al,[20] 2010	8/8	4/50	114.83 (6.25–2110.92)
Chang et al,[23] 2011	12/16	47/300	16.15 (4.99–52.22)
Thai			
Locharernkul et al,[21] 2008	6/6	8/42	52.76 (2.70–1031.31)
Tassaneeyakul et al,[22] 2010	37/42	5/42	54.76 (14.62–205.13)
Korean			
Kim et al,[26] 2011	1/7	2/485	40.25 (3.20–265.09)
Malaysian			
Then et al,[24] 2011	6/6	0/8	221.00 (3.85–12,694.65)
Chang et al,[23] 2011	12/16	47/300	16.15 (4.57–62.4)
Japanese			
Kashiwagi et al,[27] 2008	0/2	1/371	49.40 (1.59–1531.08)
Indian			
Mehta et al,[25] 2009	6/8	0/10	54.60 (2.25–1326.20)
HLA-A*3101			
Han-Chinese			
Hung et al,[16] 2006	8/31[a]	4/144	12.17 (3.6–41.2)
Japanese			
Ozeki et al,[30] 2011	37/61	47/376	9.5 (5.6–16.3)
Korean			
Kim et al,[26] 2011	13/24	50/485	10.3 (4.4–24.2)
Whites			
McCormack et al,[47] 2011	38/145	10/257	9.12 (4.03–20.65)

Abbreviation: NA, not applicable.
[a] Subjects with maculopapular exanthema and DIHS-DRESS.

extended cohorts of Han Chinese[16–20] and other Asian populations (including Thai,[21,22] Malaysian,[23,24] and Indian[25] groups). This has led the Food and Drug Administration to recommend screening HLA-B*1502 allele before starting CBZ treatment in individuals from genetically at-risk populations. However, the strong association was not replicated in other populations, including Korean, Japanese, and whites.[26–29] By contrast, HLA-A*3101 was reported to be associated with CBZ-induced hypersensitivity in populations with a low frequency of HLA-B*1502.[26,28,30] A recent study suggested that HLA-B*1502 represents a biomarker to predict the involvement of skin detachment in subjects with CBZ-induced SJS-TEN; however, HLA-A*3101 was related to CBZ-induced nonblistering hypersensitivity reactions, such as maculopapular exanthema (MPE) and DRESS.[16,31] Ethnicity seems to play an important role in the association between HLA markers and AED DHRs. Studies in white populations show that the overall rate of CBZ-related SJS-TEN is very low and estimated at 1 to 6 per 10,000 newly exposed patients. In some Asian populations, HLA-B*1502 was also observed in patients with DHRs to other AEDs such as LTG and PHT.[21] A potential protective role of HLA-B*0702 was suggested in subjects with CBZ-induced SCARs.[28] A few studies suggested other potential genetic markers associated with AED DHR. Three single nucleotide polymorphisms of the heat shock protein-70 gene cluster in white patients with CBZ-induced SCARs.[28,32] A polymorphism in the promoter region of the tumor necrosis factor α gene is also suggested as a predisposing factor for CBZ DHR.[33]

Age

Drug metabolism is usually age-dependent and an increase in reactive metabolites may result in increased susceptibility to DHRs in children compared with adults, all drugs included.[34] Messenheimer and colleagues[35] reported that LTG-induced rashes are more common in children than in adults. The incidence of SJS in patients with LTG has also been estimated to be 10 times higher in children. The occurrence of DHRs resulting in discontinuation of the offending drugs tends to be more frequent in elderly patients. Various factors, such as age-related pharmacokinetic changes, altered homeostatic mechanisms, and combined medications and diseases, affect the prevalence and severity of AED DHRs.[3] Children younger than age 12 years and adults older than age 64 years have higher risks for SCAR.[11]

Drug-Related Factors

A recent multivariate analysis suggested that a history of rash with an AED was the strongest predictor of LTG-induced rash with an odds ratio of 3.62.[36] Concurrent medications can affect the susceptibility to developing allergic DHRs. A combination of valproate with LTG (particularly in patients taking a regular starting dose of LTG) has been reported to increase the risk of LTG-induced DHR.[37] In addition, the prevalence of AED DHRs increased five times in patients with a history of AED-induced eruption.[8] Cutaneous hypersensitivity reactions are more frequent in adults with PHT, LTG, and CBZ, and less common (<1%) with other AEDs.[38]

Disease-Related Factors

Immunologic disorders, such as systemic lupus erythematosus, corticosteroid treatment, and a family history of severe skin eruptions, are risk factors for AED DHRs.[39] Causality has not been conclusively proven. However, reactivation of human herpes viruses (HHVs) 6 and 7, cytomegalovirus, and Epstein-Barr virus may occur in association with DIHS-DRESS.[40,41] Some patients with CBZ-induced DRESS had high levels of anti–HHV-6 antibodies and HHV-6 DNA copies in their sera.[42] **Box 2** is a list of potential risk factors for antiepileptic drug hypersensitivity.

Box 2
Potential risk factors for antiepileptic drug hypersensitivity

Previous history of DHRs to other AEDs

Family history of AED DHR

Younger or elderly patients

Presence of viral infections (HHV-6, HHV-7, cytomegalovirus, Epstein-Barr virus)

Head injury

HLA-B*1502 Han Chinese and Southeast Asian carriers

HLA-A*3101 European and North Asian carriers

PATHOGENESIS

The pathogenesis of AED DHRs seems to be multifactorial. There has been significant evidence for immunologic mechanisms. A sensitization period of at least 7 to 10 days is required in patients with an AED DHR, resulting in a latent period before onset of symptoms and signs of DHR. Treatment dose of AEDs is not related to the onset and severity of DHRs. Immediate type I and immune complex-mediated type III hypersensitivity reactions are less frequently associated with AEDs. Instead, most DHRs to AEDs are mediated by nonimmediate (delayed) type IV reactions in which a specific HLA allele can activate drug-specific T cells with the offending AED. HLA molecules present endogenous or processed exogenous antigens to T cells that induce an adaptive immune response. The T-cell receptor (TCR) on the effector cells recognize the complex with drug-peptide and specific HLA molecules on the antigen-presenting cell, leading to the release of immune mediators, which then initiate an AED DHR.[39,43–45]

Histopathological and immunologic findings suggest that AED DHRs are mainly mediated by adaptive immunity that involves major histocompatibility-restricted drug presentation, activation, and the clonal expansion of effector T cells.[43] CBZ and its reactive metabolites have been shown to directly activate T cells, confirming the hypothesis of direct pharmacologic interaction of drugs or metabolites with immune receptors.[45] In addition, the activated T cells from patients with CBZ-induced SJS released more than five times higher levels of interferon-γ and granulysin on CBZ stimulation compared with controls treated with gabapentin.[43] CBZ is metabolized as 30 metabolites in the human liver. A previous ex vivo experiment revealed that a high concentration of acridine (a CBZ metabolite) could trigger IL-5 production in T cells of susceptible individuals with a reduced threshold for secretion, such as individuals following a viral infection or with altered drug metabolism due to concurrent medications.[46] An altered balance between drug bioactivation and detoxification pathways may elevate levels of an AED or its reactive metabolites that bind irreversibly to cellular proteins and present to the immune system in the form of drug-modified proteins.[3]

Recent advances in pharmacogenomics studies demonstrate a strong genetic association between HLAs and specific drug-induced SCARs. A strong association between HLA-B*1502 and CBZ-induced SJS-TEN has been proven in the Han Chinese and Southeast Asian countries such as Hong Kong, Singapore, Thailand, Malaysia, and India.[15–25] However, not all carriers of HLA-B*1502 have SJS when exposed to CBZ as described above. Ko and colleagues[43] identified a specific clonotype of TCR shared by patients with CBZ-induced SJS-TEN undetected in tolerant patients. They emphasized that CBZ-specific HLA-B*1502-restricted cytotoxic T-lymphocytes shared common TCR clonotypes, recognized CBZ or peptide-HLA B*1502 complexes, and induced SJS-TEN.[43] A recent genome-wide analyses reported that HLA-A*3101 was significantly associated with CBZ-induced DHRs in Korean, Japanese, and European populations.[26,30,47] A relationship between HLA genotype and clinical phenotype of CBZ-induced DHRs determined by the extent of skin detachment was also demonstrated. The HLA-B*1502 allele showed increased sensitivity and a relative risk for CBZ-induced SJS-TEN with more extensive skin detachment, with no association in less severe reactions without detachment, such as MPE and DRESS in Han Chinese populations.[16,31]

CLINICAL FEATURES

AED DHRs may present as mild cutaneous eruptions,[8,48] such as MPE, erythema multiforme, and fixed drug eruptions, or as SCAR.[49] SCAR manifestations include

SJS-TEN, DIHS-DRESS,[50,51] AGEP,[52] and adverse reactions with overlapping clinical features.[53] The aromatic AEDs PHT, phenobarbitone, CBZ, and LTG are all classified as high-risk drugs[38,54] with a predisposition to development of SCARs following long latent periods of up to 2 to 6 weeks from initiation of the drug. They may also be a cause of organ-specific allergic DHRs, such as leukocytosis, hepatitis,[55] acute tubulointerstitial nephritis[56] or acute kidney injury, myocarditis,[57] and thyroiditis.[58]

DIAGNOSIS

Because nonimmediate DHRs to AEDs are more common than immediate reactions, skin patch tests have shown to be useful in the diagnosis of AED DHRs and are safe.[59,60] **Box 3** presents common patch test concentrations for AEDs. The positive predictive value of tests under optimal conditions are reported to be as high as 80% to 90%, depending on the drug tested, with positive tests being drug-specific (ie, CBZ and PHT) and reaction-specific (ie, DRESS). Intradermal tests with delayed readings at 48 hours or 72 hours are used in lieu of patch tests in certain centers worldwide. However, the sensitivity, specificity and predictive values to diagnose nonimmediate DHRs to AEDs have not been well studied.

In vitro tests, such as the lymphocyte transformation test (LTT) and the lymphocyte toxicity assay (LTA), are more commonly used in research centers in view of technical demands to establish and interpret these tests. The sensitivity of the LTT and the LTA are around 70% and 90%, respectively, for AEDs. In addition, the positive and negative predictive values of the tests in highly imputable cases are high.[61] Drug provocation tests should only be carried out in cases in which the history is not suggestive of AED DHRs, in-vivo or in-vitro tests are not conclusive or not available, and where the index reaction was not SCAR or an immunobullous reaction. The benefits of reaching a diagnosis of AED DHR must be carefully weighed against the risks of provoking a DHR during drug-provocation testing.[62]

Although pharmacogenetic testing for the HLA-B*1502 allele before the initiation of CBZ in ethnic Asians has become the standard of care in Hong Kong and Taiwan, and is recommended in Singapore, it remains inconclusive whether this is cost-effective to prevent SJS-TEN.[63]

MANAGEMENT

When AED DHR is suspected, the suspected AED should be stopped immediately. Mild cutaneous eruptions can be symptomatically treated and usually resolve with few sequelae.

Treatment modalities for SJS-TEN, including fluid replacement, maintenance of thermoregulation, dressings and wound debridement, ophthalmologic treatment, nutrition, and prevention and treatment of infection, apply to many different

Box 3		
Common patch test concentrations for AEDs		
Drug Name	**Concentration (weight/volume percentage) (%)**	**Vehicle**
Carbamazepine	1, 10	Petrolatum
Phenytoin	5, 10	Petrolatum
Lamotrigine	10, 50	Petrolatum
Phenobarbital	5, 10	Petrolatum

drugs and are not specific to AEDs. Despite on-going controversy about to whether high-dose intravenous immunoglobulins (IVIGs) at a dose of 2 g/kg reduces mortality in TEN,[64] up to 50% of practitioners worldwide continue to use this as the most common form of immunomodulatory therapy for TEN.[65] The evidence for IVIGs has been confounded by data predominantly from retrospective case series with variable inclusion criteria, high-risk and low-risk subjects, and subjects with TEN comprising those with SJS-TEN overlap as well. A recent systematic review and meta-analysis of the literature did not indicate any clinical benefit of IVIGs in children and adults.[66]

There is renewed interest in the use of the calcineurin inhibitor, cyclosporin,[67,68] which is the second most commonly used treatment of TEN in a worldwide survey.[64] Development of acute kidney injury due to TEN, hypovolemia, or sepsis often precludes the initiation or dose optimization of cyclosporin.

The use of systemic corticosteroids in SJS-TEN was evaluated in a case-control study based on data collected from EuroSCAR and RegiSCAR studies.[69] The previous use of corticosteroids prolonged the period of disease progression by 2.2 days (95% CI 1.1–3.2) with no influence on disease severity or mortality and delayed time to onset of SJS-TEN with exposure to high-risk drugs by 7.1 days (CI −0.2–14.5). Although there have been several case series and case reports (of which one showed histologic improvement of epidermal necrolysis on serial skin biopsies),[70] there are no controlled studies on the use of systemic corticosteroids in TEN. Although a tapering course of systemic corticosteroids is often used in the treatment of SJS[71] and DIHS,[72] there have been no controlled studies supporting this. Certain groups have recommended the use of combinations of a prolonged course of high-dose corticosteroids, IVIGs, and antivirals such as valganciclovir (if viral reactivation is confirmed) in the treatment of severe, life-threatening, or refractory visceral involvement in DIHS-DRESS.[73] AGEP is usually self-limiting, although oral corticosteroids may be useful to hasten recovery in some prolonged cases.[74]

SUMMARY AND FUTURE DIRECTION

AEDs commonly induce DHRs and sometimes result in fatal outcomes such as SCARs. CBZ, PHT, and LTG are recognized as the major culprits of AED-induced DHRs. Two HLA alleles have been suggested as potential genetic markers for CBZ DHRs in various populations: HLA-B*1502 for Han Chinese and South Asian populations, as well as HLA-A*3101 allele in European and North Asian populations. Clinical predictors, such as a history of DHRs to aromatic AEDs, family history of DHR, age, and concurrent viral infections, can be used by physicians to minimize adverse reactions to an AED. Close monitoring during the initial latent period following AED initiation should also be observed. Further investigation to understand the pathogenic mechanisms (especially in aspects of genetics and immunologic mechanisms) will provide relevant in vivo and vitro testing and new therapeutic strategies for AED DHRs.

REFERENCES

1. Gilliam F, Carter J, Vahle V. Tolerability of antiseizure medications: implications for health outcomes. Neurology 2004;63(10 Suppl 4):S9–12.
2. Perucca P, Gilliam FG. Adverse effects of antiepileptic drugs. Lancet Neurol 2012;11(9):792–802.
3. Zaccara G, Franciotta D, Perucca E. Idiosyncratic adverse reactions to antiepileptic drugs. Epilepsia 2007;48(7):1223–44.
4. Gomes ER, Demoly P. Epidemiology of hypersensitivity drug reactions. Curr Opin Allergy Clin Immunol 2005;5(4):309–16.

5. Thong BY, Tan TC. Epidemiology and risk factors for drug allergy. Br J Clin Pharmacol 2011;71(5):684–700.

6. Leeder JS. Mechanisms of idiosyncratic hypersensitivity reactions to antiepileptic drugs. Epilepsia 1998;39(Suppl 7):S8–16.

7. Reunanen M, Dam M, Yuen AW. A randomised open multicentre comparative trial of lamotrigine and carbamazepine as monotherapy in patients with newly diagnosed or recurrent epilepsy. Epilepsy Res 1996;23(2):149–55.

8. Arif H, Buchsbaum R, Weintraub D, et al. Comparison and predictors of rash associated with 15 antiepileptic drugs. Neurology 2007;68(20):1701–9.

9. Mockenhaupt M, Messenheimer J, Tennis P, et al. Risk of Stevens-Johnson syndrome and toxic epidermal necrolysis in new users of antiepileptics. Neurology 2005;64(7):1134–8.

10. Bhargava P. Anticonvulsant hypersensitivity syndrome study of 60 cases. Indian J Dermatol Venereol Leprol 2001;67(6):317–9.

11. Chan HL, Stern RS, Arndt KA, et al. The incidence of erythema multiforme, Stevens-Johnson syndrome, and toxic epidermal necrolysis. A population-based study with particular reference to reactions caused by drugs among out-patients. Arch Dermatol 1990;126(1):43–7.

12. Handoko KB, van Puijenbroek EP, Bijl AH, et al. Influence of chemical structure on hypersensitivity reactions induced by antiepileptic drugs: the role of the aromatic ring. Drug Saf 2008;31(8):695–702.

13. Alvestad S, Lydersen S, Brodtkorb E. Cross-reactivity pattern of rash from current aromatic antiepileptic drugs. Epilepsy Res 2008;80(2–3):194–200.

14. Seitz CS, Pfeuffer P, Raith P, et al. Anticonvulsant hypersensitivity syndrome: cross-reactivity with tricyclic antidepressant agents. Ann Allergy Asthma Immunol 2006;97(5):698–702.

15. Chung WH, Hung SI, Hong HS, et al. Medical genetics: a marker for Stevens-Johnson syndrome. Nature 2004;428(6982):486.

16. Hung SI, Chung WH, Jee SH, et al. Genetic susceptibility to carbamazepine-induced cutaneous adverse drug reactions. Pharmacogenet Genomics 2006; 16(4):297–306.

17. Man CB, Kwan P, Baum L, et al. Association between HLA-B*1502 allele and antiepileptic drug-induced cutaneous reactions in Han Chinese. Epilepsia 2007;48(5):1015–8.

18. Tangamornsuksan W, Chaiyakunapruk N, Somkrua R, et al. Relationship between the HLA-B*1502 allele and carbamazepine-induced Stevens-Johnson syndrome and toxic epidermal necrolysis: a systematic review and meta-analysis. JAMA Dermatol 2013;149(9):1025–32.

19. Shi YW, Min FL, Qin B, et al. Association between HLA and Stevens-Johnson syndrome induced by carbamazepine in Southern Han Chinese: genetic markers besides B*1502? Basic Clin Pharmacol Toxicol 2012; 111(1):58–64.

20. Wu XT, Hu FY, An DM, et al. Association between caebamazepine-induced cutaneous adverse reactions and the HLA-B*1502 allele among patinets in central China. Epilepsy Behav 2010;19(3):405–8.

21. Locharernkul C, Loplumlert J, Limotai C, et al. Carbamazepine and phenytoin induced Stevens-Johnson syndrome is associated with HLA-B*1502 allele in Thai population. Epilepsia 2008;49(12):2087–91.

22. Tassaneeyakul W, Tiamkao S, Jantararoungtong T, et al. Association between HLA-B*1502 and carbamazepine-induced severe cutaneous adverse drug reactions in a Thai population. Epilepsia 2010;51(5):926–30.

23. Chang CC, Too CL, Murad S, et al. Association of HLA-B*1502 allele with carbamazepine-induced toxic epidermal necrolysis and Stevens-Johnson syndrome in the multi-ethnic Malaysian population. Int J Dermatol 2011;50(2):221–4.
24. Then SM, Rani ZZ, Raymond AA, et al. Frequency of the HLA-B*1502 allele contributing to carbamazepine-induced hypersensitivity reactions in a cohort of Malaysian epilepsy patients. Asian Pac J Allergy Immunol 2011;29(3):290–3.
25. Mehta TY, Prajapati LM, Mittal B, et al. Association of HLA-B*1502 allele and carbamazepine-induced Stevens-Johnson syndrome among Indians. Indian J Dermatol Venereol Leprol 2009;75(6):579–82.
26. Kim SH, Lee KW, Song WJ, et al. Carbamazepine-induced severe cutaneous adverse reactions and HLA genotypes in Koreans. Epilepsy Res 2011;97(1–2):190–7.
27. Kashiwagi M, Aihara M, Takahashi Y, et al. Human leukocyte antigen genotypes in carbamazepine-induced severe cutaneous adverse drug response in Japanese patients. J Dermatol 2008;35(10):683–5.
28. Alfirevic A, Jorgensen AL, Williamson PR, et al. HLA-B locus in Caucasian patients with carbamazepine hypersensitivity. Pharmacogenomics 2006;7(6):813–8.
29. Lonjou C, Borot N, Sekula P, et al. A European study of HLA-B in Stevens-Johnson syndrome and toxic epidermal necrolysis related to five high-risk drugs. Pharmacogenet Genomics 2008;18(2):99–107.
30. Ozeki T, Mushiroda T, Yowang A, et al. Genome-wide association study identifies HLA-A*3101 allele as a genetic risk factor for carbamazepine-induced cutaneous adverse drug reactions in Japanese population. Hum Mol Genet 2011;20(5):1034–41.
31. Hsiao YH, Hui RC, Wu T, et al. Genotype-phenotype association between HLA and carbamazepine-induced hypersensitivity reactions: Strength and clinical correlations. J Dermatol Sci 2014;73(2):101–9.
32. Alfirevic A, Mills T, Harrington P, et al. Serious carbamazepine-induced hypersensitivity reactions associated with the HSP70 gene cluster. Pharmacogenet Genomics 2006;16(4):287–96.
33. Pirmohamed M, Lin K, Chadwick D, et al. TNF promoter region gene polymorphisms in carbamazepine-hypersensitive patients. Neurology 2001;56(7):890–6.
34. Johnson TN. The development of drug metabolising enzymes and their influence on the susceptibility to adverse drug reactions in children. Toxicology 2003;192(1):37–48.
35. Messenheimer JA, Giorgi L, Risner ME. The tolerability of lamotrigine in children. Drug Saf 2000;22(4):303–12.
36. Hirsch LJ, Weintraub DB, Buchsbaum R, et al. Predictors of Lamotrigine-associated rash. Epilepsia 2006;47(2):318–22.
37. Messenheimer J, Mullens EL, Giorgi L, et al. Safety review of adult clinical trial experience with lamotrigine. Drug Saf 1998;18(4):281–96.
38. Sassolas B, Haddad C, Mockenhaupt M, et al. ALDEN, an algorithm for assessment of drug causality in Stevens-Johnson Syndrome and toxic epidermal necrolysis: comparison with case-control analysis. Clin Pharmacol Ther 2010;88(1):60–8.
39. Pichler WJ. Delayed drug hypersensitivity reactions. Ann Intern Med 2003;139(8):683–93.
40. Hashizume H, Takigawa M. Drug-induced hypersensitivity syndrome associated with cytomegalovirus reactivation: immunological characterization of pathogenic T cells. Acta Derm Venereol 2005;85(1):47–50.

41. Seishima M, Yamanaka S, Fujisawa T, et al. Reactivation of human herpesvirus (HHV) family members other than HHV-6 in drug-induced hypersensitivity syndrome. Br J Dermatol 2006;155(2):344–9.

42. Descamps V, Valance A, Edlinger C, et al. Association of human herpesvirus 6 infection with drug reaction with eosinophilia and systemic symptoms. Arch Dermatol 2001;137(3):301–4.

43. Ko TM, Chung WH, Wei CY, et al. Shared and restricted T-cell receptor use is crucial for carbamazepine-induced Stevens-Johnson syndrome. J Allergy Clin Immunol 2011;128(6):1266–76.e11.

44. Gomez E, Torres MJ, Mayorga C, et al. Immunologic evaluation of drug allergy. Allergy Asthma Immunol Res 2012;4(5):251–63.

45. Wu Y, Sanderson JP, Farrell J, et al. Activation of T cells by carbamazepine and carbamazepine metabolites. J Allergy Clin Immunol 2006;118(1):233–41.

46. Mathieu O, Picot MC, Gelisse P, et al. Effects of carbamazepine and metabolites on IL-2, IL-5, IL-6, IL-10 and IFN-gamma secretion in epileptic patients: the influence of co-medication. Pharmacol Rep 2011;63(1):86–94.

47. McCormack M, Alfirevic A, Bourgeois S, et al. HLA-A*3101 and carbamazepine-induced hypersensitivity reactions in Europeans. N Engl J Med 2011;364(12):1134–43.

48. Mockenhaupt M. Epidemiology of cutaneous adverse drug reactions. Chem Immunol Allergy 2012;97:1–17.

49. Bastuji-Garin S, Rzany B, Stern RS, et al. Clinical classification of cases of toxic epidermal necrolysis, Stevens-Johnson syndrome, and erythema multiforme. Arch Dermatol 1993;129(1):92–6.

50. Shiohara T, Inaoka M, Kano Y. Drug-induced hypersensitivity syndrome (DIHS): a reaction induced by a complex interplay among herpesviruses and antiviral and antidrug immune responses. Allergol Int 2006;55(1):1–8.

51. Kardaun SH, Sekula P, Valeyrie-Allanore L, et al. Drug reaction with eosinophilia and systemic symptoms (DRESS): an original multisystem adverse drug reaction. Results from the prospective RegiSCAR study. Br J Dermatol 2013;169(5):1071–80.

52. Son CH, Lee CU, Roh MS, et al. Acute generalized exanthematous pustulosis as a manifestation of carbamazepine hypersensitivity syndrome. J Investig Allergol Clin Immunol 2008;18(6):461–4.

53. Matsuda H, Saito K, Takayanagi Y, et al. Pustular-type drug-induced hypersensitivity syndrome/drug reaction with eosinophilia and systemic symptoms due to carbamazepine with systemic muscle involvement. J Dermatol 2013;40(2):118–22.

54. Mockenhaupt M, Viboud C, Dunant A, et al. Stevens-Johnson syndrome and toxic epidermal necrolysis: assessment of medication risks with emphasis on recently marketed drugs. The EuroSCAR-study. J Invest Dermatol 2008;128(1):35–44.

55. Hussaini SH, Farrington EA. Idiosyncratic drug-induced liver injury: an overview. Expert Opin Drug Saf 2007;6(6):673–84.

56. Koda R, Aoyagi R, Okazaki E, et al. Acute tubulointerstitial nephritis with multiple organ involvement including fatal adrenalitis: a case report with autopsy findings. Intern Med 2012;51(20):2917–22.

57. Salzman MB, Valderrama E, Sood SK. Carbamazepine and fatal eosinophilic myocarditis. N Engl J Med 1997;336(12):878–9.

58. Gupta A, Eggo MC, Uetrecht JP, et al. Drug-induced hypothyroidism: the thyroid as a target organ in hypersensitivity reactions to anticonvulsants and sulfonamides. Clin Pharmacol Ther 1992;51(1):56–67.

59. Barbaud A, Collet E, Milpied B, et al. A multicentre study to determine the value and safety of drug patch tests for the three main classes of severe cutaneous adverse drug reactions. Br J Dermatol 2013;168(3):555–62.

60. Elzagallaai AA, Knowles SR, Rieder MJ, et al. Patch testing for the diagnosis of anticonvulsant hypersensitivity syndrome: a systematic review. Drug Saf 2009; 32(5):391–408.

61. Elzagallaai AA, Knowles SR, Rieder MJ, et al. In vitro testing for the diagnosis of anticonvulsant hypersensitivity syndrome: a systematic review. Mol Diagn Ther 2009;13(5):313–30.

62. Rerkpattanapipat T, Chiriac AM, Demoly P. Drug provocation tests in hypersensitivity drug reactions. Curr Opin Allergy Clin Immunol 2011;11(4):299–304.

63. Thong BY. Stevens-Johnson syndrome/toxic epidermal necrolysis: an Asia-Pacific perspective. Asia Pac Allergy 2013;3(4):215–23.

64. Lee HY, Lim YL, Thirumoorthy T, et al. The role of intravenous immunoglobulin in toxic epidermal necrolysis: a retrospective analysis of 64 patients managed in a specialized centre. Br J Dermatol 2013;169(6):1304–9.

65. Thong BY, Mirakian R, Castells M, et al. A world allergy organization international survey on diagnostic procedures and therapies in drug allergy/hypersensitivity. World Allergy Organ J 2011;4(12):257–70.

66. Huang YC, Li YC, Chen TJ. The efficacy of intravenous immunoglobulin for the treatment of toxic epidermal necrolysis: a systematic review and meta-analysis. Br J Dermatol 2012;167(2):424–32.

67. Singh GK, Chatterjee M, Verma R. Cyclosporine in Stevens Johnson syndrome and toxic epidermal necrolysis and retrospective comparison with systemic corticosteroid. Indian J Dermatol Venereol Leprol 2013;79(5):686–92.

68. Valeyrie-Allanore L, Wolkenstein P, Brochard L, et al. Open trial of ciclosporin treatment for Stevens-Johnson syndrome and toxic epidermal necrolysis. Br J Dermatol 2010;163(4):847–53.

69. Lee HY, Dunant A, Sekula P, et al. The role of prior corticosteroid use on the clinical course of Stevens-Johnson syndrome and toxic epidermal necrolysis: a case-control analysis of patients selected from the multinational EuroSCAR and RegiSCAR studies. Br J Dermatol 2012;167(3):555–62.

70. O'Donoghue JM, Cespedes YP, Rockley PF, et al. Skin biopsies to assess response to systemic corticosteroid therapy in early-stage TEN: case report and review of the literature. Cutis 2009;84(3):138–40, 161–2.

71. Hynes AY, Kafkala C, Daoud YJ, et al. Controversy in the use of high-dose systemic steroids in the acute care of patients with Stevens-Johnson syndrome. Int Ophthalmol Clin 2005;45(4):25–48.

72. Fernando SL. Drug-reaction eosinophilia and systemic symptoms and drug-induced hypersensitivity syndrome. Australas J Dermatol 2014;55(1):15–23.

73. Descamps V, Ben Said B, Sassolas B, et al. Management of drug reaction with eosinophilia and systemic symptoms (DRESS). Ann Dermatol Venereol 2010; 137(11):703–8 [in French].

74. Fernando SL. Acute generalised exanthematous pustulosis. Australas J Dermatol 2012;53(2):87–92.

Antiviral Drug Allergy

Brigitte Milpied-Homsi, MD[a], Ellen M. Moran, PhD[b],
Elizabeth J. Phillips, MD[b,c],*

KEYWORDS

- Altered peptide repertoire • Abacavir • Nevirapine • Antiretroviral
- Telaprevir pharmacogenomics • Human leukocyte antigen
- Major histocompatibility complex

KEY POINTS

- Antiviral drugs successful in suppressing replication of human immunodeficiency virus (HIV) and hepatitis C (HCV) are common causes of delayed drug hypersensitivities for which an increasing number have more recently been shown to be human leukocyte antigen alleles (HLA) class I and/or II–restricted and T-cell-mediated.
- HLA-B*57:01 screening before abacavir prescription to prevent abacavir hypersensitivity is an example of a translational success story whereby a marker with 100% negative predictive value has now been implemented into guideline-based routine HIV clinical practice.
- Ancillary in vivo and ex vivo laboratory tests have been useful to define the true immunologically mediated phenotype of antiviral drug hypersensitivity (eg, patch testing for abacavir); however, the lower sensitivity of these tests for severe drug hypersensitivity syndromes means that clinical diagnosis remains the gold standard to guide management.
- Most allergic syndromes associated with antiviral medications consist of mild-to-moderate delayed rash without other serious manifestations (eg, fever, mucosal involvement, blistering rash, organ impairment). In these cases, treatment can be continued with careful observation and symptomatic management, and the discontinuation rate is low.

INTRODUCTION

Pharmacologically predictable adverse drug reactions and drug interactions have been commonly associated with anti-infective drugs and, particularly, antiretroviral agents. Immunologically mediated adverse drug reactions have also been commonly

Disclosures/Conflict of Interest: None related to the content of this article.
[a] Department of Dermatology, Saint-André Hospital, Bordeaux, WA 6150, France; [b] Division of infectious diseases, Institute of Immunology and Infectious Disease, Murdoch University, Murdoch, Western Australia; [c] Division of Infectious Diseases, Vanderbilt University Medical Center, 1161 21st Avenue South, A-2200, Medical Center North, Nashville, TN 37232-2582, USA
* Corresponding author. Division of Infectious Diseases, Vanderbilt University Medical Center, 1161 21st Avenue South, A-2200, Medical Center North, Nashville, TN 37232-2582.
E-mail address: elizabeth.j.phillips@vanderbilt.edu

Immunol Allergy Clin N Am 34 (2014) 645–662
http://dx.doi.org/10.1016/j.iac.2014.04.011   immunology.theclinics.com
0889-8561/14/$ – see front matter © 2014 Elsevier Inc. All rights reserved.

described in patients receiving drugs used to treat viral infections, including those used to treat human immunodeficiency virus (HIV) and hepatitis C infection.[1–3] These hypersensitivity reactions associated with antiviral drugs can be classified by their immunologic mechanisms as well as their specific clinical manifestation or phenotype. Gell-Coombs types I–III (immediate drug allergy, antibody mediated, and immune complex mechanisms) are not commonly associated with antiviral drugs. Gell-Coombs type IV (T-cell-mediated) reactions, however, have been commonly associated with drugs used to treat viral infection.[2–4] For instance, the antiretroviral drug, abacavir (ABC), causes a hypersensitivity syndrome, which has a distinct phenotype not shared by other drugs and is characterized by fever, malaise, and gastrointestinal symptoms. Mild-to-moderate skin rash is a late manifestation of ABC hypersensitivity, which occurs in 70% of cases.[4] The antiretroviral drug, nevirapine, has been commonly associated with a delayed rash as well as more severe hypersensitivity reactions (drug reaction with eosinophilia and systemic symptoms [DRESS], also known as drug-induced hypersensitivity syndromes [DIHS], Stevens-Johnson syndrome/ toxic epidermal necrolysis [SJS/TEN], and drug-induced liver disease [DILI]).[5] Many drugs, such as the nonnucleoside reverse transcriptase inhibitor (NNRTI), efavirenz, and the anti-hepatitis C virus (HCV) NS3.4A serine protease inhibitor, telaprevir, are commonly associated with a nonspecific exanthem without systemic symptoms, which is not treatment limiting, and continued treatment is usually possible with symptom control.[5–9] More severe reactions with fever and/or mucosal and/or severe cutaneous involvement and/or internal organ (eg, liver) involvement warrant immediate discontinuation and careful clinical monitoring. A major advance in pharmacogenomics has been the discovery that many immunologically mediated drug reactions are mediated through interactions with class I and/or class II human leukocyte antigen alleles (HLA) (**Table 1**). In the case of ABC, a strong association between HLA-B*57:01 was discovered by 2 independent groups in 2002 and HLA-B*57:01 is now used as a routine screening test with a proven 100% negative predictive value, before ABC prescription to exclude those at risk.[10,11] Abacavir patch testing was also a useful research tool in this context that was used in clinical trials to identify those with true immunologically mediated ABC hypersensitivity reaction (HSR).[21–23] ABC patch testing has a diagnostic sensitivity of 87% but there is currently no in vivo or ex vivo diagnostic test for antiviral drug hypersensitivity that has a 100% sensitivity or negative predictive value, and clinical diagnosis is used as the gold standard on which future recommendations are based. Drug hypersensitivity reactions associated with nevirapine have also been associated with class I and II HLA alleles, which seem to be ethnicity-dependent and phenotype-dependent, with associations that seem currently too complex to apply as a screening strategy in routine clinical practice (see **Table 1**).[24–26] A major recent advance has been the elucidation of the science of ABC hypersensitivity, which has defined the specific mechanism by which ABC specifically interacts with HLA-B*57:01 and alters the repertoire of self-peptide ligands.[22,27,28] Based on this work, the crystal structure of ABC-bound peptide-HLA-B*57:01 has been resolved and a new mechanistic paradigm for how drugs affect T-cell-mediated reactions was defined.[29] Future applications of this work could include preclinical strategies to determine drugs at high risk to cause immunologically mediated adverse drug reactions and hence inform drug design and development.

IMMUNOPATHOGENESIS AND PHARMACOGENOMICS OF ANTIVIRAL DRUG ALLERGY

Models that have been proposed to define the immunopathogenesis of drug allergy and hypersensitivity syndromes include the prehapten/hapten hypothesis, the

Table 1
Pharmacogenomics of antiviral drugs

Clinical Phenotypes and Drug	Alleles	Populations
DRESS/DIHS		
Abacavir	B*57:01	European, African[10,11]
Nevirapine (hepatitis)	DRB1*01:01 (CD4% ≥25) and DRB1*01:02	Australian, European, South African[12–14]
Nevirapine (DRESS/DIHS with rash)	Cw*8 or Cw*8-B*14 haplotype	Italian, Japanese[15,16]
	Cw*4	White, Black, Asian Han Chinese[13,16]
	B*35	Asian[13]
	B*35:05	Asian (Thai)[15]
	B*35:01	European/Australia[17]
	CYP2B6 516 G→T+C*04	White, Black, Asian[13]
	CYP2B6 (rs2054675, rs3786547, rs3745274)	White, Black, Asian[13]
Delayed rash (nonsystemic)		
Efavirenz	DRB1*01	French[5]
Nevirapine	DRB1*01	French[5]
	Cw*04	African, Asian, European, Thai[13,18]
	B*35:05; rs1576*G CCHR1 status (GWAS)	Thai[15,16]
SJS/TEN		
Nevirapine	HLA-C*04:01	African (Malawian)[19]
	?CYP2B6 983 T→C	Mozambique[20]

pharmacologic-interaction (P-I) model, and most recently, the altered peptide repertoire model. The hapten hypothesis suggests that a drug or a reactive metabolite irreversibly binds to and covalently modifies self-proteins, leading to a neo-antigen.[27] The P-I model suggests that drugs induce T-cell activation by directly interacting with immune receptors on a pharmacologic level and noncovalently binding with HLA alleles and/or T-cell receptors.[28,30] New evidence now exists that many drugs, including the nucleoside reverse transcriptase inhibitor and antiretroviral drug ABC, mediate hypersensitivity through the altered peptide repertoire model whereby it is proposed that drugs bind noncovalently with HLA, occupy anchor sites within the antigen-binding cleft, and thereby alter the repertoire of self-peptide ligand bound and presenting to T cell, creating a form of altered T-cell immunity based on alteration of immunologic self by a drug. Multiple groups have now reproduced evidence demonstrating that ABC binds noncovalently to the F-binding pocket of HLA-B*57:01 to specific residues that define this allele and shifts the repertoire of self-peptides presented and the crystal structure of ABC bound to HLA-B*57:01 and peptide has been solved.[31–33] Because the altered peptide model does not explain why only 55% of HLA-B*57:01-positive patients experience ABC hypersensitivity, additional models are needed.[21] Other models for drug hypersensitivity include the heterologous immune model, suggesting that these reactions could be mediated by cross-reactive memory T-cell responses to chronic prevalent viruses, such as human herpes viruses (HHV) and/or mediated through restricted T-cell receptor repertoire usage as recently demonstrated for carbamazepine.[31] Reactivation of chronic persistent HHV, such as HHV 6/7, cytomegalovirus (CMV), and Epstein-Barr virus (EBV), has also been described as complications of DRESS/DIHS; however, this has not been a described feature of hypersensitivity associated with ABC or other antivirals.[34–36]

In 2002, 2 independent groups reported a strong association between the HLA class I allele, HLA-B*57:01, and ABC hypersensitivity syndrome.[10,11] The nonspecific nature of the clinical syndrome of ABC hypersensitivity characterized by fever, rash, gastrointestinal symptoms, and sometimes respiratory symptoms led to a high rate of false positive clinical diagnosis and the suggestion that the HLA-B*57:01 allele lacked sensitivity and 100% negative predictive value for ABC hypersensitivity, particularly in races with a low prevalence of HLA-B*57:01 carriage. A randomized controlled clinical trial that compared prospective HLA-B*57:01 screening versus ABC initiation without screening and used ABC patch testing (**Fig. 1**) as a co-primary endpoint to clinical diagnosis to identify true immunologically mediated ABC hypersensitivity clarified the 100% negative predictive value of HLA-B*57:01 for ABC hypersensitivity and, hence, its utility in clinical practice.[21] A follow-up study in Whites and African Americans also confirmed the generalizability of this 100% negative predictive value to non-White ethnicities.[37] Since 2008, international guidelines have recommended the use of HLA-B*57:01 screening before ABC prescription, and HLA-B*57:01 is now one of the most widely used genetic screening tests in clinical practice today.[24]

Early in the postmarketing phase of ABC's development, ABC hypersensitivity was defined as an HLA-B*57:01-restricted CD8+ T-cell-mediated reaction with long-lasting immunity, as demonstrated by patch testing and ex vivo studies.[22,38,39] The Prospective Randomized Evaluation of DNA Screening in a Clinical Trial (PREDICT-1) study demonstrated that 55% of those carrying HLA-B*57:01 will develop ABC hypersensitivity and, although to date no other HLA has been associated with ABC hypersensitivity, the mechanism of HLA-B*57:01-positive ABC tolerance has not been determined.[21] Despite this incomplete positive predictive value, ABC-specific CD8+

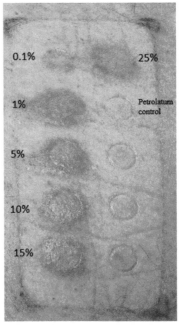

Fig. 1. ABC patch test: 24-hour reading ABC in concentrations of 0.1, 1, 5, 10, 15, and 25% in petrolatum and petrolatum control are applied to the skin and left undisturbed for 24 hours.

T-cell responses can be reproduced in 10- to 12-day culture from 100% of HLA-B*57:01-positive ABC-naive healthy blood donors.[39]

Nevirapine is a NNRTI used to treat HIV, the major treatment limiting toxicity of which is a drug hypersensitivity syndrome. The phenotypes of nevirapine hypersensitivity vary from exanthem without other symptoms, DRESS/DIHS, hepatitis (DILI), and SJS/TEN (**Fig. 2**B–D). More recently, each of these phenotypes has been associated with different class I and class II HLA associations across different ethnicities (see **Table 1**).[5,12–18] An early study in a Western Australian cohort suggested that nevirapine hypersensitivity associated with rash and hepatitis was a CD4+ T-cell-dependent HLA-DRB1*01:01-restricted process.[12]

With regards to phenotype specific class I HLA associations and nevirapine hypersensitivity syndromes this includes HLA-B*35:05 and cutaneous hypersensitivity in Southeast Asians and HLA-Cw4 in association with cutaneous phenotypes across multiple ethnicities, but, in particular, in association with CYP2B6 516 G>T in Blacks.[12] In a South African population, HLA-B*58:01 and HLA-DRB1*01:02 have recently been associated with grade 3/4 hepatitis on nevirapine, and HLA-C*04:01 was associated with SJS/TEN in a Malawian population. HLA-DRB1*01 was also previously reported with cutaneous hypersensitivity in association with nevirapine and another NNRTI, efavirenz.[5] Severe drug-induced liver injury has was reported in 3.4% of an HIV Ethiopian population started on efavirenz and associated with higher efavirenz plasma levels and CYP2B6*6 as well as advanced HIV and pretreatment liver disease. It is unclear from the report whether the hepatitis was toxic, immunologic, or a mixture of both.[40] Rash and pruritus have been associated with up to 50% or more of patients receiving combination regimens, including the direct-acting hepatitis C antiviral (NS3/4A protease inhibitor) telaprevir, resulting in treatment discontinuation in 6% of patients.[41] Severe hypersensitivity (DRESS/DIHS) or severe cutaneous adverse reactions including SJS/TEN are uncommon, occurring in less than 1% of patients.[42] A case control study of 187 telaprevir-treated patients of whom 114 had developed rash (59 severe) was conducted to explore a potential association between telaprevir rash and HLA class I and II alleles. HLA-B*44:02 and HLA-DQB1*02:02 were the top-ranked alleles associated with severe skin rash; however, these associations did not hold up after correction for multiple comparisons.[41,43]

HYPERSENSITIVITY SYNDROMES ASSOCIATED WITH ANTIRETROVIRAL TREATMENT

Those living with HIV have increased exposure to drugs more likely to cause drug hypersensitivity and immune dysregulation. Many delayed and likely T-cell-mediated drug hypersensitivity reactions have been reported to occur more commonly in HIV-infected populations. In the first decade of HIV treatment, these mainly involved drugs used to treat HIV-related infections, but now primarily include drugs used to treat HIV.[44] The most common cutaneous drug reactions in HIV-infected patients are maculopapular exanthemas (MPE). These eruptions are characterized by widespread erythematous macules and papules that usually affect the trunk and proximal extremities; these rashes are often accompanied by pruritus without fever. Initial macules and papules can be increasing in size and lead to confluence or be followed by maculopapular, pustular, or vesicular lesions. MPE usually appear between 2 and 10 weeks after primary exposure to antiretroviral therapy (ART) and within 1 to 2 days of rechallenge. Most of these exanthema are benign and resolve within 2 weeks without sequelae. The patient should be evaluated carefully for the presence of signs of severity, such as edema, skin detachment, erosions, mucosal involvement, fever or systemic symptoms that alert to a more severe drug reaction, such as DRESS/DIHS or SJS/TEN. Usually rash severity is graded

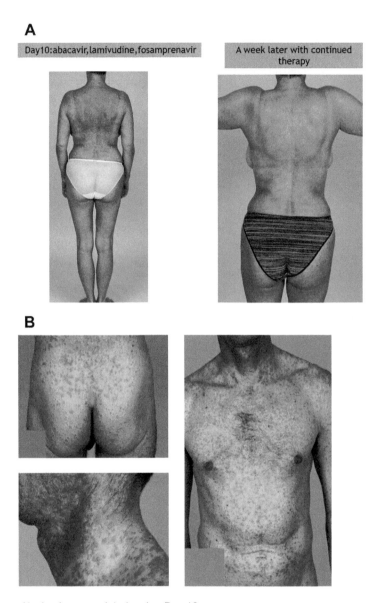

Nevirapine-associated rash – Day 10

Fig. 2. (*A*) (*left*) Patient on day 10: abacavir, lamivudine, fosamprenavir and (*right*) improvement a week later with continued therapy. (*B*) Patient displays Nevirapine-associated rash at Day 10. (*C*) Patient with Nevirapine-associated Toxic Epidermal Necrolysis. (*D*) Patient with Nevirapine-induced DRESS 15 days after the initiation of treatment. (*E*) Patients displaying Telaprevir-induced rashes of varying severity. Part A shows Grade 1 (mild): treatment is continued. Part B shows Grade 2 (moderate): treatment is continued. Part C shows Grade 3 (severe): treatment is stopped.

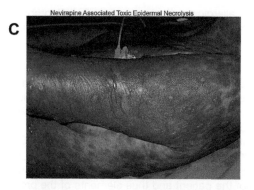

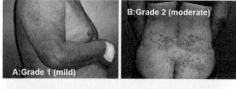

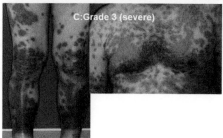

Fig. 2. (*continued*)

in 4 levels (**Box 1**). Other allergic syndromes, such as Gell-Coombs type I (IgE-mediated) reactions or delayed urticarial eruptions, are infrequently seen in association with ART.

SJS/TEN

SJS and TEN represent acute life-threatening conditions with high morbidity and mortality with an incidence estimated at 1 to 2 cases/million population/year. The histologic hallmark of these diseases is necrosis with detachment of the epidermis. Patients are classified according to the percentage of the body surface area exhibiting epidermal detachment (BSA%), which is less than 10% in SJS, more than 30% in TEN, and 10% to 30% in SJS/TEN overlap syndrome.[45,46] The mortality of SJS and TEN has recently been estimated to be about 22%,[47] correlating with the extent of detachment and age of the patient and thus elements of the prognostic score called SCORTEN[48]: seven independent risk factors: age greater than 40 years, malignancy, tachycardia greater than 120 per minute, initial BSA% greater than 10%, serum urea greater than 10 mmol per liter, serum glucose greater than 14 mmol per liter, and bicarbonate less than 20 mmol per liter. TEN usually develops 1 to 3 weeks after the administration of the responsible drug. The clinical diagnosis is based on the presence of characteristic eruptions of mucosal extensive erosions, typical targetoid lesions, erythematous confluent maculae, and bullae, with a positive Nikolsky's sign (detachment of epidermis to finger pressure). Histopathology is characterized by keratinocyte apoptosis followed by necrosis, which creates the basis for the epidermal erosion and detachment. Infection is the most common acute complication and cause of death in SJS/TEN patients. Recovery may require 3 to 6 weeks and is often followed by pigmentation disorders and pathologic scarring at mucosal sites. More than 50% of patients surviving SJS/TEN suffer from long-term complications primarily located in the eyes, such as vision loss in some cases.[44,46] To date, there is no established treatment for SJS/TEN. Symptomatic treatment (dressings, maintenance of thermoregulation, fluid and electrolyte balance, nutritional support, prevention of infections) and immediate cessation of the suspected causative drug are the key to the management of SJS/TEN. Patients benefit from being under the care of a dermatologist in an intensive care or burns unit.

Box 1
Grading of rash severity

Grade 1 (mild): localized skin eruption and/or limited skin eruption with or without pruritus

Grade 2 (moderate): diffuse eruption involving up to 50% of BSA with or without superficial skin peeling, pruritus, or mucous membrane involvement and no ulceration

Grade 3 (severe): generalized rash involving EITHER ≥50% of BSA OR rash presenting with any of the following characteristics:

- Vesicles or bullae
- Superficial ulceration of mucous membranes
- Typical or atypical target lesions
- Palpable purpura/nonblanching erythema

Grade 4 (life-threatening reactions)

- DRESS/DIHS
- SJS/TEN

DRESS/DIHS

DRESS/DIHS is a severe drug-induced adverse manifestation that occurs in most patients 2 to 6 weeks after drug administration. Clinical and biologic manifestations of DRESS are characteristic: high fever, facial edema, erythroderma followed by an exfoliative dermatitis, diffuse lymphadenopathy, eosinophilia, atypical circulating lymphocytes, and abnormal results of liver function tests. Numerous systemic manifestations may occur (hepatitis, pneumonitis, pancreatitis, renal failure, neurologic symptoms, and many others). In contrast to SJS and TEN, involvement of the mucous membranes is rare.[45,46] Reactivation of HHV, including EBV and HHV-6 and HHV-7, has been described in association with many drug-induced DRESS/DIHS syndromes, however, interestingly, not with ART-associated DRESS/DIHS. The detection of HHV-6 reactivation has even been recently proposed as a diagnostic marker for DRESS/DIHS.[27,28,30] To define more accurately the DRESS syndrome, a scoring system—the RegiSCAR scoring—has been designed to grade DRESS cases as "no," "possible," "probable," or "definite" case.[48] This condition must be recognized early to immediately stop the suspected drugs, but the persistence or aggravation of symptoms despite the discontinuation of the culprit drug is possible. Topical high-potency corticosteroids or systemic corticosteroids are usually required for a full recovery.

Cutaneous adverse drug reactions, although reported with all ART, are more prevalent with specific ART drugs and drug classes, particularly the NNRTI (**Table 2**).

PROTEASE INHIBITORS

All protease inhibitors have been associated with mild-to-moderate maculopapular rashes; these are typically observed within the first 2 weeks of treatment and are mild without need for treatment discontinuation (see **Fig. 2**A). They are uncommonly associated with severe reactions, such as DRESS/DIHS or SJS/TEN. The rate of rash in patients treated with a protease inhibitors has been recently estimated as around 5%. The newest protease inhibitors are more commonly responsible with variable rates, respectively, up to 6%, 10%, 16%, and 19% for atazanavir, tipranavir, darunavir, and fosamprenavir.[44] Darunavir and fosamprenavir are sulfa antimicrobials, and there is concern for cross-reactivity with sulfamethoxazole and other sulfa antimicrobials. For darunavir, patients with a history of sulfa antimicrobial hypersensitivity were not excluded from clinical trials.

NNRTIS

NNRTIs in clinical use include the first-generation drugs, nevirapine and efavirenz, and second-generation drugs, etravirine and rilpivirine. Cutaneous problems and hepatotoxicity are the main side effects induced by NNRTIs. In most patients, rashes are mild-to-moderate MPE that occur within the first 1 to 2 weeks of treatment and resolve with continued treatment (see **Fig. 2**B). Rashes associated with nevirapine (4%–38%) and efavirenz (4.6%–20%) are frequent (see **Table 2**). SJS/TEN has most frequently been reported with nevirapine (0.3%–1%) (see **Fig. 2**C) and less frequently with efavirenz (0·1%).[49] DRESS/DIHS syndrome is well documented with nevirapine occurring in up to 5% of patients (see **Fig. 2**D) but is uncommonly attributed to efavirenz.[50] Female sex, ethnicity (Hispanic, Chinese, and African), and individuals with higher CD4+ T-cell count and uncontrolled HIV viremia in early studies seemed to be at higher risk for nevirapine-related rash.[51] An initial 2-week lead-in period at half the recommended dose has been shown to reduce the risk of skin rashes with nevirapine by at least 50%. The prophylactic use of corticosteroids or antihistamines to prevent hypersensitivity

Table 2
Clinical manifestations and incidence of antiviral allergic syndromes

Class	Agent	Reaction	Incidence	Discontinuation
Antiretroviral treatments				
Protease inhibitors	Atazanavir	Rash	≤6%	<1%
	Darunavir	Rash	≤10%	<1%
		SJS/TEN/DIHS/DRESS	<1%	100%
	Fosamprenavir	Rash	≤19%	<1%
		Moderate-severe	—	<1%
	Lopinavir/ Ritonavir	Rash	2%	<1%
	Tipranavir	Rash	≤10%	<1%
NNRTIs	Efavirenz	Rash	4.6%–20%	<2%
		SJS/TEN	0.1%	100%
		DRESS/DIHS	—	—
	Etravirine	Rash	≤10%	<2%
		DRESS/DIHS, SJS/TEN	<0.1%	100%
	Nevirapine	Rash	4%–38%	6%
		DRESS/DIHS	Up to 5%	100%
		SJS/TEN	0.3%–1%	—
	Rilpivirine	Rash	2%	<1%
Fusion inhibitors	Enfuvirtide	Hypersensitivity reaction	<1%	Mostly for subcutaneous reactions, not HSR
NRTIs	Tenofovir	Rash	5%–7%	<1%
	Abacavir	Hypersensitivity reaction (fever, gastrointestinal symptoms, rash in 70%)	5%–8%	100%, hypotension, severe morbidity on rechallenge
		Rash only	3%	<1%
	Emtricitabine	Pruritus, rash	17%–30%	<1%
Integrase inhibitors	Raltegravir	Pruritus, diaphoresis, rash	2%–7%	<1%
		DRESS/DIHS/SJS/TEN	<1%	100%
CCR5 inhibitors	Maraviroc	Pruritus	3.8%	<1%
Direct-acting hepatitis C treatments	Telaprevir	Mild to moderate eczematous rash	50%	<10%
		DRESS/DIHS	5%	100%
		SJS/TEN	<1%	—

reactions to nevirapine has not been shown to be of benefit and may even increase risk.[52,53] Risk factors for efavirenz-induced rash are less well-described. Nevirapine-associated hypersensitivity syndromes have a pharmacogenomic basis and have been associated with various class I and II HLA alleles as described above.

Etravirine is the first of the second-generation NNRTIs that has showed efficacy in controlling HIV replication in treatment-experienced patients, in combination with other active agents. In clinical trials, rash was reported in 16.9% of the etravirine-treated patients compared with 9.3% in placebo (see **Table 2**). Most rashes were of mild or moderate severity, occurring within the first few weeks of treatment (median 14 days) and resolved with continued treatment (only 2.2% of patients discontinued etravirine). In clinical trials, women developed more rash than men. There was no relationship between rash and etravirine pharmacokinetic exposure, CD4+ T-cell count, nor history of other NNRTI-related rash. DRESS/DIHS and SJS/TEN were reported in less than 0.1% of the etravirine-treated patients during clinical trials. In 2009, the manufacturer issued a drug warning regarding the safety of etravirine in light of postmarketing reports of severe skin and hypersensitivity reactions. Cases included life-threatening and fatal reports of DRESS/DIHS and SJS/TEN.[54] Another second-generation NNRTI, rilpivirine, has been associated with a low incidence (2%) of mild-to-moderate rash in clinical trials (see **Table 2**).[55]

FUSION INHIBITORS

Enfuvirtide was the first of a class of antiretroviral medications called fusion inhibitors and the only one currently available as an injectable formulation. Most cutaneous side effects are injection site reactions. Hypersensitivity reaction has an incidence rate of less than 1% of patients in clinical trials.[56]

NUCLEOSIDE REVERSE TRANSCRIPTASE INHIBITORS

Nucleoside reverse transcriptase inhibitors (NRTIs) were the first medication approved for the treatment of HIV. Currently, the nucleoside analogues commonly used as part of combination ART include Lamivudine (2′,3′-dideoxy-3′-thiacytidine, commonly called 3TC), emtricitabine (3TC), tenofovir (nucleotide analogue), and ABC. Because of the inconvenience of dosing and long-term toxicities, Zidovudine (INN)/azidothymidine (AZT), Didanosine (2′,3′-dideoxyinosine, ddl, DDI), and Stavudine (2′,3′-didehydro-2′,3′-dideoxythymidine, d4T) are currently much less commonly used in the developed world. Rash has been less commonly associated with tenofovir and a hypersensitivity syndrome has been rarely reported (see **Table 2**).[44]

ABC

ABC can be associated with a drug hypersensitivity syndrome that is distinct from DRESS/DIHS. In early studies, ABC hypersensitivity was reported to occur within the first 6 weeks of exposure, although most cases occur in the second week of first exposure at a median of 8 to 9 days. It is characterized by fever, malaise, gastrointestinal symptoms, and internal organ involvement in approximately 5% to 8% of patients who begin therapy with ABC.[4]

The syndrome can be accompanied by a mild-to-moderate rash in 70% of patients with ABC hypersensitivity and is associated with severe hypotension and possible death on rechallenge, in contrast to the complete abrogation of symptoms 72 hours after withdrawal of the drug. Once the hypersensitivity syndrome reaction has been diagnosed, ABC therapy should be discontinued immediately and permanently. Corticosteroids, given prophylactically, do not seem to reduce the severity or frequency of the ABC hypersensitivity syndrome.[53] There is a strong association with ABC hypersensitivity and the presence of the HLA-B*57:01 allele[7,8,57] and genetic testing to prevent ABC HSR is currently one of the best examples of integrating pharmacogenetic testing into clinical practice. Mild-to-moderate rash without other symptoms of ABC hypersensitivity is known to occur in 3% of those starting ABC. This MPE is not known to be associated with HLA-B*57:01 and is not treatment limiting. SJS/TEN has only rarely been suspected in association with ABC therapy.[58] ABC patch testing (see **Fig. 1**) has been used as a research tool to identify true immunologically mediated ABC hypersensitivity; however, it has a diagnostic sensitivity of 87% and in view of the severe rechallenge reactions (hypotension, shock) that have occurred in patients with ABC hypersensitivity on second exposure to ABC, a negative patch test alone should never be used as the sole basis for ABC reintroduction.[23,24,59]

Emtricitabine

Emtricitabine is used to prevent the replication of HIV and hepatitis B virus. The skin rashes most commonly reported in emtricitabine trials were pruritus, maculopapular rash, urticaria, vesiculobullous, and pustular rash, observed in 17% to 30% of the patients. These reactions were mild or moderate; only 1% of the patients discontinued treatment because of rash (see **Table 2**).[44]

INTEGRASE INHIBITORS

Most rash events in raltegravir-treated subjects in the clinical trials were mild to moderate in intensity, and no discontinuations were reported. However, many of the rash events have been confounded by the use of concomitant medications associated, such as NNRTIs, ABC, and Protease inhibitors. More recently, there have been cases of raltegravir-associated DRESS/DIHS and SJS/TEN with 3 separate case publications of raltegravir-associated DRESS/DIHS syndrome all in women of African descent.[60–62] A newly approved integrase inhibitor, dolutegravir, has not been associated with rash.

INHIBITORS OF THE CCR5 CHEMOKINE RECEPTOR

Maraviroc is the first human chemokine receptor 5 (CCR5) co-receptor antagonist approved for HIV treatment. Information about the cutaneous adverse events and hypersensitivity syndromes associated with maraviroc is scarce; however, pruritus occurred in 3.8% of the patients receiving maraviroc in clinical trials (see **Table 2**).[63]

HYPERSENSITIVITY SYNDROMES ASSOCIATED WITH TREATMENT OF HCV

HCV is a major global health problem with an estimated 170 million people chronically infected.[64] It may lead to chronic liver disease, cirrhosis, and hepatocellular carcinoma, with high morbidity and mortality.[65] Standard combination treatment with pegylated interferon-α (PegIFN) and ribavirin (RBV) results in a virological response in only about 45% of patients.[66] New direct-acting antiviral drugs, such as telaprevir and boceprevir that are inhibitors of the HCV NS3.4A serine protease, have thus become of great interest for improving the efficacy of anti-HCV treatment. Telaprevir has been recently developed for the treatment of chronic genotype 1 HCV infection in combination with RBV and PegIFN.[67] Telaprevir-associated rash has occurred in up to 50% or more of the patients on combination treatment with RBV and PegIFN since its first evaluation in clinical studies (see **Fig. 2**E, **Table 2**). More than 90% of these eruptions are mild and moderate eczematous dermitits (grades 1 and 2) that does not require telaprevir discontinuation and are usually well controlled by antihistamine therapy, emollients, and topical steroids (see **Fig. 2**E).[2] Approximately 5% of these skin eruptions are potentially severe with cases of DRESS/DIHS and SJS/TEN reported.[8,9,41] There has been no association between the pharmacokinetics of PegIFN, RBV, and telaprevir and incidence of rash.[41] The safety data of the combination of boceprevir with PegIFN and RBV were assessed in phase 2 and 3 placebo-controlled clinical trials. The most common adverse events observed were anemia, dysgeusia, and cutaneous side effects. Rashes were noted in 14% to 22% of cases and dry skin in 18% to 22% of cases, which was noted more significantly compared with PegIFN and RBV alone in treatment-experienced patients; however, no patient receiving boceprevir discontinued the treatment because of skin eruption.[68] Severe cutaneous syndromes are uncommon with boceprevir, with one recently published case of DRESS/DIHS associated with boceprevir.[69] For mild-to-moderate skin rash without systemic symptoms or mucosal involvement, appropriate skin-care management usually facilitates continuation of antiviral therapy (see **Table 2**),[70] which emphasizes the importance of close collaboration between dermatologists and hepatologists.

DIAGNOSIS AND TREATMENT

The diagnosis and treatment of drug hypersensitivity to antivirals, as per any drugs, are still largely based on clinical assessment of the specific syndrome involved. As per other drugs, the presence of mild-to-moderate rash without systemic symptoms, or internal organ or mucosal involvement, is commonly associated with many antiviral drugs. Given the need to continue uninterrupted antiretroviral and hepatitis C treatment, it is reasonable in these mild cases to continue treatment with careful observation with the expectation that the rash will remit, although the mechanism of immunologic tolerance is not clear.

Desensitization or graded reintroduction of drug has also been used to reintroduce an antiviral whereby the original reaction consisted of an isolated mild-to-moderate skin rash.[8] ABC patch testing showed great utility as a research tool in the PREDICT-1 and Study of Hypersensitivity to Abacavir and Pharmacogenetic Evaluation (SHAPE) studies to define the specific syndrome of immunologically mediated ABC hypersensitivity.[11,21] From the PREDICT-1 study, the diagnostic sensitivity of ABC patch testing was 87%, giving it one of the highest sensitivities of patch testing for drug hypersensitivity. However, given the severity and potential for morbidity and mortality associated with rechallenge with ABC in patients who have already experienced ABC hypersensitivity syndrome, patch testing alone should never be used as the basis for rechallenge and clinical judgment should always take precedent.[71] In general, patch testing has shown diagnostic utility for other drug hypersensitivity syndromes, such as DRESS/DIHS, acute generalized exanthematous pustulosis (AGEP), and fixed drug eruption, and less so for SJS/TEN; however, in general, the sensitivity of patch testing for drugs other than ABC has been less than 50% and is very drug-specific.[72,73] Patch testing for syndromes such as DRESS/DIHS/SJS/TEN for specific antivirals such as nevirapine appears to have low sensitivity and utility.[59,72] For efavirenz, a type of photoallergic dermatitis has been described and there have been case reports of positive photopatch, whereby the drug is applied for 48 hours followed by low-dose ultraviolet A application for 24 hours.[73–75] More recently, direct-acting drugs against hepatitis C, such as telaprevir, have been associated with a very high incidence of delayed rash; however, treatment is largely supportive and most patients do not have associated systemic symptoms or signs and can continue treatment.[41] Specific ex vivo tests such as ELISpot have reproducibly shown γ-interferon responses to the parent drug for several years after the acute ABC hypersensitivity reaction, but seem less reliable for other drugs, such as nevirapine, whereby responses have been shown to wane quickly over months to years. In general, the management of antiviral drug hypersensitivity is similar to other drugs and includes use of prednisone or other immunosuppressants in cases of DRESS/DIHS with severe organ involvement of SJS/TEN, respectively. The long half-life of nevirapine is a risk factor for poor outcome associated with SJS/TEN, and nevirapine should be stopped immediately after onset of symptoms/signs suggestive of SJS/TEN.[76]

HLA-B*57:01 has had great utility as a screening test with 100% negative predictive value generalizable across different ethnicities to identify patients at risk to develop ABC hypersensitivity.[21,77,78] The complexity of HLA associations across different phenotypes and ethnicities with other drugs such as nevirapine is such that currently HLA testing has limited utility as a screening strategy to prevent nevirapine hypersensitivity syndromes before nevirapine prescription.

SUMMARY AND FUTURE DIRECTIONS

Antiviral drugs are common causes of delayed T-cell-mediated drug reactions for which the immunopathogenesis has been more recently defined to be largely HLA class I and/or class II restricted and T-cell-mediated. Fortunately, most of these reactions are benign and consist of a mild-to-moderate delayed skin rash, which is not treatment limiting and resolved with continued dosing. Although these drugs may share structure, such as a shared sulfa antimicrobial group in the case of darunavir and fosamprenavir, or shared mechanism of action and propensity to develop skin rash, as for the HIV NNRTI, clinical and immunologic cross-reactivity between antiviral drugs is uncommon in clinical practice. The association between HLA-B*57:01 and ABC hypersensitivity represents an successful example of where a genetic marker with 100% negative predictive value and generalizable across different ethnicities has been used as a screening test in the routine clinical setting to prevent a specific antiviral drug hypersensitivity syndrome. Many other HLA class I and II associations have been described between various phenotypes of nevirapine hypersensitivity, which have shed further light on the immunopathogenesis of antiviral hypersensitivity syndromes; however, the complexity of these associations and the lack of generalizability across all ethnicities make it unlikely they these will be used in the routine clinical setting. A paradigm shift has occurred in the science of drug hypersensitivity with definition of the crystal structure of ABC bound to peptide-HLA-B*57:01 and evidence for an altered peptide model of drug hypersensitivity. From recent research, it is likely that this altered peptide repertoire model applies to many other phenotypes of severe T-cell-mediated drug reactions, including DIHS/DRESS and SJS/TEN.[24,27] The altered peptide repertoire model does not explain why in general only a small fraction of patients carrying a specific HLA class I and/or II risk allele will develop a drug hypersensitivity syndrome and other models are needed. Some evidence now exists to suggest that hypersensitivity reactions to drugs like ABC, where symptoms can occur within 1 to 2 days of first exposure, may occur secondary to a pre-existing memory T-cell response. This pre-existing memory T-cell response may be targeted against a prevalent persistent viral pathogen, such a human herpes virus representing a heterologous immune model of drug hypersensitivity. The convergence of structural, biochemical, and functional immunologic approaches to define interactions between antiviral drugs and HLA molecules offers promise for being able to predict drug hypersensitivity risk in the preclinical stage of drug development and positively impact the efficacy, safety, and efficiency of antiviral drug development and design.

REFERENCES

1. Vilar FJ, Naisbitt DJ, Park BK, et al. Mechanisms of drug hypersensitivity in HIV-infected patients: the role of the immune system. J HIV Ther 2003;8(2):42–7.
2. Cacoub P, Bourliere M, Lubbe J, et al. Dermatological side effects of hepatitis C and its treatment: patient management in the era of direct-acting antivirals. J Hepatol 2012;56(2):455–63.
3. Phillips E, Mallal S. Drug hypersensitivity in HIV. Curr Opin Allergy Clin Immunol 2007;7(4):324–30.

4. Clay PG. The abacavir hypersensitivity reaction: a review. Clin Ther 2002;24(10): 1502–14.
5. Vitezica ZG, Milpied B, Lonjou C, et al. HLA-DRB1*01 associated with cutaneous hypersensitivity induced by nevirapine and efavirenz. AIDS 2008;22(4): 540–1.
6. Sherman KE. Managing adverse effects and complications in completing treatment for hepatitis C virus infection. Top Antivir Med 2012;20(4):125–8.
7. Torii H, Sueki H, Kumada H, et al. Dermatological side-effects of telaprevir-based triple therapy for chronic hepatitis C in phase III trials in Japan. J Dermatol 2013;40(8):587–95.
8. Phillips EJ, Kuriakose B, Knowles SR. Efavirenz-induced skin eruption and successful desensitization. Ann Pharmacother 2002;36(3):430–2.
9. Roujeau JC, Mockenhaupt M, Tahan SR, et al. Telaprevir-related dermatitis. JAMA Dermatol 2013;149(2):152–8.
10. Hetherington S, Hughes AR, Mosteller M, et al. Genetic variations in HLA-B region and hypersensitivity reactions to abacavir. Lancet 2002;359(9312):1121–2.
11. Mallal S, Nolan D, Witt C, et al. Association between presence of HLA-B*5701, HLA-DR7, and HLA-DQ3 and hypersensitivity to HIV-1 reverse-transcriptase inhibitor abacavir. Lancet 2002;359(9308):727–32.
12. Martin AM, Nolan D, James I, et al. Predisposition to nevirapine hypersensitivity associated with HLA-DRB1*0101 and abrogated by low CD4 T-cell counts. AIDS 2005;19(1):97–9.
13. Yuan J, Guo S, Hall D, et al. Toxicogenomics of nevirapine-associated cutaneous and hepatic adverse events among populations of African, Asian, and European descent. AIDS 2011;25(10):1271–80.
14. Phillips EB, Sanne I, Lederman M, et al. Associations between HLA-DRBA*0102, HLA-B*5801 and hepatotoxicity in patients who initiated nevirapine containing regimens in South Africa. 18th Conference on retroviruses and opportunistic infections. Boston, February 27–March 1, 2011. Paper #949.
15. Chantarangsu S, Mushiroda T, Mahasirimongkol S, et al. HLA-B*3505 allele is a strong predictor for nevirapine-induced skin adverse drug reactions in HIV-infected Thai patients. Pharmacogenet Genomics 2009;19(2):139–46.
16. Chantarangsu S, Mushiroda T, Mahasirimongkol S, et al. Genome-wide association study identifies variations in 6p21.3 associated with nevirapine-induced rash. Clin Infect Dis 2011;53(4):341–8.
17. Phillips E, Lucas M, Keane N, et al. HLA-B*35 is associated with nevirapine hypersensitivity in the contemporary western Australian HIV cohort study. Eur Ann Allergy Clin Immunol 2010;42:48.
18. Likanonsakul S, Rattanatham T, Feangvad S, et al. HLA-Cw*04 allele associated with nevirapine-induced rash in HIV-infected Thai patients. AIDS Res Ther 2009; 6:22.
19. Carr DF, Chaponda M, Jorgensen AL, et al. Association of human leukocyte antigen alleles and nevirapine hypersensitivity in a Malawian HIV-infected population. Clin Infect Dis 2013;56(9):1330–9.
20. Ciccacci C, Di Fusco D, Marazzi MC, et al. Association between CYP2B6 polymorphisms and Nevirapine-induced SJS/TEN: a pharmacogenetics study. Eur J Clin Pharmacol 2013;69(11):1909–16.
21. Mallal S, Phillips E, Carosi G, et al. HLA-B*5701 screening for hypersensitivity to abacavir. N Engl J Med 2008;358(6):568–79.
22. Phillips EJ, Wong GA, Kaul R, et al. Clinical and immunogenetic correlates of abacavir hypersensitivity. AIDS 2005;19(9):979–81.

23. Phillips EJ, Sullivan JR, Knowles SR, et al. Utility of patch testing in patients with hypersensitivity syndromes associated with abacavir. AIDS 2002;16(16): 2223–5.
24. Pavlos R, Mallal S, Phillips E. HLA and pharmacogenetics of drug hypersensitivity. Pharmacogenomics 2012;13(11):1285–306.
25. Rive CM, Bourke J, Phillips EJ. Testing for drug hypersensitivity syndromes. Clin Biochem Rev 2013;34(1):15–38.
26. Pavlos R, Mallal S, Ostrov D, et al. Fever, rash, and systemic symptoms: understanding the role of virus and HLA in severe cutaneous drug allergy. J Allergy Clin Immunol Pract 2014;2(1):21–33.
27. Pichler W, Yawalkar N, Schmid S, et al. Pathogenesis of drug-induced exanthems. Allergy 2002;57(10):884–93.
28. Adam J, Pichler WJ, Yerly D. Delayed drug hypersensitivity: models of T-cell stimulation. Br J Clin Pharmacol 2011;71(5):701–7.
29. Pompeu YA, Stewart JD, Mallal S, et al. The structural basis of HLA-associated drug hypersensitivity syndromes. Immunol Rev 2012;250(1):158–66.
30. Pichler WJ, Beeler A, Keller M, et al. Pharmacological interaction of drugs with immune receptors: the p-i concept. Allergol Int 2006;55(1):17–25.
31. Illing PT, Vivian JP, Dudek NL, et al. Immune self-reactivity triggered by drug-modified HLA-peptide repertoire. Nature 2012;486(7404):554–8.
32. Norcross MA, Luo S, Lu L, et al. Abacavir induces loading of novel self-peptides into HLA-B*57: 01: an autoimmune model for HLA-associated drug hypersensitivity. AIDS 2012;26(11):F21–9.
33. Ostrov DA, Grant BJ, Pompeu YA, et al. Drug hypersensitivity caused by alteration of the MHC-presented self-peptide repertoire. Proc Natl Acad Sci U S A 2012;109(25):9959–64.
34. Kano Y, Shiohara T. The variable clinical picture of drug-induced hypersensitivity syndrome/drug rash with eosinophilia and systemic symptoms in relation to the eliciting drug. Immunol Allergy Clin North Am 2009;29(3):481–501.
35. Shiohara T, Inaoka M, Kano Y. Drug-induced hypersensitivity syndrome (DIHS): a reaction induced by a complex interplay among herpesviruses and antiviral and antidrug immune responses. Allergol Int 2006;55(1):1–8.
36. Tohyama M, Hashimoto K, Yasukawa M, et al. Association of human herpesvirus 6 reactivation with the flaring and severity of drug-induced hypersensitivity syndrome. Br J Dermatol 2007;157(5):934–40.
37. Saag M, Balu R, Phillips E, et al. High sensitivity of human leukocyte antigen-b*5701 as a marker for immunologically confirmed abacavir hypersensitivity in white and black patients. Clin Infect Dis 2008;46(7):1111–8.
38. Martin AM, Nolan D, Gaudieri S, et al. Predisposition to abacavir hypersensitivity conferred by HLA-B*5701 and a haplotypic Hsp70-Hom variant. Proc Natl Acad Sci U S A 2004;101(12):4180–5.
39. Chessman D, Kostenko L, Lethborg T, et al. Human leukocyte antigen class I-restricted activation of CD8+ T cells provides the immunogenetic basis of a systemic drug hypersensitivity. Immunity 2008;28(6):822–32.
40. Yimer G, Amogne W, Habtewold A, et al. High plasma efavirenz level and CYP2B6*6 are associated with efavirenz-based HAART-induced liver injury in the treatment of naive HIV patients from Ethiopia: a prospective cohort study. Pharmacogenomics J 2012;12(6):499–506.
41. Chen ST, Wu PA. Severe cutaneous eruptions on telaprevir. J Hepatol 2012; 57(2):470–2.

42. Teixeira R, Nascimento YD, Crespo D. Safety aspects of protease inhibitors for chronic hepatitis C: adverse events and drug-to-drug interactions. Braz J Infect Dis 2013;17(2):194–204.

43. Advisory Committee Briefing Document for NDA 201-917 Telaprevir 375 mg tablets In: Members APAC, ed.

44. Borras-Blasco J, Navarro-Ruiz A, Borras C, et al. Adverse cutaneous reactions associated with the newest antiretroviral drugs in patients with human immunodeficiency virus infection. J Antimicrob Chemother 2008;62(5):879–88.

45. Roujeau JC, Stern RS. Severe adverse cutaneous reactions to drugs. N Engl J Med 1994;331(19):1272–85.

46. Bastuji-Garin S, Rzany B, Stern RS, et al. Clinical classification of cases of toxic epidermal necrolysis, Stevens-Johnson syndrome, and erythema multiforme. Arch Dermatol 1993;129(1):92–6.

47. Mockenhaupt M, Viboud C, Dunant A, et al. Stevens-Johnson syndrome and toxic epidermal necrolysis: assessment of medication risks with emphasis on recently marketed drugs. The EuroSCAR-study. J Invest Dermatol 2008; 128(1):35–44.

48. Bastuji-Garin S, Fouchard N, Bertocchi M, et al. SCORTEN: a severity-of-illness score for toxic epidermal necrolysis. J Invest Dermatol 2000;115(2):149–53.

49. Fagot JP, Mockenhaupt M, Bouwes-Bavinck JN, et al. Nevirapine and the risk of Stevens-Johnson syndrome or toxic epidermal necrolysis. AIDS 2001;15(14): 1843–8.

50. Colebunders R, Vanwolleghem T, Meurrens P, et al. Efavirenz-associated Stevens-Johnson syndrome. Infection 2004;32(5):306–7.

51. de Maat MM, ter Heine R, Mulder JW, et al. Incidence and risk factors for nevirapine-associated rash. Eur J Clin Pharmacol 2003;59(5–6):457–62.

52. Knobel H, Miro JM, Domingo P, et al. Failure of a short-term prednisone regimen to prevent nevirapine-associated rash: a double-blind placebo-controlled trial: the GESIDA 09/99 study. J Acquir Immune Defic Syndr 2001;28(1):14–8.

53. Wit FW, Wood R, Horban A, et al. Prednisolone does not prevent hypersensitivity reactions in antiretroviral drug regimens containing abacavir with or without nevirapine. AIDS 2001;15(18):2423–9.

54. Croxtall JD. Etravirine: a review of its use in the management of treatment-experienced patients with HIV-1 infection. Drugs 2012;72(6):847–69.

55. Molina JM, Clumeck N, Redant K, et al. Rilpivirine vs. efavirenz in HIV-1 patients with baseline viral load 100,000 copies/ml or less: week 48 phase III analysis. AIDS 2013;27(6):889–97.

56. Emerson CR, Post JJ, Workman C. A delayed hypersensitivity reaction to enfuvirtide after rechallenge. Int J STD AIDS 2009;20(4):288–9.

57. Phillips E, Keane N, Blyth C, et al. Both HLA Class I restricted CD8+ and Class II restricted CD4+T cells are implicated in the pathogenesis of nevirapine hypersensitivity. In: 51st Interscience Conference of Antimicrobial Agents and Chemotherapy. Chicago; 2011.

58. Karlin E, Phillips E. Genotyping for severe drug hypersensitivity. Curr Allergy Asthma Rep 2014;14(3):418.

59. Phillips EJ, Mallal SA. Pharmacogenetics of drug hypersensitivity. Pharmacogenomics 2010;11(7):973–87.

60. Perry ME, Almaani N, Desai N, et al. Raltegravir-induced Drug Reaction with Eosinophilia and Systemic Symptoms (DRESS) syndrome—implications for clinical practice and patient safety. Int J STD AIDS 2013;24(8):639–42.

61. Loulergue P, Mir O. Raltegravir-induced DRESS syndrome. Scand J Infect Dis 2012;44(10):802–3.

62. Zhang KS, Modi GM, Hsu S. DRESS syndrome associated with raltegravir. Dermatol Online J 2011;17(8):14.

63. Babiker ZO, Douthwaite ST, Collier LE, et al. Real-life outcomes of maraviroc-based regimens in HIV-1-infected individuals. J Int Assoc Provid AIDS Care 2013;12(1):12–4.

64. Lauer GM, Walker BD. Hepatitis C virus infection. N Engl J Med 2001;345(1): 41–52.

65. Lee MH, Yang HI, Lu SN, et al. Chronic hepatitis C virus infection increases mortality from hepatic and extrahepatic diseases: a community-based long-term prospective study. J Infect Dis 2012;206(4):469–77.

66. Hoofnagle JH, Seeff LB. Peginterferon and ribavirin for chronic hepatitis C. N Engl J Med 2006;355(23):2444–51.

67. Hezode C, Forestier N, Dusheiko G, et al. Telaprevir and peginterferon with or without ribavirin for chronic HCV infection. N Engl J Med 2009;360(18):1839–50.

68. Ascione A. Boceprevir in chronic hepatitis C infection: a perspective review. Ther Adv Chronic Dis 2012;3(3):113–21.

69. Samain A, Duval-Modeste AB, Joly P, et al. First case of drug rash eosinophilia and systemic symptoms due to boceprevir. J Hepatol 2014;60(4):891–3.

70. Dupin N, Mallet V, Carlotti A, et al. Severe skin rash in case of readministration of telaprevir in a patient who previously experienced a non severe rash. Hepatology 2012;55(6):2042–3.

71. Weiss ME. Recognizing drug allergy. How to differentiate true allergy from other adverse drug reactions. Postgrad Med 2005;117(5):32–6, 39.

72. Shear NH, Milpied B, Bruynzeel DP, et al. A review of drug patch testing and implications for HIV clinicians. AIDS 2008;22(9):999–1007.

73. Furue M. Photosensitive drug eruption induced by efavirenz in a patient with HIV infection. Intern Med 2004;43(7):533.

74. Yoshimoto E, Konishi M, Takahashi K, et al. The first case of efavirenz-induced photosensitivity in a Japanese patient with HIV infection. Intern Med 2004;43(7): 630–1.

75. Treudler R, Husak R, Raisova M, et al. Efavirenz-induced photoallergic dermatitis in HIV. AIDS 2001;15(8):1085–6.

76. Pollard RB, Robinson P, Dransfield K. Safety profile of nevirapine, a nonnucleoside reverse transcriptase inhibitor for the treatment of human immunodeficiency virus infection. Clin Ther 1998;20(6):1071–92.

77. Hughes DA, Vilar FJ, Ward CC, et al. Cost-effectiveness analysis of HLA B*5701 genotyping in preventing abacavir hypersensitivity. Pharmacogenetics 2004; 14(6):335–42.

78. Schackman BR, Scott CA, Walensky RP, et al. The cost-effectiveness of HLA-B*5701 genetic screening to guide initial antiretroviral therapy for HIV. AIDS 2008;22(15):2025–33.

Allergic Contact Dermatitis from the Vehicle Components of Topical Pharmaceutical Products

R. An Goossens, Pharm, PhD

KEYWORDS

- Allergic contact dermatitis • Iatrogenic • Topical pharmaceutical products
- Excipients • Preservatives • Fragrances

KEY POINTS

- The different categories in which the most important allergens can be classified are excipients, preservative agents, antioxidants, and fragrance components.
- The most frequently encountered allergens among the excipients are wool alcohols, propylene glycol, sorbitan oleate esters, and cetyl- en stearyl alcohol.
- The most frequently encountered allergens among the preservative agents are thimerosal, parabens, benzoic acid, and mercurials.
- The most frequently encountered allergens among the antioxidants are ethylene diamine (complexing agent) and (bi) sulfites.
- The most frequently encountered allergens among the fragrance components found in topical drugs are essential oils.

INTRODUCTION

The local application of pharmaceutical products may induce allergic and photo-allergic contact dermatitis (and, in some cases, skin reactions after systemic administration of the allergen or a chemically related compound), contact urticaria (immediate-type reactions), irritation, and systemic adverse effects caused by drug absorption. This article will only discuss allergic contact dermatitis.

ALLERGIC CONTACT DERMATITIS FROM TOPICAL PHARMACEUTICAL PRODUCTS

Topical pharmaceutical products are, in general, applied to diseased or inflamed skin, the barrier function of which is often incapacitated, leading to enhanced skin penetration of the applied chemicals. In such cases, even weak allergens are able to induce

The author has nothing to disclose.
Contact Allergy Unit, Department of Dermatology, University Hospital, Katholieke Universiteit Leuven, Kapucijnenvoer 33, Leuven B-3000, Belgium
E-mail address: An.Goossens@uz.kuleuven.ac.be

Immunol Allergy Clin N Am 34 (2014) 663–670
http://dx.doi.org/10.1016/j.iac.2014.04.010
0889-8561/14/$ – see front matter © 2014 Elsevier Inc. All rights reserved.

immunology.theclinics.com

sensitization. Hence, contact allergy to topical pharmaceutical products is common, particularly in subjects suffering from stasis eczema and/or leg ulcers, perianal dermatitis, and otitis externa, but also in individuals with irritant and/or other pre-existing eczematous conditions.[1–4]

NATURE OF THE CONTACT ALLERGENS

The contact allergens in topical pharmaceutical products concern active principles and vehicle components. Not only products such as creams, ointments, and solutions, but also wound dressings may be involved.

This article will concentrate on the vehicle components. **Box 1** gives the number of cases with positive patch-test reactions to vehicle components of topical pharmaceutical products (ie, excipients, preservative agents, and fragrances). The allergens have been identified in a total population of 17,367 patients tested between 1990 and 2013, of whom 2513 (14.5%) presented with an allergic iatrogenic contact dermatitis.

The different categories in which the most important allergens can be classified are listed in **Box 1**.[1,2]

Excipients

Excipients include wool alcohols (eg, eucerin and lanolin), propylene glycol, sorbitan oleate esters, and cetyl- en stearyl alcohol. **Fig. 1** shows a positive reaction to isopropyl myristate. **Fig. 2** shows clinical symptoms and positive patch-test reaction to cetyl alcohol in a 15-month-old atopic baby, due to its presence in a pharmaceutical cream.

Preservative Agents

Preservative agents include thimerosal, parabens, benzoic acid, mercurial, and benzalkonium chloride. **Fig. 3**: shows contact dermatitis from a combination preparation containing a local antibiotic and corticosteroid caused by the preservative potassium sorbate (sorbic acid also positive).

Antioxidants

Antioxidants include ethylene diamine (complexing agent), previously the main allergen in a combined antimycotic/antibiotic/anti-inflammatory widely used cream, (bi) sulfites (test substance sodium metabisulfite),[5] and butylhydroxyanisole.

Perfume Components

Previously these were often present in historical wound-healing preparations, but they actually are still used in many preparations, including nonsteroidal anti-inflammatory products, which for example contain lavender, geranium-, or other essential oils. Indeed, in a previous study, the author could demonstrate that 10% of the topical pharmaceutical products in Belgium were found to contain fragrance components.[6] **Fig. 4** shows allergic contact dermatitis from fragrance components, including lavender oil in a nonsteroidal anti-inflammatory product.

Wound dressings

In general, wound dressings mainly contain higher molecular (polymeric) compounds that are less likely to induce sensitization, and thus seem to be safer than the previously used creams and ointments; however, some additives, particularly in hydrocolloids, such as modified colophony or antioxidants, may still be the allergenic culprits.[7,8]

Box 1
Allergic contact dermatitis from excipients (ie, vehicle components, preservatives, and fragrances in topical pharmaceutical products) (K.U. Leuven, 1990–2013)

Nr + Cases	Allergens
Vehicle components	
354	Wool alcohols
146	Propylene glycol
132	Sorbitan sesquioleate
77	Cetyl alcohol
66	Nonoxynol 9
21	Lauraminoxide
14	Benzyl alcohol
12	Polyethylene glycol
12	Olive oil
10	Stearyl alcohol
9	Sodium sulforicinate
8	Modified colophonium
7	Sesame oil
7	Isopropyl myristate
5	Glycerol monostearate
4	Triethanolamine
4	Polyethyleneglycol stearate
4	Hexylene glycol
3	Polysorbate 60
3	Polyethylene glycol glyceryl 20 oleaat
2	Sorbitan monolaurate
2	Polysorbate 80
2	Petrolatum
2	Eucerin
2	Almond oil (sweet)
2	Lactic acid
2	Laureth-9
2	Propyleneglycol monostearate
2	Beeswax
1	Polyethyleneglycol distearate
1	Hydroxyethylmethylacrylate
1	Butylene glycol
1	Glyceryl rosinate
1	Cetearyl glucoside
1	Myristyl alcohol
1	Castor oil
1	Diethanolamine
1	Ethyleneglycol monostearate
Preservative agents	
81	Thiomersal
65	Parabens
33	Benzoic acid
27	Phenylmercuriborate
26	Benzalkonium chloride
15	Chlorocresol
12	Sorbic acid
10	Imidazolidinylurea
10	Formaldehyde
9	Potassium sorbate
5	Phenylmercurinitrate
3	Fenoxyethanol
3	Diazolidinylurea
1	Quaternium 15
1	Propyl gallate
1	Phenylmercutiacetate

Antioxidants	
62	Ethylenediamine
38	Sodium metabisulfite
21	Butylhydroxyanisole
4	Disodium Edetate (EDTA)
2	Butylhydroxytoluene
Fragrances[a]	
88	Fragrance-mix I[b]
68	Balsam of Peru
31	Lavender oil
15	Perfume
10	Geranium oil
8	Orange flower oil
6	Eucalyptus oil
4	Terpineol
4	Fragrance-mix II[b]
3	Pine tree oil
2	Thyme oil
2	Niaouli oil
2	Rose oil
1	Jasmin oil
1	Clove oil
1	Nutmeg oil
1	Rosemary oil

14,367 subjects patch tested, 2514 with iatrogenic dermatitis.

[a] Some of these component are also used for other purposes than perfuming (eg, for their antiseptic properties).

[b] Markers for fragrance allergy tested in the baseline series.

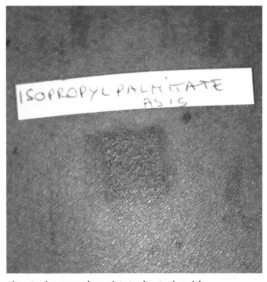

Fig. 1. Positive reaction to isopropyl myristate (tested as is).

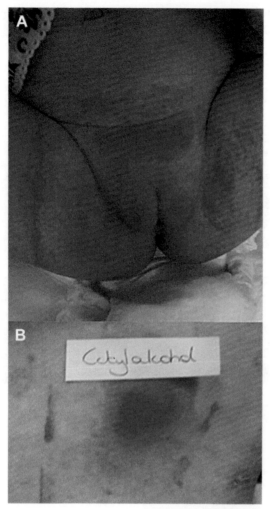

Fig. 2. (*A, B*) Clinical symptoms and positive patch-test reaction to cetyl alcohol in a 15-month-old atopic baby, due to its presence in a pharmaceutical cream.

DIAGNOSIS OF ALLERGIC CONTACT DERMATITIS

Patch (or epicutaneous) testing is the universally accepted method for the detection of causative agents. The test conditions for most of the contact allergens can be found in the literature.[9] Testing with the topical products used is also highly recommended; open and semiopen or semiocclusive tests,[10] use tests,[11] and repeated open application tests (ROATs)[12] are useful additional methods to identify the culprits.

Patch-Tests

Allergens, usually incorporated in petrolatum (sometimes also another vehicle), are applied in round or square chambers, which are mounted on adhesive tape, on the

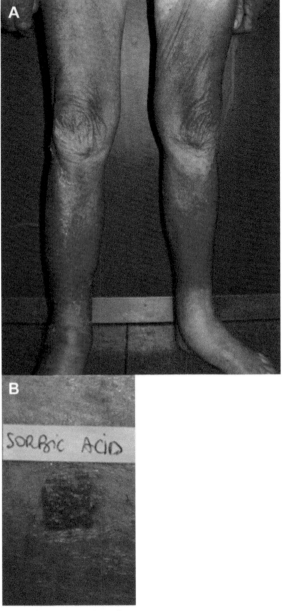

Fig. 3. (*A, B*) Allergic contact dermatitis from a combination preparation containing a local antibiotic and corticosteroid due to the preservative potassium sorbate (sorbic acid also positive).

upper back of the patients during 2 days. The readings of the test results are performed about 20 minutes after removal of the patches and again after 3 or 4 days (sometimes later). Allergen identification for a patient with a possible contact allergy to topical pharmaceutical products is performed by means of patch testing with the

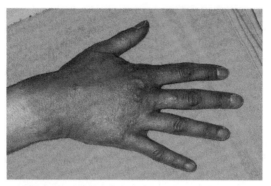

Fig. 4. Allergic contact dermatitis from fragrance components, including lavender oil in a nonsteroidal anti-inflammatory product.

standard series, specific pharmaceutical series, the product itself, and all of its ingredients. Sometimes dilution series are used to detect the sensitivity level of the patient and to determine the relevance with regard to the actual use situation.

Open and Semiopen (or Semiocclusive) Tests

These tests are useful modifications for topical pharmaceutical products that have an irritation potential. With an open test, the substance is applied uncovered on the upper arm or upper back twice a day during at least 2 days (without washing the test site).

A semiocclusive test consists of 1 application, with a cotton swab on about 1 cm^2 of the upper back, of a minute amount of a test material, which is left to dry completely, and covered with acrylate paper tape. The readings are performed after 2, 3, or 4 days. Diluted products (eg, 1%–2% aqueous) can also be tested this way.[10]

Use Tests and ROATs

Patch tests are vastly different from normal use conditions; therefore, tests can be completed by provocative use testing of sensitized subjects.[11,12]

With ROATs, about 0.1 mL of test material is applied twice daily to the flexor aspect of the forearm near the cubital fossa, to an area approximately 5 × 5 cm. The results are read after 1 week, but sometimes ROATs need to be performed up to 21 days, especially with low-concentrated allergens, in order to reveal an allergic reaction.

REFERENCES

1. Brandão FM, Goossens A. Ingredients of the vehicles, in topical drugs, chapter 38. In: Johansen JD, Frosch PJ, Lepoittevin JP, editors. Textbook of contact dermatitis. 5th edition. Berlin; Heidelberg (Germany): Springer-Verlag; 2011. p. 595–600.
2. Goosens A, Medeiros S. Allergic contact dermatitis from topical medicaments. Expert Rev Dermatol 2008;3:37–42.
3. Barbaud A, Collet E, Le Coz CJ, et al. Contact allergy in chronic leg ulcers: results of a multicentre study carried out in 423 patients and proposal for an updated series of patch tests. Contact Dermatitis 2009;60:279–87.
4. White IR. "Preservatives", in cosmetics and skin care products, chapter 32. In: Johansen JD, Frosch PJ, Lepoittevin JP, editors. Textbook of contact dermatitis. 5th edition. Berlin; Heidelberg (Germany): Springer-Verlag; 2011. p. 595–600.

5. Garcia-Gavin J, Parente J, Goossens A. Allergic contact dermatitis caused by sodium metabisulfite: a challenging allergen. A case series and literature review. Contact Dermatitis 2012;67(5):260–9.

6. Nardelli A, D'Hooghe E, Drieghe J, et al. Allergic contact dermatitis from fragrance components in specific topical pharmaceutical products in Belgium. Contact Dermatitis 2009;60(6):303–13.

7. Motolese A, Capriata S, Simonelli M. Contact sensitivity to 'advanced' wound dressings in 116 patients with leg ulcers. Contact Dermatitis 2009;60:107.

8. Pereira TM, Flour M, Goossens A. Allergic contact dermatitis from modified colophonium in wound dressings. Contact Dermatitis 2007;56:5.

9. dr Groot AC. Patch testing: test concentrations and vehicles for 4350 chemicals. Wapserveen: de Groot; 2008.

10. Goossens A. Semi-open (or semi-occlusive) tests. In: Lachapelle JM, Bruze M, Elsner PU, editors. Patch testing tips: recommendations form the ICDRG. Heidelberg (Germany); Berlin: Springer; 2014. p. 123–7.

11. Robinson MK, Stotts J, Danneman PJ, et al. A risk assessment process for allergic contact sensitization. Food Chem Toxicol 1989;27:479–89.

12. Hannuksela M, Salo H. The repeated open application test (ROAT). Contact Dermatitis 1986;14:221–7.

Place of Excipients in Systemic Drug Allergy

Annick Barbaud, MD, PhD*

KEYWORDS

- Excipients • Sulfites • Carboxymethylcellulose • Sodium benzoate • Vaccines
- Insulin

KEY POINTS

- Overdiagnosis of vaccine allergy is common and is considered as a major public health problem.
- The diagnosis of allergy to vaccine is complex and is often retained due to fear of severe anaphylactic reactions. However, most of the patients labeled as allergic to a vaccine tolerate a subsequent injection of the vaccine without clinical reaction. This is particularly the case of patients developing local reactions or delayed benign skin rashes.
- Regarding patients with a history suggestive of an immediate IgE-mediated hypersensitivity, a complete workup is mandatory. It will be primarily based on skin tests and/or specific IgE measurements.
- In the vast majority of cases, the vaccines can be administered using adapted protocols, even if the allergy tests are positive.
- Some vaccines' administrations carry a relatively high risk of severe anaphylactic reactions and should always be performed by well-trained physicians and emergency equipment must be readily available.

An excipient is an inert substance added to a drug to change dissolution or the kinetics of absorption, improve stability, influence palatability, or create a distinctive appearance. Also called additives, they are preservatives, emulsifiers, stabilizers, or thickeners. Drug hypersensitivity reactions (DHR) to them may lead to a false-positive diagnosis of DHRs to the specific active principle.

Allergic contact dermatitis to drug excipients has been more thoroughly studied (see article in this issue by Goossens) than DHRs related to excipients in drugs administered systemically. We only discuss the most frequent of the latter.

No funding source supported the work.

Conflict of Interest: None declared.

Dermatology and Allergy Department, Brabois Hospital, University Hospital of Nancy, Lorraine University, Rue du Morvan, Vandoeuvre les Nancy 54500, France

* Dermatology Department, University Hospital of Nancy, Pole des Specialités Medicales, Brabois Hospital, Universite de Lorraine, 6 Rue du Morvan, Vandoeuvre les Nancy 54500, France.

E-mail address: a.barbaud@chu-nancy.fr

Immunol Allergy Clin N Am 34 (2014) 671–679

http://dx.doi.org/10.1016/j.iac.2014.04.006

0889-8561/14/$ – see front matter © 2014 Elsevier Inc. All rights reserved.

immunology.theclinics.com

BENZYL ALCOHOL

When used as a preservative, benzyl alcohol can cause sensitization by contact with topical ointments but also by a systemic way. Two case reports illustrate this. Shmunes[1] has reported a case of allergy to benzyl alcohol used as a preservative in a solution of sodium tetradecyl sulfate, an agent used in sclerotherapy for varicose veins. A 16-year-old girl had immediate sensation of substernal burning and pleuritic pain associated with pruritus of the arms and legs after cyanocobalamin injections, with a vitamin B12 preparation containing benzyl alcohol (0.9%).[2] Prick test results were negative, but intradermal tests gave immediate positive results in testing 3 different cyanocobalamin brands containing benzyl alcohol and also with benzyl alcohol diluted at 0.009%.

CARBOXYMETHYLCELLULOSE

Carboxymethylcellulose (also called *carmellose* or *croscarmellose*, *sodium carboxymethylcellulose*, and *E466*) is a hydrophilic derivative of cellulose used in injectable preparations as a suspending agent to promote solubilization of compounds with poor water solubility; it is also present in tablets as binder, glidant, and antiadherent, as active principle in bulk laxatives and as an additive in food products. The immediate hypersensitivity of croscarmellose is primarily reported after intra-articular infiltration of corticosteroids[3–7] but also with a generic furosemide.[8]

In immediate reactions to injectable drugs containing carboxymethylcellulose, it is reported that oral administration of carboxymethylcellulose is well tolerated owing to its weak absorption through the digestive tract.[3,9]

However, carboxymethylcellulose anaphylaxis has been reported after contact with gut mucosa during barium enema.[10,11]

In immediate hypersensitivity to carboxymethylcellulose, prick tests and intradermal tests can have positive results, and immunoglobulin E (IgE) has been identified using dot-blot analysis but could not be specific.[10,11] Bigliardi and colleagues[7] have emphasized the value of the cellular antigen stimulation test.

For patients with a suspicion of carboxymethylcellulose sensitization, it is recommended to perform prick tests with carboxymethylcellulose, then, to determine if there is an oral tolerance to carboxymethylcellulose, to continue with an oral provocation test. Prick tests can be done with carboxymethylcellulose at 5 mg/mL[7] and can be positive at lower concentrations.[4]

Positive results have been reported using intradermal tests (IDT) with carboxymethylcellulose at 0.005 or 0.01 mg/mL.[7,10,11] Unfortunately, currently, we do not have any more available injectable forms of carboxymethylcellulose for performing IDT. Therefore, performing IDT with the responsible drugs containing carboxymethylcellulose is the only alternative.

Bigliardi and colleagues[7] suggest performing an oral provocation test with carboxymethylcellulose to exclude a reaction to small oral doses of this widely used carbohydrate. But patients allergic to carboxymethylcellulose usually do not react to the oral application of a small amount of carboxymethylcellulose typically present in food and tablets.

Three cases of systemic delayed hypersensitivity to carboxymethylcellulose have been reported with maculopapular rash.[12] This delayed sensitization can mimic multiple sensitizations to different drug classes. In such cases, prick tests and intradermal tests can have positive results on their delayed readings, there is no oral tolerance to carboxymethylcellulose, and there are no cross-reactions with hydroxypropylcellulose.

DYES

The relevance of hypersensitivity to dyes among all drug hypersensitivities remains unclear. According to Bhatia,[13] among 2210 patients exposed to tartrazine-containing drugs, 83 (3.8%) had adverse reactions, and the symptoms subsided within 24 to 48 hours of stopping the drug. None of the patients showed allergy to non–tartrazine-containing brands. Swerlick and Campbell[14] reported on 11 patients with chronic, unexplained pruritic skin disorders that have responded to medication changes centered around avoidance of dyes, particularly FD&C Blue No. 1 (bright blue) and Blue No. 2 (indigo carmine). Therapies were switched back to the lighter-colored tablets or a dye-free liquid form (doxepin), and the dermatitis promptly resolved.

Twenty-four hours after beginning an iron oral treatment (ferrous sulfate, Sunset Yellow FC&C No. 6 (E110 = orange disperse 3), erythrosine (E127), titanium dioxide (E171), and methyl methacrylate), a 43-year-old woman had a severe facial erythema with itching and skin edema.[15] It could be considered a flare up of a previous professional contact dermatitis. After patch tests, slight facial erythema was observed 6 hours after the application, and the patient had positive patch tests for orange disperse 3 (Sunset Yellow), para-phenylenediamine, and nickel sulfate after 48 hours. The authors supposed that she had become sensitized to these substances during her former occupation as a hairdresser. A single-blind, placebo-controlled oral challenge was made, with ferrous sulfate eliciting facial itching and erythema and no reaction with ferric propionate.

On the other hand, yellow dye tartrazine was supposed to be a potential cause of exacerbations of asthma, allergic rhinitis and urticaria in atopic patients. But, in 26 atopic patients, a double-blind, placebo-controlled, crossed-over challenge with 35 mg of tartrazine was done, and no significant cutaneous, respiratory, or cardiovascular reactions were seen when compared with placebo.[16]

In a unicenter, retrospective study, 102 subjects with suspected tartrazine-induced acute urticaria/angioedema had a placebo-controlled challenge with 5 mg of tartrazine.[17] Among them, only one patient had a positive oral provocation test result. The authors suggested that all patients who have had adverse reactions that could be attributed to tartrazine should also be carefully evaluated for other possible causes.

In case of hypersensitivity reactions supposedly caused by dyes, only a provocation test can prove the responsibility of these excipients.

POVIDONE

Povidone (PVP, polyvinylpyrrolidone) is a mixture of synthetic polymers with molecular weights between 10,000 and 70,000 Da, comparable to those of the plasma proteins.

Michavila-Gomez and colleagues[18] reported one case with an anaphylactic reaction occurring in a 4-year old boy after using a prednisolone oral solution with povidone. The result of prick test with pure noniodinated povidone (25 mg/mL) was positive, and the result of oral provocation test carried out with methylprednisolone at 20 mg was negative. A relapse occurred when the child orally received cefuroxime axetil with povidone K30. From the literature, the authors collected other cases in children caused by PVP associated with flubendazol or in a formulation containing paracetamol. In adults, there are cases involving the intra-articular administration of drugs containing corticosteroid and PVP or after the administration of contrast medium containing PVP. One case with acetaminophen-containing tablets was also reported by Rönnau and colleagues.[19]

Methods for testing PVP are not standardized. There are some reports with positive results in performing prick tests with PVP, with solution of povidone iodine, or with the formulation of the responsible drug and another formulation with another excipient, positive scratch test, or intracutaneous provocation tests with injectable forms of the responsible drugs.

SODIUM BENZOATE

Sodium benzoate (E211) has been implicated in the onset of some types of food-induced asthma, urticaria, or anaphylaxis. It is found in anticough syrups, vitamin preparations, heparin, or antibiotic syrups.

Recently, a high frequency of sodium benzoate hypersensitivity has been reported in children with cutaneous reactions occurring during the amoxicillin plus clavulanic acid suspension intake.[20] Single-blind oral provocation tests with amoxicillin plus clavulanic acid, sodium benzoate, and placebo were performed in 89 children with cutaneous reactions while taking the antibiotic suspension and in 20 sex- and age-matched controls who had chronic idiopathic urticaria. Sodium benzoate was administered at 2 doses up to 150 mg and 250 mg depending on the body weight (15–40 kg or 41–50 kg). Ten children (11%) had reactions after the provocation test with sodium benzoate with tolerance to amoxicillin plus clavulanic acid, and 3 children had positive reactions to both the excipient and the active drug. The provoking cumulative dose of sodium benzoate was usually 150 mg (9 of 13), and 4 patients had a positive response to 50 mg of sodium benzoate.

Some investigators suggest that because benzoates are structurally similar to acetyl salicylic acid (aspirin), they may act on eicosanoid production, so Mori and colleagues[20] suggest that it would also be good to check acetyl salicylic acid tolerance in children reacting to sodium benzoate. These results suggest that benzoate hypersensitivity should be investigated in children manifesting reactions to drugs containing it, once an allergy status in relation to the antibiotic is excluded or confirmed.

SULFITES

Sulfites are sulfur dioxide salts that are widely used as antioxidants in food and drugs. In the pharmaceutical industry, they are mainly used in local anesthetic solutions, including those containing epinephrine and most of the available solutions of epinephrine; in some injectable antibiotics, corticosteroids, dopamine, isoproterenol, and propofol; and in ancient bronchodilator inhalational agents. By systemic exposure, most adverse reactions have been reported with sulfites contained in food. They occur primarily in asthmatic patients and induce exacerbation of asthma, pruritus, urticaria, angioedema, flush, or even hypotension.

With drugs, sulfites have been found to cause paradoxical worsening of asthma exacerbations when old bronchodilator inhalational agents were used after injection of local anesthetic agents containing sulfites or epinephrine. They are suspected to be responsible for angioedema, urticaria, and for the reactivation of an occupational-related contact dermatitis (flare up of a contact allergy).[21]

A few cases of asthma exacerbations have been reported caused by sulfites in drugs such as corticosteroids, local anesthetics, gentamicin, metoclopramide, doxycycline and vitamin B complex, or propofol.[22,23]

The mechanism involved in adverse reactions after a systemic exposure to sulfites remains unclear and may be a multifactorial process: inadequate sulfite oxidase activity, non–IgE-induced mast cell degranulation. Prick tests and intradermal tests with sulfite have no value; that of oral challenge tests is better but is not well standardized and potentially dangerous in sulfite-sensitive asthmatics. Recently, it has been observed in vitro that sodium sulfite significantly and dose-dependently suppressed Th1-type immune response, which could play a central role in the precipitation of allergy symptoms by modulating cytokine profiles toward a Th2-type pattern.[23]

Sensitization to sulfites contained in drugs seems to be rare and must be considered mainly in patients with asthma. However, provocation test with the suspected drug and with sulfites can show hypersensitivity to this excipient. As emphasized by Vally and colleagues,[22] most of the commercially available preparations of adrenaline contain metabisulfite. However, even in patients with serious sulfite sensitivity, the benefit from adrenaline is considered to outweigh the risk of sulfite exposure associated with use of adrenaline in an emergency.

NONIONIC POLYETHOXYLATED SURFACTANTS

Nonionic polyethoxylated surfactants, polysorbate 80 (PS80, E433, Tween 80, polyoxyethylene sorbitan monooleate), and Cremophor-EL (CrEL = polyoxyethylated castor oil in 50% ethanol) activate the complement system in vitro in normal human serum and plasma. They are more efficient reactogens than their structural homolog, Tween-20. Cremophor-EL and Tween-80 activate the complement system in similar extent. Therapeutic side effects, such as acute hypersensitivity and systemic immunostimulation, caused by intravenous medicines containing polyethoxylated detergents, can be attributed to complement activation-derived inflammatory mediators.[24]

Serious forms of hypersensitivity reactions have been reported several medicines containing nonionic polyethoxylated surfactants, including paclitaxel with CrEL, docetaxel, or erythropoietin with PS80.[25,26] Premedication regimens and longer infusion times lowered the incidence of reactivity. If tolerance remains poor, rapid desensitization by a standardized 12-step protocol has been reported as safe and effective.[26]

EXCIPIENTS IN VACCINES
Aluminum-Induced Granuloma

Sulfate and aluminum phosphate hydroxide are used as adjuvants in numerous vaccines and in solutions for subcutaneous allergen immunotherapy. Aluminum sensitization caused by vaccinal solutions results in the appearance of nodules at the injection site, which usually regress after a few weeks or months.[27,28]

In some cases, the granulomas persist for years. These cases have been reported after vaccination or subcutaneous allergen immunotherapy.[27] These patients can experience flare ups at the nodule site, especially if they are exposed to aluminum again, either by injection of a solution with aluminum or by using antiperspirants containing aluminum salts.

Histologic assessment is not necessary because, when performed, a poorly circumscribed infiltration of lymphocytes into the hypodermis can be observed, sometimes reaching the deeper dermis, with a crown shape circling the cicatricial sclerosis. Staining with pentahydroxyflavone can be used to detect fluorescent intramacrophagic aluminum particles.

Diagnostic confirmation can be made by revealing the sensitization to aluminum by positivity to the patch test with an aluminum extract or in using an empty aluminum-made Finn Chamber cupule. Patch tests with aluminum extracts are inconsistently positive in patients who have granulomas at the site of injection.

In sensitized subjects, the use of antiperspirants, deodorants, or topics containing aluminum salts should be discouraged. Subcutaneous allergen immunotherapy with aeroallergens containing aluminum is contraindicated. For vaccinal solutions that do not exist without aluminum, the injections should be deep enough to limit the exposure to aluminum.[27,28]

Antibiotics in Vaccines

Several vaccines are subjected to processing with antibiotics during the manufacturing process. Although these antibiotics (neomycin, streptomycin, kana-mycin, Aureomycin) may be present in a vaccine solution, they were never implicated in vaccine allergy (see Caubet-Ponvert in this issue).

Egg Protein and Vaccines

Some vaccinal preparations, such as measles, seasonal flu, yellow-fever, rabies, tick-borne encephalitis and some influenza A H1N1 vaccines, are made on chicken egg embryos or fibroblasts of chicken embryos.[27]

For the flu vaccine, the prick test is of no interest when determining if tests for vaccinal solutions help in patients with egg allergies.[29] In patients with serious anaphy-lactic reactions to egg proteins (asthma or anaphylactic shock), some investigators proposed carrying out the vaccination through a 2-step protocol under hospital super-vision: a first injection at 10% of the dose, and 30 minutes later, if well tolerated, a sec-ond injection at 90%.

For any patient suspected to be allergic to eggs, the following points should be taken into account:

- If eggs are consumed and well tolerated: it is possible to vaccinate without any particular precaution
- If egg consumption leads to minor allergic manifestations: vaccinate and follow up after 30 minutes
- If there is a suspicion of egg allergy but eggs have never been consumed: perform a prick test with egg proteins and adapt the vaccine to the intensity of the response to these tests
- In case of proven egg allergy (positive prick tests), and severe or uncontrolled asthma or history of anaphylaxis: the risk-to-benefit ratio should be evaluated, the maximal ovalbumin concentration authorized in the vaccinal solution should be verified, and vaccination should be performed under hospital supervision, possibly by a 2-step protocol (10%, and 30 minutes later, 90%).

Contamination from the Media Used for Recombinant Vaccines

Engerix B is the only hepatitis B vaccine prepared from *Saccharomyces cerevisiae*. A female patient with a history of food allergy to yeast suffered an anaphylactic shock with the first injection of Engerix B.[27] Prick tests were positive with the vaccine and yeasts, which implied that the triggering agents were anti-*Saccharomyces* IgE. Vac-cine adverse effects are rare in yeast-sensitive individuals.[30]

Gelatin

This protein derivative of animal collagen, the component most widely used in manufacturing drug capsules, is sometimes used as an excipient in injectable solu-tions. Gelatin is well tolerated when used as an excipient, unlike what is observed when it is used as a plasma expander. Contained in some vaccines, gelatins induced an anaphylactic reaction with antichickenpox injection in a 4-year-old child who had a previous food allergy to gelatinous candies; an anaphylactic reaction has also been seen in some cases with the mumps-measles-rubella vaccine.[27,31,32] Among 366 Japanese patients who presented hypersensitivity reactions after mumps-measles-rubella vaccination with 0.2% gelatin, anti-gelatin IgE was detected in 25 of the 27 (93%) subjects with anaphylaxis.[32]

EXCIPIENTS IN INSULIN

The prevalence of allergic reactions to insulin products appears to be approximately 2%, and less than one-third of these events has been considered related to the insulin itself. Other reactions occur because of the preservatives added to insulin, including metacresol, protamine, and zinc.

Metacresol

Localized reactions at the injection site can be accompanied by positive patch tests to metacresol.[33,34]

Three cases of delayed-type hypersensitivity reactions to meta-cresol were reported with systemic symptoms, including nausea, headache, sweating, and diarrhea. In only one of the 3 cases erythematous burning lesions at the injection sites were present on the day after the subcutaneous administration of insulin.[35] Delayed reactions improved after they were treated with human insulin free of metacresol.

Protamine

Protamine is a low-molecular-weight polycationic protein purified from testes and sperm of salmon. It is used in the treatment of cardiovascular disorders to neutralize the effects of heparin and also as an adjuvant in insulin. In this latter use, it could induce localized delayed reactions or urticaria. Protamine reactions could be triggered by allergic or nonimmunologic mechanisms through an activation of the classical complement pathway.[35,36]

Chu and colleagues[36] reported one case of a fatal allergic reaction possibly associated with protamine administration in a patient with a history of allergy to fish and to protamine-containing insulin. Some investigators have recommended the dose of antiprotamine IgE.[37]

Zinc Oxide

Delayed-onset allergic reactions localized at the site of insulin injection or systemic urticaria associated with zinc have been reported.[38] In a patient who had generalized urticaria with face edema and dyspnea after each injection of zinc-containing insulin, a prick test done with zinc chloride (5 mg/mL), displayed positive results with a local reaction and also a laryngeal tickling and a transient urticaria.[39]

SUMMARY

Hypersensitivity reactions to excipients contained in drugs are rare but can be severe or confusing. With regard to generic versus brand drug, often the ingredients are different; for each DHR, we recommend that the physician exercises caution in considering which brand drug or generic was administered and in listing all medicine components and not only the active drug.

REFERENCES

1. Shmunes E. Allergic dermatitis to benzylalcohol in an injectable solution. Arch Dermatol 1984;120:1200–1.

2. Turvey SE, Cronin B, Arnold AD, et al. Adverse reactions to vitamin B12 injections due to benzylalcohol sensitivity: successful treatment with intranasal cyanocobalamin. Allergy 2004;59:1023–4.

3. Rival-Tringali AL, Gunera-Saad N, Berard F, et al. Tolerance de la carboxymethylcellulose par voie orale chez deux malades ayant developpe une anaphylaxie a la carboxymethylcellulose injectable. Ann Dermatol Venereol 2008; 135:402–6.

4. Laing ME, Fallis B, Murphy GM. Anaphylactic reaction to intralesional corticosteroid injection. Contact Dermatitis 2007;57:132–3.

5. Field S, Falvey E, Barry J, et al. Type 1 hypersensitivity reaction to carboxymethylcellulose following intra-articular triamcinolone injection. Contact Dermatitis 2009;61:302–3.

6. Grims RH, Kranke B, Aberer W. Pitfalls in drug allergy skin testing: false-positive reactions due to (hidden) additives. Contact Dermatitis 2006;54:290–4.

7. Bigliardi PL, Izakovic J, Weber JM, et al. Anaphylaxis to the carbohydrate carboxymethylcellulose in parenteral corticosteroid preparations. Dermatology 2003;207:100–3.

8. Mumoli N, Cei M, Luschi R, et al. Allergic reaction to Croscarmellose sodium used as excipient of a generic drug. QJM 2011;104:709–10.

9. Bircher AJ, Izakovic J. Oral tolerance of carboxymethylcellulose in patients with anaphylaxis to parenteral carboxymethylcellulose. Ann Allergy Asthma Immunol 2004;92:580–1.

10. Dumond P, Franck P, Morisset M, et al. Pre-lethal anaphylaxis to carboxymethylcellulose confirmed by identification of specific IgE–review of the literature. Eur Ann Allergy Clin Immunol 2009;41:171–6.

11. Muroi N, Mori S, Ono S, et al. Allergy to carboxymethylcellulose. Allergy 2002;57: 1212–3.

12. Barbaud A, Waton J, Pinault AL, et al. Cutaneous adverse drug reactions due to delayed sensitization to carboxymethylcellulose. Contact Dermatitis 2011;64: 294–7.

13. Bhatia MS. Allergy to tartrazine in psychotropic drugs. J Clin Psychiatry 2000;61: 473–6.

14. Swerlick RA, Campbell CF. Medication dyes as a source of drug allergy. J Drugs Dermatol 2013;12:99–102.

15. Rogkakou A, Guerra L, Scordamaglia A, et al. Severe skin reaction due to excipients of an oral iron treatment. Allergy 2007;62:334–5.

16. Pestana S, Moreira M, Olej B. Safety of ingestion of yellow tartrazine by double-blind placebo controlled challenge in 26 atopic adults. Allergol Immunopathol (Madr) 2010;38:142–6.

17. Nettis E, Colanardi MC, Ferrannini A, et al. Suspected tartrazine-induced acute urticaria/angioedema is only rarely reproducible by oral rechallenge. Clin Exp Allergy 2003;33:1725–9.

18. Michavila-Gomez AV, Moreno-Palanques MA, Ferrer-Vazquez M, et al. Anaphylactic reaction to povidone secondary to drug ingestion in a young child. Allergol Immunopathol (Madr) 2012;40:259–61.

19. Rönnau AC, Wulferink M, Gleichmann E, et al. Anaphylaxis to polyvinylpyrrolidone in an analgesic preparation. Br J Dermatol 2000;143:1055–8.

20. Mori F, Barni S, Pucci N, et al. Cutaneous adverse reactions to amoxicillin-clavulanic acid suspension in children: the role of sodium benzoate. Curr Drug Saf 2012;7:87–91.

21. Simon RA. Sulfite sensitivity. Ann Allergy 1986;56:281–8.

22. Vally H, Misso NL, Madan V. Clinical effects of sulphite additives. Clin Exp Allergy 2009;39:1643–51.
23. Schroecksnadel S, Jenny M, Fuchs D. Sensitivity to sulphite additives. Clin Exp Allergy 2010;40:688–9.
24. Weiszhár Z, Czúcz J, Révész C, et al. Complement activation by polyethoxylated pharmaceutical surfactants: Cremophor-EL, Tween-80 and Tween-20. Eur J Pharm Sci 2012;45:492–8.
25. Limaye S, Steele RH, Quin J, et al. An allergic reaction to erythropoietin secondary to polysorbate hypersensitivity. J Allergy Clin Immunol 2002;110:530.
26. Castells MC, Tennant NM, Sloane DE, et al. Hypersensitivity reactions to chemotherapy: outcomes and safety of rapid desensitization in 413 cases. J Allergy Clin Immunol 2008;122:574–80.
27. Barbaud A, Deschildre A, Waton J, et al. Hypersensitivity and vaccines: an update. Eur J Dermatol 2013;23:135–41.
28. Bergfors E, Trollfors B, Inerot A. Unexpectedly high incidence of persistent itching nodules and delayed hypersensitivity to aluminium in children after the use of adsorbed vaccines from a single manufacturer. Vaccine 2003;22:64–9.
29. Roukens AH, Vossen AC, van Dissel JT, et al. Reduced intradermal test dose of yellow fever vaccine induces protective immunity in individuals with egg allergy. Vaccine 2009;27:2408–9.
30. DiMiceli L, Pool V, Kelso JM, et al, V.A.E.R.S. Team. Vaccination of yeast sensitive individuals: review of safety data in the US vaccine adverse event reporting system (VAERS). Vaccine 2006;24:703–7.
31. Kelso JM, Jones RT, Yunginger JW. Anaphylaxis to measles, mumps, and rubella vaccine mediated by IgE to gelatin. J Allergy Clin Immunol 1993;91:867–72.
32. Nakayama T, Aizawa C, Kuno-Sakai H. A clinical analysis of gelatin allergy and determination of its causal relationship to the previous administration of gelatin-containing acellular pertussis vaccine combined with diphtheria and tetanus toxoids. J Allergy Clin Immunol 1999;103:321–5.
33. Clerx V, Van Den Keybus C, Kochuyt A, et al. Drug intolerance reaction to insulin therapy caused by metacresol. Contact Dermatitis 2003;48:162–3.
34. Kim D, Baraniuk J. Delayed-type hypersensitivity reaction to the meta-cresol component of insulin. Ann Allergy Asthma Immunol 2007;99:194–5.
35. Ghazavi MK, Johnston GA. Insulin allergy. Clin Dermatol 2011;29:300–5.
36. Chu YQ, Cai LJ, Jiang DC, et al. Allergic shock and death associated with protamine administration in a diabetic patient. Clin Ther 2010;32:1729–32.
37. Bollinger ME, Hamilton RG, Wood RA. Protamine allergy as a complication of insulin hypersensitivity: a case report. J Allergy Clin Immunol 1999;104:462–5.
38. Gin H, Aubertin J. Generalized allergy due to zinc and protamine in insulin preparation treated with insulin pump. Diabetes Care 1987;10:789–90.
39. Ben Ammar I, Ksouri H, Trabelsi N, et al. Generalized allergy due to zinc in insulin treated with zinc-free insulin. Acta Diabetol 2012;49:239–41.

In Vitro Diagnosis of Immediate IgE-Mediated Drug Hypersensitivity
Warnings and (Unmet) Needs

Astrid P. Uyttebroek, MD, Vito Sabato, MD, Chris H. Bridts, MLT, Didier G. Ebo, MD, PhD*

KEYWORDS

- Basophil activation • Drug provocation • Flow cytometry • IgE
- Immediate drug allergy

KEY POINTS

- Immediate drug hypersensitivity reaction (DHR) constitutes an important health condition, with serious consequences of inadequate diagnosis. In this article, some of the most important, but certainly not all, issues related to in vitro diagnosis of IgE-mediated allergies are discussed.
- Correct development and validation of novel tests need sufficient numbers of appropriately identified patients and (exposed) control individuals. It is likely that collaborative studies are necessary to meet these requirements.
- These studies should adopt standardized and harmonized clinical and laboratory protocols, to avoid erroneous inclusions that might impede appropriate clinical validation of the assays.
- Although basophil activation testing in drug allergy might seem to be still in its infancy, with increasing original applications over the last years and with increasing employment, we can expect the assay to enter mainstream clinical use, especially for DHR that cannot readily or correctly be diagnosed by other means.
- In vitro diagnostics will benefit from expanded and novel insights and understandings in drug chemical reactivity, protein binding, biotransformation, degradation, identification of (cross-reactive) drug antigenic determinants, and deeper understanding of sensitization routes. DHR remains a conundrum, because knowledge in these areas remains sparse and ignorance great. Collective efforts should be undertaken to activate fundamental and clinical investigations.

The authors have nothing to disclose.
V. Sabato is a Clinical Researcher of the Research Foundation-Flanders (FWO: 1700614N). D.G. Ebo is a Senior Clinical Researcher of the FWO (1800614N).
Department of Immunology, Allergology, Rheumatology, Faculty of Medicine and Health Science, Antwerp University Hospital, University of Antwerp, Antwerp 2610, Belgium
* Corresponding author. Department of Immunology, Allergology, Rheumatology, Faculty of Medicine and Health Science, University of Antwerp, Campus Drie Eiken T5.95, Universiteitsplein 1, Antwerpen 2610, Belgium.
E-mail address: immuno@uantwerpen.be

Immunol Allergy Clin N Am 34 (2014) 681–689
http://dx.doi.org/10.1016/j.iac.2014.04.007
0889-8561/14/$ – see front matter © 2014 Elsevier Inc. All rights reserved.

INTRODUCTION

Challenges in in vitro immediate drug hypersensitivity reaction (DHR) diagnosis lie in the development and validation of reliable assays enabling safe and correct identification of all incriminated agents and potential alternatives for the future. Although drug provocation tests (DPT) are considered as the gold standard for drug hypersensitivity diagnosis, DPT are hampered by the risk of severe, life-threatening reactions and might be contraindicated (ie, patients taking β-blockers or angiotensin-converting enzyme inhibitors) or not possible for obvious reasons (ie, hypersensitivity to neuromuscular blocking agents [NMBA]). Besides, even DPT do not show absolute predictive values.[1] Hitherto, diagnostic DPT have not entered mainstream clinical practice.

Therefore, diagnosis of immediate DHR usually starts with a thorough history complemented with skin tests or in vitro quantification of (commercially available) specific IgE (sIgE) antibodies when an IgE-mediated mechanism with activation of mast cells and basophils is suspected.[2]

However, only a few drug-sIgE assays are available, and most of them have not been thoroughly clinically validated. In addition, immediate DHR with release of mediators by mast cells and basophils does not per se always involve crosslinking of the high affinity IgE receptor (FcεRI), but might also result from various alternative mechanisms that cannot be depicted by traditional sIgE assays, reinforcing the requirement for the development and validation of additional cellular tests such as basophil activation assays, because these tests can also be informative for immediate DHR independent from IgE. Starting from our clinical priorities and experience, the objective of this article is to identify some misconceptions, shortcomings, and unmet needs in in vitro immediate DHR diagnosis and to emphasize different obstacles that might hamper correct validation and harmonization of sIgE quantification and cellular tests. Undoubtedly, as with any subject still beset by many questions, alternative interpretations, hypotheses, or explanations expressed here may not find universal acceptance.

QUANTIFICATION OF SIGE ANTIBODIES

There are different automated in vitro techniques to quantify serum sIgE antibodies. However, unlike protein allergens, for routine application of immunoassays to drug-sIgE antibodies, the current situation is characterized by a limited availability of well-validated drug-specific tests. The only drug-specific IgE assays that are readily accessible comprise penicilloyl G (c1), penicilloyl V (c2), ampicilloyl (c5) and amoxicilloyl (c6) determinants, cephaclor (c7), chlorhexidine (c8, antiseptic), chymopapain (c209), (bovine) gelatin (c74), human (c73), bovine (c71) and porcine (c70) insulin, morphine (c260, marker for sensitization to tertiary and quaternary substituted ammonium determinants), pholcodine (c261) and suxamethonium (c202), which are commercially available from Thermo Fisher Scientific, Uppsala, Sweden. In addition, and for research purposes only, adrenocorticotropic hormone, atracurium, bacitracin, carboplatin, cefamandole, cefoxitin, cefotaxime, cefuroxime, cisplatinum, mepivacaine, methylprednisolone-21-succinate, nafamostat (4-guanidinobenzoic acid), oxaliplatin, penicillin minor determinants (eg, penicillanyl), propyphenazone, protamine, rocuronium, and tetanus toxoid are offered via the Thermo Fisher Scientific special allergen service. However, as exemplified in the introductory paragraph, most of these assays have not been sufficiently clinically validated, mainly as a result of the unavailability of sufficient numbers of accurately phenotyped patients and exposed control individuals.

Probably the most studied sIgE tests are those for β-lactam antibiotics. The most used antibiotics of this class in clinical practice consist of monocyclic molecules, such as monobactams, and bicyclic molecules, such as penicillins and clavams, cephalosporin, and carbapenems. The European Network for Drug Allergy recommends for safety reasons to perform serum sIgE assays in patients with a history of immediate penicillin hypersensitivity in addition to skin test in the allergologic workup.[3]

Although IgE assays show a generally low sensitivity (12.50%–50%), several cases of positive sIgE results in immediate reactions with negative skin test have been described.[4–7] However, not only sensitivity but also specificity of commercial available tests are far from ideal, for reasons such as increased total IgE and immunologic cross-reactivity.[8,9] For example, Fontaine and colleagues,[4] who compared DPT and skin testing, observed sIgE to β-lactam antibiotics to yield a specificity between 83.30% and 100%.

Because patients with positive sIgE results are generally precluded from DPT, improvement of these techniques is mandatory to avoid erroneous overdiagnosis of penicillin allergy. Another important issue in the diagnostic approach of IgE-mediated β-lactam allergy is the assessment of cross-reactivity and identification of safe alternatives. However, the currently available drug-sIgE assays do not contribute significantly in the prediction of the clinical outcome.

Another representative example showing the potential and limitations of drug-specific IgE immunoassays is the morphine solid-phase assay. Morphine, by virtue of its overtly accessible single tertiary N-methyl ammonium group, is readily recognized by sera from most, but certainly not all, patients who reacted to curarizing NMBA. Moreover, morphine solid-phase immunoassays have been reported to be superior to NMBA-specific assays for the detection of NMBA-reactive sIgE antibodies.[10–12] One of these immunoassays is available as the ImmunoCAP Allergen c260 Morphine (Thermo Fisher Scientific); the package leaflet indicates that the test is an alternative quaternary ammonium marker to suxamethonium and is intended for use as a diagnostic tool in NMBA-induced anaphylaxis. However, several issues should be addressed here. First, the morphine solid phase might not identify all patients allergic to NMBA, particularly to benzylisoquinolines, such as atracurium, cis-atracurium, and mivacurium.[10,12] The excellent sensitivity that applies to suxamethonium and rocuronium allergy cannot simply be extrapolated to benzylisoquinolines. Second, attention needs to be drawn to a prevalence of IgE reactivity to morphine between 1% and 10% in individuals without NMBA allergy.[11–13] Although the morphine solid-phase test might be a valuable backup to equivocal and negative skin tests in highly suggestive cases, caution is advised on too loose application of these assays and thoughtless interpretation of positive sIgE results. This situation could not only result in overestimation of NMBA allergy with unnecessary avoidance measures but, more seriously, could also entail dramatic consequences by overlooking alternative diagnoses. From the earliest days of application, it was obvious that NMBA-reactive and substituted ammonium-reactive sIgE antibody tests should not be used in isolation to diagnose curare allergy, but as a supplement to skin tests,[14,15] and should never be used to predict NMBA allergy in primary prevention. Mutatis mutandis, this recommendation applies to opiate allergy, because patients showing sIgE reactivity in the morphine solid-phase assay generally have negative basophil activation tests (BATs) and provocation tests for morphine or structurally closely related compounds such as codeine (**Fig. 1**).[16] Although frequently found in sera from allergic patients, especially with rocuronium and suxamethonium allergy, there is no compelling evidence that these morphine sIgE antibodies underlie allergic reactions to this opiate. Nevertheless, it seems that in the ninth French survey (2005–2007),[17] 12 patients had their diagnosis of NMBA allergy established by an isolated positive sIgE result to a quaternary ammonium, and 13 patients were identified as morphine allergic.

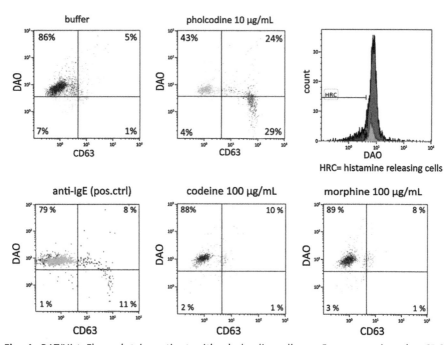

Fig. 1. BAT/HistaFlow plot in patient with pholcodine allergy. Representative plot CD63 appearance and histamine release in response to buffer, anti-IgE as a positive control, pholcodine 10 μg/mL, and the structurally almost similar opiates codeine 100 mg/mL and morphine 100 μg/mL. Di-amino-oxidase (DAO) (Sigma Aldrich, Saint Louis, MO, USA); pos.ctrl, positive control. (*From* Leysen J, De WL, Sabato V, et al. IgE-mediated allergy to pholcodine and cross-reactivity to neuromuscular blocking agents: lessons from flow cytometry. Cytometry B Clin Cytom 2013;84:69; with permission.)

Generally, in the absence of clinical validation, manufacturers have traditionally been recommending a positive cutoff of 0.35 kUA/L for serologic assessment of allergen-specific IgE. However, this threshold might not be interchangeable between different techniques and may not be appropriate for correct diagnosis. Different studies indicate that predefined and usually arbitrarily chosen decision thresholds for determination of sensitivity, specificity, and predictive values should be abandoned.[11,18] All possible combinations that can be achieved by changing the cutoff value of the test can be summarized using a single parameter, the area under the receiver operating characteristic (ROC) curve. In addition, the ROC technique enables comparison of different tests and can be used to optimize threshold values with regard to a given prevalence in the target population and cost ratio of false-negative and false-positive results.[19,20] Obviously, it is recommended to calculate drug-specific decision thresholds for other diagnostic methods, such as the BAT.

sIgE results can also be affected by the preparation of the drug solid-phase conjugates. For example, it has been shown that solid-phase assays prepared by alkali treatment of some cephalosporins might lack the potential allergenic R2 side chain, because of the lability of their dihydrothiazine ring.[21] Such tests not only could potentially put patients at risk of anaphylaxis if allergy was falsely excluded but could also fail to correctly predict cross-reactivity with other β-lactam antibiotics. Therefore, it is mandatory to detail the preparation and conjugation processes when reporting on a new drug-specific solid-phase assay.

CELLULAR TESTS

Before considering the potentials and shortcomings of cellular tests, it should be remembered that the signs and symptoms of an IgE-mediated reaction are a direct consequence of cross-linking of adjacent IgE/FcεRI complexes present on the membrane of basophils and mast cells with triggering of almost immediate release of various preformed mediators such as histamine, tryptase, and platelet activating factor. In addition, newly synthesized mediators such as different leukotrienes and cytokines are also released. However, release of these quantifiable mediators does not per se reflect an IgE/FcεRI-mediated mechanism but might also result from various alternative means of mast cell activation (eg, via anaphylatoxins [C5a, C3a]) or direct mast cell degranulation, as seen with opioids, NMBAs, iodinated contrast media, quinolones, and vancomycin. Although for many the reference test for effector cell activation remains the basophilic histamine release test, the technique has never really entered mainstream application.[22] The foundations of modern BAT research and practice were laid about 2 decades ago,[23] and in the meantime, BAT has largely supplanted histamine release tests. The principles and applications of BAT are detailed elsewhere.[24] BAT relies on flow cytometric identification and quantification of alterations of specific activation or degranulation markers on the surface membrane or inside the basophils. These changes can be detected and quantified on a single-cell level using specific monoclonal antibodies conjugated to particular laser-excitable fluorochromes. Alternative methods to assess antigen-specific in vitro basophil activation imply quantification of phosphorylation of intracellular signaling molecules[25,26] and quantification of the intracellular histamine content by an enzyme affinity method.[27] During the last decade, an increasing number of studies have shown that flow cytometric analysis and quantification of in vitro activated basophils can be a reliable instrument in the diagnostic management of immediate DHR (for review, see Refs.[28,29]). BAT not only allows safe simultaneous testing of different compounds, including active components as well as excipients and additives, but also enables tailoring safe alternatives for the future. BAT can be complementary to skin tests, and BAT results might have more clinical relevance than sIgE data.[16,30–32] Likely, this observation reflects the underlying processes in the different tests. SIgE tests simply measure the interaction between the epitope(s) of the drug (or related compound) and the paratope(s) of the antibody, whereas BAT and skin tests depict drug-induced cross-linking of membrane-bound sIgE, with subsequent degranulation and release of mediators, thereby more closely mirroring the in vivo situation. Moreover, for drugs such as opioids, BAT might help to discriminate between genuine allergy and nonspecific release of mediators by mast cells.[16] Alternatively, because cross-linking of sIgE/FcεRI is not an absolute prerequisite for basophil activation and degranulation, the technique might also be valuable to document IgE-independent immediate DHR.

Another example of the potential of BAT is allergy toward quinolones, a family of synthetic antibiotics based on a the 4-quinolone and 1,8-naphthyridine nuclei. These drugs can cause severe allergies, often after first exposure; moxifloxacin is the most important culprit.[33] Diagnosis of quinolone allergy is not straightforward. Although several attempts have been undertaken to prepare different quinolone conjugates, there are still no well-validated drug-specific sIgE assays readily available, and controversy has arisen about the specificity of some methods.[34] Quinolone skin testing is also associated with uncertainties, and positive skin responses to various quinolones have been reported in individuals without overt quinolone allergy. Because questions remain concerning the relevance and applicability of sIgE and skin tests in quinolone allergy, several groups have pinned their hopes on BAT. Studies have reported divergent findings with respect to the sensitivity of the test. The literature and our own preliminary experiments seem to indicate that (some) quinolones might induce basophil degranulation that goes completely undetected in traditional CD63-based assay. Using this readout, only Aranda and colleagues,[35] and not Seitz and colleagues[36] or Lobera and colleagues,[37] managed to show in vitro basophil activation. The reasons for this observation remain elusive. However, the more consistent results with CD203c[38,39] could indicate that basophil degranulation in response to quinolones results from an alternative (IgE-independent) pathway.

BAT provides the physician with a novel instrument in the diagnosis of DHR. However, additional trials are required to further optimize and validate the technique, to avoid skepticism and cynicism and to allow its entry in to mainstream diagnostic use. These studies should address several points. First, as with any study of this nature, a major difficulty could be to accurately identify sufficient numbers of well-phenotyped patients and to compose an appropriate exposed control group. In this context, medical history can be inaccurate and even misleading, because it relies on the patients' or relatives' recollection, appreciation, and description of events. For example, a maculopapular exanthema as seen in cell-mediated type IV reactions toward penicillins could easily be mistaken for an urticaria observed in the context of an IgE-mediated type I reaction. The same holds true for urticaria induced by an infectious agent. Pharmacologic adverse events erroneously described or interpreted as DHR can also profoundly affect the outcome. These validation studies, ideally, should enroll only patients with a well-established and unequivocal (doctor-based) diagnosis of DHR. In this context, not all apparently allergic reactions are truly immunologic in nature or even drug induced. For example, various drugs such as opioids, iodinated contrast media, vancomycin, and quinolones can elicit direct mast cell (and basophil) degranulation, whereas nonsteroidal antiinflammatory drugs can mimic drug allergy via a redirection of mediator synthesis and intake of angiotensin-converting enzyme inhibitors can trigger angioedema caused by accumulation of bradykinin. Moreover, because of the absolute necessity of collaborative inputs from clinic and laboratory, studies would need clearly harmonized practice parameters and standardized procedures and should be performed in specialized/dedicated allergy clinics/centers for drug allergy testing and management. From a recent World Allergy Organization survey on diagnostic procedures and therapies in drug allergy,[40] it seems that such centers are available in only about 60% of the participating countries. This harmonized collaborative approach should not only help to circumvent the issues of small numbers and inadequate diagnosis but also identify other confounders that might seriously affect the outcome. Perhaps one of the most relevant examples to show this point is the highly disputed proposal to apply BAT in hypersensitivity to nonsteroidal antiinflammatory drugs. A likely explanation for this dispute could be the occurrence of IgE-mediated reactions to the pyrazolone-derived nonsteroidal antiinflammatory drugs. Proponents of this proposal have generally been applying BAT for allergic reactions to metamizol[41] and dipyrone,[42] whereas critics of the proposal studied pyrazolones,[43] and mostly other compounds such as diclofenac[44,45] and salicylic acid.[45,46]

Second, small chemicals, such as drugs, might elicit highly heterogeneous and less pronounced in vitro basophil responses, compared with large protein allergens. Therefore, it will be critical to identify optimal allergen-specific stimulation conditions, which cannot always be extrapolated from studies with histamine and leukotriene release tests or from tests with (structurally or pharmacologically) related compounds. For example, stimulation conditions for aminosteroid myorelaxants might not apply for benzylisoquinolines, and vice versa. These optimized conditions might differ according to the applied technique (whole blood vs purified leukocytes, CD63 vs CD203c).

Third, as previously exemplified for quantification of sIgE, arbitrarily chosen thresholds should be abandoned but drug-specific decision cutoffs should be applied. Moreover, the decision threshold might not be interchangeable for the different readouts. For example, data obtained for the appearance of surface CD63 might not be extrapolated to the upregulation of CD203c.

Fourth, about 5% to 10% of patients are not responsive to BAT (ie, they do not react to positive control stimulation). In such patients, it becomes impossible to interpret negative allergen stimulation, and the test is valueless as a diagnostic tool. Whether repeating the test in such patients is merited requires to be established, but results and conclusions of studies that do not mention nonresponders should be interpreted carefully. Other reasons for false-negative results are inappropriate storage of cells, incorrect stimulation conditions (eg, with cytotoxic drugs or cytotoxic concentrations), concomitant drug intake,[47] or postponement of testing.[42,48,49] However, many of these issues remain poorly studied.

REFERENCES

1. Demoly P, Romano A, Botelho C, et al. Determining the negative predictive value of provocation tests with beta-lactams. Allergy 2010;65:327–32.
2. Ebo DG, Leysen J, Mayorga C, et al. The in vitro diagnosis of drug allergy: status and perspectives. Allergy 2011;66:1275–86.
3. Torres MJ, Blanca M, Fernandez J, et al. Diagnosis of immediate allergic reactions to beta-lactam antibiotics. Allergy 2003;58:961–72.
4. Fontaine C, Mayorga C, Bousquet PJ, et al. Relevance of the determination of serum-specific IgE antibodies in the diagnosis of immediate beta-lactam allergy. Allergy 2007;62:47–52.
5. Silva R, Cruz L, Botelho C, et al. Immediate hypersensitivity to penicillins with negative skin tests–the value of specific IgE. Eur Ann Allergy Clin Immunol 2009;41:117–9.
6. Qiao HL, Li Z, Yang J, et al. Hypersensitivity reactions to penicillins: studies in a group of patients with negative benzylpenicillin G skin test. J Clin Pharm Ther 2009;34:249–54.
7. Hjortlund J, Mortz CG, Skov PS, et al. Diagnosis of penicillin allergy revisited: the value of case history, skin testing, specific IgE and prolonged challenge. Allergy 2013;68:1057–64.
8. Macy E, Goldberg B, Poon KY. Use of commercial anti-penicillin IgE fluorometric enzyme immunoassays to diagnose penicillin allergy. Ann Allergy Asthma Immunol 2010;105:136–41.
9. Johansson SG, Adedoyin J, van Hage M, et al. False-positive penicillin immunoassay: an unnoticed common problem. J Allergy Clin Immunol 2013;132:235–7.
10. Fisher MM, Baldo BA. Immunoassays in the diagnosis of anaphylaxis to neuromuscular blocking drugs: the value of morphine for the detection of IgE antibodies in allergic subjects. Anaesth Intensive Care 2000;28:167–70.
11. Ebo DG, Venemalm L, Bridts CH, et al. Immunoglobulin E antibodies to rocuronium: a new diagnostic tool. Anesthesiology 2007;107:253–9.
12. Laroche D, Chollet-Martin S, Leturgie P, et al. Evaluation of a new routine diagnostic test for immunoglobulin E sensitization to neuromuscular blocking agents. Anesthesiology 2011;114:91–7.
13. Florvaag E, Johansson SG, Oman H, et al. Prevalence of IgE antibodies to morphine. Relation to the high and low incidences of NMBA anaphylaxis in Norway and Sweden, respectively. Acta Anaesthesiol Scand 2005;49:437–44.

14. Fisher MM, Baldo BA. The incidence and clinical features of anaphylactic reactions during anesthesia in Australia. Ann Fr Anesth Reanim 1993;12:97–104.
15. Pham NH, Baldo BA, Puy RM. Studies on the mechanism of multiple drug allergies. Structural basis of drug recognition. J Immunoassay Immunochem 2001;22:47–73.
16. Leysen J, De Witte L, Sabato V, et al. IgE-mediated allergy to pholcodine and cross-reactivity to neuromuscular blocking agents: lessons from flow cytometry. Cytometry B Clin Cytom 2013;84:65–70.
17. Dong SW, Mertes PM, Petitpain N, et al. Hypersensitivity reactions during anesthesia. Results from the ninth French survey (2005-2007). Minerva Anestesiol 2012;78:868–78.
18. Ebo DG, Stevens WJ, Bridts CH, et al. Latex-specific IgE, skin testing, and lymphocyte transformation to latex in latex allergy. J Allergy Clin Immunol 1997; 100:618–23.
19. Plebani M, Borghesan F, Basso D, et al. Receiver-operating characteristic (ROC) curves: a fundamental tool for improving the clinical usefulness of in vitro IgE tests. Allergy 1996;51:407–11.
20. Greiner M, Pfeiffer D, Smith RD. Principles and practical application of the receiver-operating characteristic analysis for diagnostic tests. Prev Vet Med 2000;45:23–41.
21. Pham NH, Baldo BA. Beta-lactam drug allergens: fine structural recognition patterns of cephalosporin-reactive IgE antibodies. J Mol Recognit 1996;9:287–96.
22. Demoly P, Lebel B, Arnoux B. Allergen-induced mediator release tests. Allergy 2003;58:553–8.
23. Knol EF, Mul FP, Jansen H, et al. Monitoring human basophil activation via CD63 monoclonal antibody 435. J Allergy Clin Immunol 1991;88:328–38.
24. Ebo DG, Hagendorens MM, Bridts CH, et al. In vitro allergy diagnosis: should we follow the flow? Clin Exp Allergy 2004;34:332–9.
25. Ebo DG, Dombrecht EJ, Bridts CH, et al. Combined analysis of intracellular signalling and immunophenotype of human peripheral blood basophils by flow cytometry: a proof of concept. Clin Exp Allergy 2007;37:1668–75.
26. Aerts NE, Dombrecht EJ, Bridts CH, et al. Simultaneous flow cytometric detection of basophil activation marker CD63 and intracellular phosphorylated p38 mitogen-activated protein kinase in birch pollen allergy. Cytometry B Clin Cytom 2009;76:8–17.
27. Ebo DG, Bridts CH, Mertens CH, et al. Analyzing histamine release by flow cytometry (HistaFlow): a novel instrument to study the degranulation patterns of basophils. J Immunol Methods 2012;375:30–8.
28. Hausmann OV, Gentinetta T, Bridts CH, et al. The basophil activation test in immediate-type drug allergy. Immunol Allergy Clin North Am 2009;29:555–66.
29. Leysen J, Sabato V, Verweij MM, et al. The basophil activation test in the diagnosis of immediate drug hypersensitivity. Expert Rev Clin Immunol 2011;7: 349–55.
30. Gamboa PM, Garcia-Aviles MC, Urrutia I, et al. Basophil activation and sulfidoleukotriene production in patients with immediate allergy to betalactam antibiotics and negative skin tests. J Investig Allergol Clin Immunol 2004;14:278–83.
31. Ebo DG, Bridts CH, Hagendorens MM, et al. Flow-assisted diagnostic management of anaphylaxis from rocuronium bromide. Allergy 2006;61:935–9.
32. Pinnobphun P, Buranapraditkun S, Kampitak T, et al. The diagnostic value of basophil activation test in patients with an immediate hypersensitivity reaction to radiocontrast media. Ann Allergy Asthma Immunol 2011;106:387–93.

33. Jones SC, Budnitz DS, Sorbello A, et al. US-based emergency department visits for fluoroquinolone-associated hypersensitivity reactions. Pharmacoepidemiol Drug Saf 2013;22:1099–106.

34. Baldo BA, Pham NH. Drug allergy. clinical aspects, diagnosis, mechanisms, structure-activity relationships. New York: Springer; 2013.

35. Aranda A, Mayorga C, Ariza A, et al. In vitro evaluation of IgE-mediated hypersensitivity reactions to quinolones. Allergy 2011;66:247–54.

36. Seitz CS, Brocker EB, Trautmann A. Diagnostic testing in suspected fluoroquinolone hypersensitivity. Clin Exp Allergy 2009;39:1738–45.

37. Lobera T, Audicana MT, Alarcon E, et al. Allergy to quinolones: low cross-reactivity to levofloxacin. J Investig Allergol Clin Immunol 2010;20:607–11.

38. Ben SB, Berard F, Bienvenu J, et al. Usefulness of basophil activation tests for the diagnosis of IgE-mediated allergy to quinolones. Allergy 2010;65:535–6.

39. Rouzaire P, Nosbaum A, Denis L, et al. Negativity of the basophil activation test in quinolone hypersensitivity: a breakthrough for provocation test decision-making. Int Arch Allergy Immunol 2012;157:299–302.

40. Thong BY, Mirakian R, Castells M, et al. A World Allergy Organization international survey on diagnostic procedures and therapies in drug allergy/hypersensitivity. World Allergy Organ J 2011;4:257–70.

41. Gamboa PM, Sanz ML, Caballero MR, et al. Use of CD63 expression as a marker of in vitro basophil activation and leukotriene determination in metamizol allergic patients. Allergy 2003;58:312–7.

42. Gomez E, Blanca-Lopez N, Torres MJ, et al. Immunoglobulin E-mediated immediate allergic reactions to dipyrone: value of basophil activation test in the identification of patients. Clin Exp Allergy 2009;39:1217–24.

43. Couto M, Gaspar A, Piedade S, et al. IgE-mediated metamizol allergy and the usefulness of the cellular allergen stimulation test. Eur Ann Allergy Clin Immunol 2012;44:113–6.

44. Malbran A, Yeyati E, Rey GL, et al. Diclofenac induces basophil degranulation without increasing CD63 expression in sensitive patients. Clin Exp Immunol 2007;147:99–105.

45. Bavbek S, Ikinciogullari A, Dursun AB, et al. Upregulation of CD63 or CD203c alone or in combination is not sensitive in the diagnosis of nonsteroidal anti-inflammatory drug intolerance. Int Arch Allergy Immunol 2009;150:261–70.

46. Celik GE, Schroeder JT, Hamilton RG, et al. Effect of in vitro aspirin stimulation on basophils in patients with aspirin-exacerbated respiratory disease. Clin Exp Allergy 2009;39:1522–31.

47. Majlesi Y, Samorapoompichit P, Hauswirth AW, et al. Cerivastatin and atorvastatin inhibit IL-3-dependent differentiation and IgE-mediated histamine release in human basophils and downmodulate expression of the basophil-activation antigen CD203c/E-NPP3. J Leukoc Biol 2003;73:107–17.

48. Fernandez TD, Torres MJ, Blanca-Lopez N, et al. Negativization rates of IgE radioimmunoassay and basophil activation test in immediate reactions to penicillins. Allergy 2009;64:242–8.

49. Kvedariene V, Kamey S, Ryckwaert Y, et al. Diagnosis of neuromuscular blocking agent hypersensitivity reactions using cytofluorimetric analysis of basophils. Allergy 2006;61:311–5.

In Vitro Diagnosis of Delayed-type Drug Hypersensitivity

Mechanistic Aspects and Unmet Needs

Dean J. Naisbitt, PhD*, Ryan G. Nattrass, MR,
Monday O. Ogese, MR

KEYWORDS

- Delayed-type drug hypersensitivity • T lymphocytes • Hapten hypothesis
- PI hypothesis • Altered peptide repertoire hypothesis

KEY POINTS

- For the effective diagnosis of delayed-type drug hypersensitivity, our laboratory currently uses the lymphocyte transformation test (LTT) and a panel of enzyme-linked immunosorbent spot assays selected from interferon gamma, interleukin (IL)-4, IL-5, IL-13, IL-17, IL-22, Fas ligand, tumor necrosis factor alpha, granzyme B, and perforin (individual panels depend on the volume of blood available and the nature of the clinical reaction).
- The availability of multiple readouts has improved clinicians' ability to diagnose reactions.
- Most studies published to date originate from well-defined test and control patient groups.
- We are currently collecting samples longitudinally from patients with cystic fibrosis exposed to β-lactam to characterize markers of the effector and regulatory immune response in hypersensitive and tolerant patients.
- A component of this analysis is a detailed assessment of the sensitivity and specificity of the LTT for the diagnosis of β-lactam hypersensitivity.

INTRODUCTION

The term delayed-type drug hypersensitivity reaction is used loosely to describe a myriad of clinical syndromes caused by a variety of different drugs. Characterization of mechanisms is difficult because the same drug has the potential to activate different arms of the adaptive immune system via diverse chemical pathways. Layered on top

The authors have nothing to disclose.
The Centre for Drug Safety Science is supported by the Medical Research Council (grant no. G0700654).
Department of Clinical and Molecular Pharmacology, MRC Centre for Drug Safety Science, University of Liverpool, Sherrington Building, Ashton Street, Liverpool L69 3GE, England
* Corresponding author.
E-mail address: dnes@liv.ac.uk

Immunol Allergy Clin N Am 34 (2014) 691–705
http://dx.doi.org/10.1016/j.iac.2014.04.009   immunology.theclinics.com

of this is the recent discovery of human leukocyte antigen (HLA) molecules as important susceptibility factors for certain reactions.

The only common aspect in all forms of delayed-type hypersensitivity reaction is the drug-specific activation of T lymphocytes. In contrast, effector T-cell responses to drugs are not detected in tolerant controls. Researchers in specialist facilities have used these observations to develop test systems that detect the drug-specific activation of T cells and, in certain circumstances, the applicability of the test for patient diagnosis has been assessed. Despite this, diagnostic tests are not yet available for routine use in the clinic. Thus, this article (1) briefly summarizes the cellular and chemical basis of delayed-type drug hypersensitivity, highlighting, when appropriate, gaps in current knowledge (**Table 1**); and (2) reviews the in vitro assays that are currently available for the diagnosis of drug hypersensitivity.

DRUG HYPERSENSITIVITY REACTIONS: DEFINITION AND OVERVIEW OF CLINICAL SYNDROMES

Drug hypersensitivity can be defined simply as a serious adverse drug reaction with an immunologic cause, to an otherwise safe and effective therapeutic agent.[1] Many delayed-type reactions manifest in the skin. Reactions vary in severity from self-limiting maculopapular eruptions to life-threatening Stevens-Johnson syndrome/toxic epidermal necrolysis. Pichler expanded the classic Gell and Coombs[2] classification through the categorization of delayed-type cutaneous reactions into 4 groups according to the phenotype and function of drug-responsive T cells (**Table 2**).[3] The discovery of drug-responsive T cells from patients with delayed liver and kidney reactions to drugs including flucloxacillin,[4] disulfiram,[5] Augmentin (Katy Saide, 2014), and isoniazid (Toru Usui, 2014) indicates that noncutaneous reactions should also be categorized as a form of delayed-type drug hypersensitivity reaction. Thus, we have expanded Pichlers'[3] classification to include reactions targeting kidney and liver. However, this

Table 1
Pathways of drug-specific T-cell activation: main supporting experimental evidence and unmet needs

Hypothesis	Main Experimental Observation	Unmet Needs
Hapten	Drug (metabolite)-protein adducts activate T cells	Chemical characterization of hapten-peptide conjugates naturally eluted off MHC and demonstration that they act as T-cell antigens Identification of drug metabolite–modified proteins that contain T-cell stimulatory peptide sequences
Pharmacologic interaction	Chemically inert drugs stimulate T cells in a readily reversible manner	Demonstration that activated T cells cause clinical reactions in patients and/or experimental models of drug-induced tissue injury
Altered self-peptide repertoire	Indirect T-cell activation by abacavir through MHC binding and alteration of the repertoire of self-peptides displayed on MHC molecules	Assessment of whether the altered self-peptide repertoire pathway can be used to describe the activation of T cells by other drugs

Abbreviation: MHC, major histocompatibility complex.

Table 2
Clinical and immunologic features of delayed-type drug hypersensitivity reactions

Clinical Reaction	Normal Time to Onset	Principal Drug-specific T-cell Response	Additional Features	Key References
Maculopapular exanthema	4–14 d	Th2-secreting CD4+ T cells	Account for many delayed-type drug hypersensitivity reactions, often associated with an eosinophilic inflammation. Self-limiting after drug withdrawal	77,78
Drug rash with eosinophilia and systemic symptoms	2–6 wk	CD4+ and CD8+ T cells secreting IFN-γ and IL-5	Multiple organs are damaged, viral reactivation often observed, and viral-specific T cells may be involved in the disease pathogenesis. Mortality approximately 10%	64,66,79
Pustular eruptions (eg, acute generalized exanthematous pustulosis)	<24 h–30 d	CD4 and CD8+ T cells secreting IL-8	Neutrophil infiltration is a common characteristic in pustules. Mortality approximately 5%	80,81
Bullous eruptions (eg, Stevens-Johnson syndrome)	1–3 wk	Cytotoxic CD8+ T cells, NK T cells	Blistering lesions leading to extensive skin detachment. Killing mediated by FasL, granzyme B, and granulysin. Fatality rate more than 30% for toxic epidermal necrolysis	46,82,83
Abacavir hypersensitivity	3–14 d	Cytotoxic CD8+ T cells	All patch-test-confirmed patients express HLA-B*57:01. Only reaction that does not involve CD4+ T-cell help. Genetic testing for B*57:01 prevents hypersensitivity	57–59,61
Liver reactions	7 d++; frequently >80 d	Cytotoxic CD4+ and CD8+ T cells[a]	Broad spectrum of clinical syndromes. In flucloxacillin reactions, T cells express gut-homing chemokine receptors	4,84,85
Kidney reactions	1–3 wk	CD4+ T cells secreting heterogeneous cytokine pattern[a]	T cells do not secrete cytotoxic molecules, indicating they orchestrate a local inflammatory response in the target organ	5

Abbreviations: IFN, interferon; IL, interleukin; NK, natural killer.
[a] Data limited to 1 or 2 mechanistic studies focusing on a limited number of drugs.

classification is still outdated because it does not encompass new T-cell populations including Th9, Th17, Th22, and T_{reg}.

ACTIVATION OF DRUG-RESPONSIVE T CELLS

T cells are activated through the interaction of a major histocompatibility complex (MHC)–associated peptide with a specific T-cell receptor. In the appropriate cytokine microenvironment, the activated T cells divide and differentiate into multiple effector populations. In terms of drug hypersensitivity, the drug must in some way mimic the actions of the MHC-associated antigenic peptide.

There are currently 3 hypotheses that describe the way in which drugs act as antigens to activate T cells: the hapten hypothesis, the pharmacologic interaction (PI) concept, and the altered self-peptide repertoire hypothesis. Each hypothesis has been reviewed in detail elsewhere (**Fig. 1**)[6–8]; this article briefly describes the

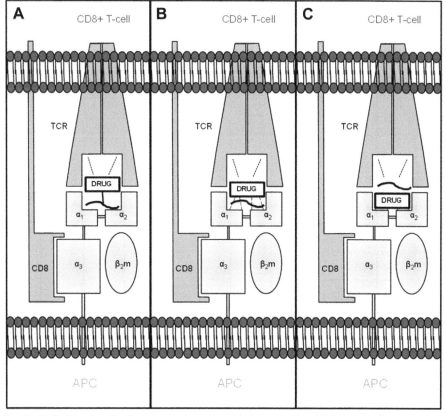

Fig. 1. CD8+ T-cell activation via hapten, PI, and altered self-peptide repertoire pathways. (A) Hapten hypothesis. The peptide embedded in the MHC-I molecule is covalently bound and altered by a protein-reactive drug (eg, flucloxacillin), creating an antigen. (B) Pi concept. The drug (sulfamethoxazole, carbamazepine) is capable of binding directly to MHC and/or the T-cell receptor. (C) Altered peptide repertoire hypothesis. The drug is capable of binding directly to a particular MHC class molecule, allowing for presentation of altered self-peptides to CD8+ T cells (eg, only abacavir to date).

experimental evidence using T cells from drug hypersensitive patients and/or drug-naive human donors that supports each hypothesis. This information will aid the later discussion of the limitations of existing in vitro diagnostic assays.

HAPTEN HYPOTHESIS

The hapten hypothesis states that low-molecular-weight chemicals must form stable adducts with endogenous proteins to be able to induce an immune response. The hypothesis evolved from groundbreaking studies by Landsteiner and Jacobs,[10] who were able to correlate direct reactivity of the dinitrohalobenzenes with sensitization potential.[9,10] The hapten concept is still considered the primary pathway by which chemical sensitizers cause allergic contact dermatitis.[11] Protein-reactivity screens represent an important tool for the identification of skin sensitizers.[12,13]

The hapten hypothesis is also used to describe the chemical basis of delayed-type β-lactam hypersensitivity reactions. The β-lactam nucleus binds irreversibly to amino acid residues within the active site of penicillin binding proteins (a group of bacteria cell wall proteins with high affinity for the β-lactam antibiotics), preventing cross-linking of the nascent peptidoglycan layer and disrupting bacterial cell wall synthesis. However, this intrinsic reactivity leads to covalent modification of other endogenous proteins, especially at lysine residues. Such drug-protein adducts are thought to be involved in a variety of adverse events including hypersensitivity.[14–18] However, under cell culture conditions, adduct formation by the β-lactam antibiotics is extremely protein selective. All of the drugs analyzed to date (penicillin G, amoxicillin, flucloxacillin, piperacillin) modify extracellular protein, but essentially ignore cellular protein.[4,19–21] This protein selectivity is restricted to the β-lactam antibiotics; other reactive chemicals and drug metabolites modify multiple cellular and extracellular proteins.[22–28] Using mass spectrometric methods, we identified albumin as the major protein modified by β-lactam antibiotics and defined the profile of drug-protein conjugation at specific lysine residues with respect to dose and incubation time. Because human serum albumin accounts for most serum-bound penicilloyl groups in vivo, we also considered it a suitable model for investigating the chemistry underlying β-lactam adduct formation in patients. The β-lactam antibiotics piperacillin and flucloxacillin were bound in vivo to the same lysine residues that are modified in vitro.[20,29] These data confirm that drug-protein adducts are formed in exposed patients and hence have the potential to be recognized by the hosts' immune system.

β-Lactam antibiotics stimulate CD4+ and CD8+ T cells from hypersensitive patients to proliferate and secrete a diverse cytokine secretion profile.[30–35] Several studies have shown that β-lactam antibiotics conjugated directly to MHC molecules, and synthetic β-lactam–albumin constructs stimulate T cells from hypersensitive patients and drug-naive donors.[19,20,36,37] Furthermore, penicillin peptide conjugates that have been designed to fit in specific MHC molecules have been shown to stimulate penicillin-responsive T cells[38]; this proves that human T cells from hypersensitive patients are activated via a hapten mechanism.

Most drugs are not directly protein reactive (reactivity is designed out during drug development); however, protein adducts may form as a consequence of metabolic activation. Many drugs associated with a high incidence of drug hypersensitivity reaction form reactive intermediates, providing circumstantial evidence that they are involved in the disease pathogenesis. To study whether drug metabolites selectively activate T cells several groups have focused on patients with sulfamethoxazole hypersensitivity. Sulfamethoxazole is metabolized via a hydroxylamine intermediate to a nitroso metabolite, which binds readily to cysteine groups on protein.[23,25,39] The synthetic nitroso metabolite is a potent T-cell sensitizer in rodents[25,40,41] and in vitro human T-cell priming assays.[42,43] Furthermore, nitroso sulfamethoxazole–responsive T cells have been isolated from the blood and skin of 100% of hypersensitive patients presenting with reactions varying in severity from maculopapular eruptions to toxic epidermal necrolysis.[44–47] A recent analysis found that more than 80% of drug-antigen–specific T cells from sulfamethoxazole-hypersensitive patients are activated with the nitroso metabolite.[44] Moreover, in sulfamethoxazole-hypersensitive patients with cystic fibrosis, the T-cell response is directed exclusively against the nitroso metabolite.[48,49] Sulfamethoxazole hypersensitivity is one of only a few examples in which a synthetic metabolite is available that can be incorporated into in vitro studies. Detection of T-cell responses to the parent compound (discussed later) does not exclude the presence of drug metabolite–specific T cells.

There is an unmet need for identification of drug metabolite–modified proteins that contain T-cell–stimulatory peptide sequences.

THE PI HYPOTHESIS

The PI hypothesis states that drugs do not need to bind covalently to protein to become immunogenic and that some drugs can bind directly to MHC to activate T cells.[8,50] This concept was devised through experimentation with human peripheral blood mononuclear cells and drug-specific T-cell clones from hypersensitive patients. The primary observation from these experiments was that T cells are reactive against a variety of drugs that do not bind covalently to protein.[51] This concept is not compatible with a hapten mechanism. More detailed analysis revealed that the T cells were activated rapidly via an MHC-restricted, processing-independent pathway.[52–56] Because reactive metabolites of most drugs associated with a high incidence of hypersensitivity are not widely available, most in vitro assays currently used to diagnose drug hypersensitivity rely on the direct activation of drugs via a PI mechanism.

ALTERED SELF-PEPTIDE REPERTOIRE HYPOTHESIS

Several drugs and chemicals have been shown to activate T cells via hapten and PI mechanisms. In contrast, only 1 drug (abacavir) has been shown to activate T cells indirectly through MHC binding and alteration of the repertoire of peptides that are ultimately displayed on the surface of antigen-presenting cells. Abacavir hypersensitivity is atypical in that skin test–confirmed reactions are only seen in individuals carrying the risk allele HLA-B*57:01[57]; furthermore, the drug interacts exclusively with B*57:01 to activate CD8+ T cells.[58–61] In all other forms of drug hypersensitivity reaction (including reactions strongly associated with HLA risk alleles), drug-specific CD4+ and CD8+ T cells are detectable and those that have been studied interact with multiple MHC molecules.

Elegant, integrated, structural, modeling, and biological studies describe the interaction of abacavir with endogenous HLA-B*57:01 and show that the binding interaction changes the confirmation of the peptide binding cleft, altering the repertoire of peptides displayed on the cell surface.[58–60] These data imply that preexisting peptide-specific T cells are activated indirectly by abacavir through the display of cross-reacting altered self-peptides.

DIAGNOSIS OF DELAYED-TYPE DRUG HYPERSENSITIVITY REACTIONS

Diagnosis of delayed-type drug hypersensitivity is extremely difficult in the clinical setting. In vitro tests are not routinely available and hence assessment of causality is usually based on a clinician's assessment of the relationship between drug intake and the time to onset of the adverse reaction. Because T cells are involved in the pathogenesis of all forms of delayed-type reaction, the ideal in vitro test would use a small volume of a patient's blood to detect a drug-antigen–specific T-cell response as a marker of sensitization.

The lymphocyte transformation test (LTT; also known as the lymphocyte proliferation assay) is the most established assay in this category (**Box 1**). The assay is based on incubation of freshly isolated peripheral blood mononuclear cells from hypersensitive patients (and drug-exposed tolerant controls) with titrated concentrations of the suspect drug. A stimulation index (counts per minute [cpm] in drug-treated wells/cpm in vehicle control wells) of 2 or 3 or more indicates a drug-specific T-cell response and can be used for causality assessment if other drugs render a negative result.

A PubMed (http://www.ncbi.nlm.nih.gov) database search (December 2013) using the terms drug hypersensitivity and lymphocyte transformation test generates 633 results. Many of the articles describe the successful application of the test for the diagnosis of drug hypersensitivity. In a detailed retrospective analysis of 923 probable/definite patients with drug hypersensitive, the LTT had a sensitivity (ie, percentage of hypersensitive patients with a positive LTT result) and specificity (ie, percentage of drug-exposed tolerant patients with a negative LTT result) of 78% and 85%, respectively.[62] More recently, Pichler and Tilch[63] cited a sensitivity of 60% to 70% for the diagnosis of β-lactam hypersensitivity. In our own retrospective analysis of β-lactam hypersensitivity in patients with cystic fibrosis, we found similar results, with the sensitivity of the assay being 76% when patients receiving oral steroids were excluded from the analysis.[19,20] Specificity was close to 0%. In a separate cohort (patients with different forms of cutaneous hypersensitivity exposed to carbamazepine and lamotrigine) we again used the LTT for diagnosis and found a sensitivity of more than 80%.[64–67] So the questions are: (1) why is the LTT not applied more widely in the clinical setting, and (2) what can be done to overcome the issues restricting its use. The main limitations of the LTT in its current form are discussed here.

- Technical limitations
    1. The assay relies on the availability of freshly isolated peripheral blood mononuclear cells and/or a cryopreservation facility if assays are to be conducted at a later date.
    2. A researcher must be trained in cell isolation, sterile technique, and cell culture methods.

Box 1
LTT

The LTT measures the proliferation of memory T cells to a particular drug to which a patient has been exposed and provides an insight into the pathomechanism of the reactions. It has a high specificity with various drugs including the β-lactam antibiotics, sulfonamides, anticonvulsants and p-phenylenediamine. Sensitivity depends on the chemical properties of the drug.

The assay is performed using peripheral blood mononuclear cells isolated from sensitized patients over a density gradient. Cells (1.5×10^5, 100 μL) are cultured in triplicate in a 96-well U-bottomed microtiter plate with various concentrations of the culprit drug or drugs using tetanus toxoid and cell culture medium as positive and negative controls respectively at 37°C, 5% CO_2 for 6 days. [^{3}H]-thymidine (0.5 μCi) is added during the final 16 hours of the incubation and T-cell proliferation evaluated using a scintillation counter. Lymphocyte proliferation is expressed as stimulation index, which is the ratio of the proliferative response with and without the drug.

3. Incorporation of the drug into the assay in an appropriate form is technically demanding. The sensitivity/specificity analysis discussed earlier focuses on a small number of compounds for which T-cell stimulatory concentrations have been defined over many years, largely through trial and error. For example:
   a. Sulfonamides are solubilized in phosphate-buffered saline (PBS) at a high pH and diluted into medium before use. T cells are activated between 0.5 and 2 mM. Sulfonamide metabolites are dissolved in small quantities of dimethylsulfoxide (DMSO) before use. T cells are activated at low μM concentrations; 100 μM is toxic.
   b. Anticonvulsants, such as carbamazepine, form a suspension in a PBS/DMSO (10%) mixture. Following dilution the drug is solubilized and concentrations of 50 to 400 μM activate T cells.
   c. β-Lactam antibiotics dissolve directly in culture medium. T cells are activated at 0.5 to 4 mM.

The protocol used for new chemicals/drugs generates a stock concentration using small quantities of DMSO, which is then serially diluted (2-fold or 3-fold dilutions) starting with a concentration that causes approximately 25% peripheral blood cell death. When sufficient cells are available, 7 concentrations of the drug are assessed.

- Interpretation of the results
  1. A stimulation index of 5 or more detected at 2 or more drug concentrations is considered in our laboratory as strongly positive. However, stimulation index results of 50 and more are seen regularly. In these patients, the positive LTT is reproducible and detectable over a period of several years. The outcome of the test is less clear when the LTT yields a stimulation index of 1.5 to 3. On repeated testing of the same individual, the result varies between these parameters. Thus, the relevance of the results is difficult to interpret without additional testing, namely T-cell cloning and analysis of drug-responses (**Box 2**).
  2. The quantity of [^{3}H]thymidine incorporated in control cells is extremely variable. This variation is apparent when (1) samples from different donors and (2) repeated samples from same donor are analyzed. It is therefore difficult to conclude whether a donor with high counts in control wells (eg, 3000–5000 cpm) and a stimulation index of 3 to 4 is more strongly sensitized to the drug than a donor with low counts in control wells (eg, 200–500 cpm) and a stimulation index of 10.
- Mechanistic limitations
  1. Negative data in specific patient cohorts:
     a. The pathogenesis of Stevens-Johnson syndrome/toxic epidermal necrolysis involves the activation of drug-specific T cells. However, the LTT is negative in many patients (even to drugs that yield positive results in patients with other forms of hypersensitivity),[68,69] which may be because CD8+ T cells that do not proliferate readily are the primary effector cells in this patient group.[70] By changing the end point of the LTT to a functional marker of T-cell activation (discussed later) more sensitive assays are being developed for diagnosis.
     b. Negative LTT data are obtained using cells from patients with flucloxacillin-induced liver injury.[4] In these patients, sensitization to the drug was confirmed through analysis of flucloxacillin-specific peripheral blood mononuclear cell cytokine release and the generation of drug-responsive T-cell clones.

Box 2
Other assays that detect antigen-specific T cells

- Flow cytometry

    Flow cytometry is a technique used for the determination of multiple phenotypic parameters. Cell surface markers of T-cell activation (eg, CD69 CD25, CD40L, CD71, and HLA-DR [HLA D related]) can be used to measure drug-specific T-cell populations. Flow cytometry can also be used to evaluate T-cell proliferative responses. Cells are first stained with the fluorescent dye carboxyfluorescein diacetate succinimidyl ester (CFSE), which interacts with the amino group of intracellular protein. The intensity of CFSE is reduced by half following each cell division. Hence, the dividing population of antigen-specific T cells can be evaluated.

- Intracellular cytokine staining

    Intracellular cytokine staining is a flow cytometry–based assay that evaluates the cytokine profile of activated cells. The method can detect cytokines secreted by different subsets of T cells following antigen stimulation. Drug-stimulated and control peripheral blood mononuclear cells are treated with either monensin or Brefeldin A to block Golgi-mediated transport. This process results in an accumulation of intracellular cytokines, thereby enhancing the cytokine signal obtained by flow cytometry. Cells are stained with anticytokine antibodies alongside antibodies against cell surface antigens in order to evaluate defined cell populations.

- Multiplex (Luminex) assays

    Multiplex assays are expensive but are able to quantify soluble proteins secreted by a given cell population. Multiplex assays provide an accurate, quick, and efficient method to analyze multiple cytokines secreted from antigen-specific T cells. They are flow cytometry–based assays in which beads with known spectral characteristics are bound to particular capture antibodies and mixed with the cell suspension of interest. Using the spectral properties of fluorescent proteins conjugated to beads, the concentrations of specific proteins in each sample can be determined relative to a standard curve.

- T-cell cloning

    T-cell cloning provides a valuable alternative to detect drug-specific T cells when other assays discussed earlier yield negative results. Cloning is performed by limiting dilution followed by repetitive mitogen stimulation. Several hundred single cell populations are generated and antigen-specificity assessed by culturing irradiated Epstein-Barr virus–transformed B cells with antigen and the clones (5×10^4/well; 200 µL) for 48 hours. Proliferation can be measured by the addition of [^{3}H]thymidine. Clones with a stimulation index of greater than 2 are expanded and then characterized in terms of cellular phenotype and function.

---

    c. The LTT has limited value in the diagnosis of drug hypersensitivity in patients with acute reactions, possibly because the drug-responsive T cells are preactivated during the acute reaction or located primarily in the tissue. Polak and colleagues[71] recently showed that the combined analysis of interferon gamma (IFN-γ) and interleukin (IL)-4 offers potential compared with the LTT for diagnosis in the acute setting.

2. Interpretation of a negative LTT result is extremely difficult because it is currently impossible to include all forms of drug antigen in the test. As mentioned earlier, the assay is almost always performed using the parent drug alone.

To improve the sensitivity of the LTT for the diagnosis of delayed-type hypersensitivity reactions, the main strategy has been to alter the readout used to detect the drug-specific activation of T cells. Flow cytometry–based methods have been developed to measure the number of dividing T cells (carboxyfluorescein diacetate succinimidyl ester staining[33]), increased expression of surface markers of T-cell activation (eg, CD69,[72] CD107a[73]), and cytokine production[68] in drug-treated and vehicle-treated peripheral blood mononuclear cell cultures (see **Box 2**). When used in combination, these assays have an advantage compared with the LTT because the readouts provide information on the nature of the drug-specific T-cell response. However, because the frequency of drug-specific T cells in hypersensitive patients' blood can be as low as 1 in 5000,[33] flow cytometry–based methods lack sensitivity to accurately diagnose drug hypersensitivity reactions. Flow cytometry methods are more valuable for mechanistic studies in which it is easier to established drug-specific T-cell lines and clones for assessment of phenotype and function.

The enzyme-linked immunosorbent spot (ELIspot) methodology has been developed to quantify the number of cytokine/cytolytic molecule–secreting cells in antigen-stimulated peripheral blood mononuclear cell cultures. The method is antibody based (**Box 3**) but has the advantage that low numbers of drug-specific T cells can be detected. IFN-γ ELIspot has been used to analyze the presence of drug-specific T cells in 23 amoxicillin-hypersensitive patients presenting with delayed-type maculopapular eruptions.[32] The assay could detect drug-specific T-cell precursors as low as 1:30,000, allows the detection of cross-reacting drugs, and (3) is more sensitive than the LTT. ELIspot assays have recently been used to detect drug-specific T cells in the acute setting[71] and in retrospective patients presenting with a range of conditions including Stevens-Johnson syndrome,[68,74] drug-induced liver injury,[4] and abacavir hypersensitivity. In each of these studies, the LTT had a low sensitivity because proliferating T cells were not readily detectable.

A cautionary note is that a single ELIspot readout cannot be used to detect all drug-specific T cells. This point is clearly shown (1) in our recent analysis of abacavir-specific T-cell clones that kill target cells through the release of either FasL or granzyme B,[75] and (2) during the application of a human T-cell priming assay to identify contact chemical allergens based on IFN-γ and tumor necrosis factor alpha (TNF-α) readouts.[76]

Box 3
ELIspot assay

ELIspot assay is a quick, highly sensitive, and precise technique applied to the detection of low-frequency cytokine-secreting T cells following antigen stimulation. This type of assay provides an insight into the biological function of the T cells that mediate drug hypersensitivity reactions as well as quantification of specific cytokine-secreting T cells. Activated T cells can secrete an array of cytokines as well as other effector molecules like granzyme, perforin, and Fas ligand. ELIspot kits are available to detect a wide range of proteins; a panel of assays can be conducted simultaneously to characterize the nature of the drug-specific response.

The assay is performed by coating nitrocellulose plates with a capture antibody of choice and incubating them overnight at 4°C. The following day, wells are washed and blocked before use. Peripheral blood mononuclear cells (5×10^5 to 1×10^6) are then cultured with various concentrations of the culprit drug or drugs using Phytohaemagglutinin (PHA) and culture medium as positive and negative controls respectively at 37°C in 5% CO_2. Plates are developed after 48 hours according to the manufacturer's instructions. Spots (representing cytokine-secreting cells) are visualized by the addition of nitro-blue tetrazolium and 5-bromo-4-chloro-3'-indolyphosphate (BCIP/NBT) substrate. When thoroughly dried, the plate is counted on an ELIspot reader. Results are expressed as either spot-forming units per million cells or as a stimulation index relative to control.

SUMMARY

For the effective diagnosis of delayed-type drug hypersensitivity, our laboratory currently uses the LTT and a panel of ELIspot assays selected from IFN-γ, IL-4, IL-5, IL-13, IL-17, IL-22, FasL, TNF-α, granzyme B, and perforin (individual panels depend on the volume of blood available and the nature of the clinical reaction). The availability of multiple readouts has improved our ability to diagnose reactions. However, most studies published to date, originate from well-defined test and control patient groups. We are currently collecting samples longitudinally from patients with cystic fibrosis exposed to β-lactam to characterize markers of the effector and regulatory immune response in hypersensitive and tolerant patients. A component of this analysis is a detailed assessment of the sensitivity and specificity of the LTT for the diagnosis of β-lactam hypersensitivity.

REFERENCES

1. Pichler WJ, Naisbitt DJ, Park BK. Immune pathomechanism of drug hypersensitivity reactions. J Allergy Clin Immunol 2011;127(Suppl 3):S74–81.
2. Gell PG, Coombs RR, editors. Clinical aspects of immunology. Oxford (United Kingdom): Blackwell; 1963.
3. Pichler WJ. Delayed drug hypersensitivity reactions. Ann Intern Med 2003; 139(8):683–93.
4. Monshi MM, Faulkner L, Gibson A, et al. Human leukocyte antigen (HLA)-B*57:01-restricted activation of drug-specific T cells provides the immunological basis for flucloxacillin-induced liver injury. Hepatology 2013;57(2):727–39.
5. Spanou Z, Keller M, Britschgi M, et al. Involvement of drug-specific T cells in acute drug-induced interstitial nephritis. J Am Soc Nephrol 2006;17(10): 2919–27.
6. Uetrecht J, Naisbitt DJ. Idiosyncratic adverse drug reactions: current concepts. Pharmacol Rev 2013;65(2):779–808.
7. Illing PT, Vivian JP, Purcell AW, et al. Human leukocyte antigen-associated drug hypersensitivity. Curr Opin Immunol 2013;25(1):81–9.
8. Pichler WJ. Consequences of drug binding to immune receptors: immune stimulation following pharmacological interaction with immune receptors (T-cell receptor for antigen or human leukocyte antigen) with altered peptide-human leukocyte antigen or peptide. Dermatologica Sinica 2013;31(4):181–90.
9. Ashby J, Basketter DA, Paton D, et al. Structure activity relationships in skin sensitization using the murine local lymph node assay. Toxicology 1995; 103(3):177–94.
10. Landsteiner K, Jacobs J. Studies on the sensitization of animals with simple chemical compounds. J Exp Med 1935;61:643–56.
11. Martin SF, Esser PR, Schmucker S, et al. T-cell recognition of chemicals, protein allergens and drugs: towards the development of in vitro assays. Cell Mol Life Sci 2010;67(24):4171–84.
12. Gerberick GF, Troutman JA, Foertsch LM, et al. Investigation of peptide reactivity of pro-hapten skin sensitizers using a peroxidase-peroxide oxidation system. Toxicol Sci 2009;112(1):164–74.
13. Gerberick F, Aleksic M, Basketter D, et al. Chemical reactivity measurement and the predictive identification of skin sensitisers. The report and recommendations of ECVAM Workshop 64. Altern Lab Anim 2008;36(2):215–42.
14. Chang C, Mahmood MM, Teuber SS, et al. Overview of penicillin allergy. Clin Rev Allergy Immunol 2012;43(1–2):84–97.

15. Pullen H, Wright N, Murdock JM. Hypersensitivity to the penicillins. Lancet 1968; 1(7551):1090.
16. Batchelor FR, Dewdney JM, Gazzard D. Penicillin allergy: the formation of the penicilloyl determinant. Nature 1965;206:362–4.
17. Levine BB, Ovary Z. Studies on the mechanism of the formation of the penicillin antigen. III. The N-(D-alpha-benzylpenicilloyl) group as an antigenic determinant responsible for hypersensitivity to penicillin G. J Exp Med 1961;114:875–904.
18. Levine BB. Studies on the mechanism of the formation of the penicillin antigen. I. Delayed allergic cross-reactions among penicillin G and its degradation products. J Exp Med 1960;112:1131–56.
19. El-Ghaiesh S, Monshi MM, Whitaker P, et al. Characterization of the antigen specificity of T-cell clones from piperacillin-hypersensitive patients with cystic fibrosis. J Pharmacol Exp Ther 2012;341(3):597–610.
20. Whitaker P, Meng X, Lavergne SN, et al. Mass spectrometric characterization of circulating and functional antigens derived from piperacillin in patients with cystic fibrosis. J Immunol 2011;187(1):200–11.
21. Meng X, Jenkins RE, Berry N, et al. Direct evidence for the formation of diastereoisomeric benzylpenicilloyl haptens from benzylpenicillin and benzylpenicillenic acid in patients. J Pharmacol Exp Ther 2011;338:841–9.
22. Castrejon JL, Lavergne SN, El-Sheikh A, et al. Metabolic and chemical origins of cross-reactive immunological reactions to arylamine benzenesulfonamides: T-cell responses to hydroxylamine and nitroso derivatives. Chem Res Toxicol 2010;23(1):184–92.
23. Callan HE, Jenkins RE, Maggs JL, et al. Multiple adduction reactions of nitroso sulfamethoxazole with cysteinyl residues of peptides and proteins: implications for hapten formation. Chem Res Toxicol 2009;22(5):937–48.
24. Sanderson JP, Naisbitt DJ, Farrell J, et al. Sulfamethoxazole and its metabolite nitroso sulfamethoxazole stimulate dendritic cell costimulatory signaling. J Immunol 2007;178(9):5533–42.
25. Naisbitt DJ, Farrell J, Gordon SF, et al. Covalent binding of the nitroso metabolite of sulfamethoxazole leads to toxicity and major histocompatibility complex-restricted antigen presentation. Mol Pharmacol 2002;62(3):628–37.
26. Megherbi R, Kiorpelidou E, Foster B, et al. Role of protein haptenation in triggering maturation events in the dendritic cell surrogate cell line THP-1. Toxicol Appl Pharmacol 2009;238(2):120–32.
27. Pickard C, Louafi F, McGuire C, et al. The cutaneous biochemical redox barrier: a component of the innate immune defenses against sensitization by highly reactive environmental xenobiotics. J Immunol 2009;183(11):7576–84.
28. Pickard C, Smith AM, Cooper H, et al. Investigation of mechanisms underlying the T-cell response to the hapten 2,4-dinitrochlorobenzene. J Invest Dermatol 2007;127(3):630–7.
29. Jenkins RE, Meng X, Elliott VL, et al. Characterisation of flucloxacillin and 5-hydroxymethyl flucloxacillin haptenated HSA in vitro and in vivo. Proteomics Clin Appl 2009;3(6):720–9.
30. Hertl M, Geisel J, Boecker C, et al. Selective generation of CD8+ T-cell clones from the peripheral blood of patients with cutaneous reactions to beta-lactam antibiotics. Br J Dermatol 1993;128:619–26.
31. Sachs B, Erdmann S, Malte Baron J, et al. Determination of interleukin-5 secretion from drug-specific activated ex vivo peripheral blood mononuclear cells as a test system for the in vitro detection of drug sensitization. Clin Exp Allergy 2002;32(5):736–44.

32. Rozieres A, Hennino A, Rodet K, et al. Detection and quantification of drug-specific T cells in penicillin allergy. Allergy 2009;64(4):534–42.
33. Beeler A, Engler O, Gerber BO, et al. Long-lasting reactivity and high frequency of drug-specific T cells after severe systemic drug hypersensitivity reactions. J Allergy Clin Immunol 2006;117(2):455–62.
34. Brugnolo F, Annunziato F, Sampognaro S, et al. Highly Th2-skewed cytokine profile of beta-lactam-specific T cells from nonatopic subjects with adverse drug reactions. J Immunol 1999;163(2):1053–9.
35. Mauri-Hellweg D, Zanni M, Frei E, et al. Cross-reactivity of T cell lines and clones to beta-lactam antibiotics. J Immunol 1996;157(3):1071–9.
36. Brander C, Mauri-Hellweg D, Bettens F, et al. Heterogeneous T cell responses to beta-lactam-modified self-structures are observed in penicillin-allergic individuals. J Immunol 1995;155(5):2670–8.
37. Nhim C, Delluc S, Halgand F, et al. Identification and frequency of circulating CD4(+) T lymphocytes specific to benzylpenicillin in healthy donors. Allergy 2013;68(7):899–905.
38. Padovan E, Mauri-Hellweg D, Pichler WJ, et al. T cell recognition of penicillin G: structural features determining antigenic specificity. Eur J Immunol 1996;26: 42–8.
39. Manchanda T, Hess D, Dale L, et al. Haptenation of sulfonamide reactive metabolites to cellular proteins. Mol Pharmacol 2002;62(5):1011–26.
40. Naisbitt DJ, Gordon SF, Pirmohamed M, et al. Antigenicity and immunogenicity of sulphamethoxazole: demonstration of metabolism-dependent haptenation and T-cell proliferation in vivo. Br J Pharmacol 2001;133(2):295–305.
41. Farrell J, Naisbitt DJ, Drummond NS, et al. Characterization of sulfamethoxazole and sulfamethoxazole metabolite-specific T-cell responses in animals and humans. J Pharmacol Exp Ther 2003;306(1):229–37.
42. Faulkner L, Martinsson K, Castelazo AS, et al. The development of in vitro culture methods to characterize primary T cell responses to drugs. Toxicol Sci 2012;127:150–8.
43. Engler OB, Strasser I, Naisbitt DJ, et al. A chemically inert drug can stimulate T cells in vitro by their T cell receptor in non-sensitised individuals. Toxicology 2004;197(1):47–56.
44. Castrejon JL, Berry N, El-Ghaiesh S, et al. Stimulation of human T cells with sulfonamides and sulfonamide metabolites. J Allergy Clin Immunol 2010;125(2): 411–8.e4.
45. Schnyder B, Burkhart C, Schnyder-Frutig K, et al. Recognition of sulfamethoxazole and its reactive metabolites by drug-specific CD4+ T cells from allergic individuals. J Immunol 2000;164(12):6647–54.
46. Nassif A, Bensussan A, Boumsell L, et al. Toxic epidermal necrolysis: effector cells are drug-specific cytotoxic T cells. J Allergy Clin Immunol 2004;114(5): 1209–15.
47. Elsheikh A, Lavergne SN, Castrejon JL, et al. Drug antigenicity, immunogenicity, and costimulatory signaling: evidence for formation of a functional antigen through immune cell metabolism. J Immunol 2010;185(11):6448–60.
48. Elsheikh A, Castrejon L, Lavergne SN, et al. Enhanced antigenicity leads to altered immunogenicity in sulfamethoxazole-hypersensitive patients with cystic fibrosis. J Allergy Clin Immunol 2011;127(6):1543–51.e3.
49. Lavergne SN, Whitaker P, Peckham D, et al. Drug metabolite-specific lymphocyte responses in sulfamethoxazole allergic patients with cystic fibrosis. Chem Res Toxicol 2010;23(6):1009–11.

50. Yun J, Adam J, Yerly D, et al. Human leukocyte antigens (HLA) associated drug hypersensitivity: consequences of drug binding to HLA. Allergy 2012;67: 1338–46.

51. Mauri-Hellweg D, Bettens F, Mauri D, et al. Activation of drug-specific CD4+ and CD8+ T cells in individuals allergic to sulfonamides, phenytoin, and carbamazepine. J Immunol 1995;155(1):462–72.

52. Burkhart C, von Greyerz S, Depta JP, et al. Influence of reduced glutathione on the proliferative response of sulfamethoxazole-specific and sulfamethoxazole-metabolite-specific human CD4+ T-cells. Br J Pharmacol 2001;132(3):623–30.

53. Zanni MP, von Greyerz S, Schnyder B, et al. HLA-restricted, processing- and metabolism-independent pathway of drug recognition by human alpha beta T lymphocytes. J Clin Invest 1998;102(8):1591–8.

54. Schnyder B, Mauri-Hellweg D, Zanni M, et al. Direct, MHC-dependent presentation of the drug sulfamethoxazole to human alphabeta T cell clones. J Clin Invest 1997;100(1):136–41.

55. Wuillemin N, Adam J, Fontana S, et al. HLA haplotype determines hapten or p-i T cell reactivity to flucloxacillin. J Immunol 2013;190(10):4956–64.

56. Keller M, Lerch M, Britschgi M, et al. Processing-dependent and -independent pathways for recognition of iodinated contrast media by specific human T cells. Clin Exp Allergy 2010;40(2):257–68.

57. Mallal S, Phillips E, Carosi G, et al. HLA-B*5701 screening for hypersensitivity to abacavir. N Engl J Med 2008;358(6):568–79.

58. Illing PT, Vivian JP, Dudek NL, et al. Immune self-reactivity triggered by drug-modified HLA-peptide repertoire. Nature 2012;486(7404):554–8.

59. Ostrov DA, Grant BJ, Pompeu YA, et al. Drug hypersensitivity caused by alteration of the MHC-presented self-peptide repertoire. Proc Natl Acad Sci U S A 2012;109(25):9959–64.

60. Norcross MA, Luo S, Lu L, et al. Abacavir induces loading of novel self-peptides into HLA-B*57: 01: an autoimmune model for HLA-associated drug hypersensitivity. AIDS 2012;26(11):F21–9.

61. Chessman D, Kostenko L, Lethborg T, et al. Human leukocyte antigen class I-restricted activation of CD8+ T cells provides the immunogenetic basis of a systemic drug hypersensitivity. Immunity 2008;28(6):822–32.

62. Nyfeler B, Pichler WJ. The lymphocyte transformation test for the diagnosis of drug allergy: sensitivity and specificity. Clin Exp Allergy 1997;27:175–81.

63. Pichler WJ, Tilch J. The lymphocyte transformation test in the diagnosis of drug hypersensitivity. Allergy 2004;59(8):809–20.

64. Wu Y, Farrell J, Pirmohamed M, et al. Generation and characterization of antigen-specific CD4+, CD8+, and CD4+CD8+ T-cell clones from patients with carbamazepine hypersensitivity. J Allergy Clin Immunol 2007;119(4): 973–81.

65. Wu Y, Sanderson JP, Farrell J, et al. Activation of T cells by carbamazepine and carbamazepine metabolites. J Allergy Clin Immunol 2006;118(1):233–41.

66. Naisbitt DJ, Britschgi M, Wong G, et al. Hypersensitivity reactions to carbamazepine: characterization of the specificity, phenotype, and cytokine profile of drug-specific T cell clones. Mol Pharmacol 2003;63(3):732–41.

67. Naisbitt DJ, Farrell J, Wong G, et al. Characterization of drug-specific T cells in lamotrigine hypersensitivity. J Allergy Clin Immunol 2003;111(6):1393–403.

68. Porebski G, Pecaric-Petkovic T, Groux-Keller M, et al. In vitro drug causality assessment in Stevens-Johnson syndrome - alternatives for lymphocyte transformation test. Clin Exp Allergy 2013;43(9):1027–37.

69. Porebski G, Gschwend-Zawodniak A, Pichler WJ. In vitro diagnosis of T cell-mediated drug allergy. Clin Exp Allergy 2011;41(4):461–70.
70. Nassif A, Bensussan A, Dorothee G, et al. Drug specific cytotoxic T-cells in the skin lesions of a patient with toxic epidermal necrolysis. J Invest Dermatol 2002; 118(4):728–33.
71. Polak ME, Belgi G, McGuire C, et al. In vitro diagnostic assays are effective during the acute phase of delayed-type drug hypersensitivity reactions. Br J Dermatol 2013;168(3):539–49.
72. Beeler A, Zaccaria L, Kawabata T, et al. CD69 upregulation on T cells as an in vitro marker for delayed-type drug hypersensitivity. Allergy 2008;63(2):181–8.
73. Zawodniak A, Lochmatter P, Yerly D, et al. In vitro detection of cytotoxic T and NK cells in peripheral blood of patients with various drug-induced skin diseases. Allergy 2010;65(3):376–84.
74. Fu M, Gao Y, Pan Y, et al. Recovered patients with Stevens-Johson syndrome and toxic epidermal necrolysis maintain long-lived IFN-gamma and sFasL memory response. PLoS One 2012;7(9):e45516.
75. Bell CC, Faulkner L, Martinsson K, et al. T-cells from HLA-B*57:01+ human subjects are activated with abacavir through two independent pathways and induce cell death by multiple mechanisms. Chem Res Toxicol 2013;26(5):759–66.
76. Richter A, Schmucker SS, Esser PR, et al. Human T cell priming assay (hTCPA) for the identification of contact allergens based on naive T cells and DC–IFN-gamma and TNF-alpha readout. Toxicol In Vitro 2013;27(3):1180–5.
77. Yawalkar N, Pichler WJ. Pathogenesis of drug-induced exanthema. Int Arch Allergy Immunol 2001;124(1–3):336–8.
78. Yawalkar N, Shrikhande M, Hari Y, et al. Evidence for a role for IL-5 and eotaxin in activating and recruiting eosinophils in drug-induced cutaneous eruptions. J Allergy Clin Immunol 2000;106(6):1171–6.
79. Picard D, Janela B, Descamps V, et al. Drug reaction with eosinophilia and systemic symptoms (DRESS): a multiorgan antiviral T cell response. Sci Transl Med 2010;2(46):46ra62.
80. Schaerli P, Britschgi M, Keller M, et al. Characterization of human T cells that regulate neutrophilic skin inflammation. J Immunol 2004;173(3):2151–8.
81. Britschgi M, Steiner UC, Schmid S, et al. T-cell involvement in drug-induced acute generalized exanthematous pustulosis. J Clin Invest 2001;107(11): 1433–41.
82. Wei CY, Chung WH, Huang HW, et al. Direct interaction between HLA-B and carbamazepine activates T cells in patients with Stevens-Johnson syndrome. J Allergy Clin Immunol 2012;129(6):1562–9.e5.
83. Ko TM, Chung WH, Wei CY, et al. Shared and restricted T-cell receptor use is crucial for carbamazepine-induced Stevens-Johnson syndrome. J Allergy Clin Immunol 2011;128:1266–76.e11.
84. Mennicke M, Zawodniak A, Keller M, et al. Fulminant liver failure after vancomycin in a sulfasalazine-induced DRESS syndrome: fatal recurrence after liver transplantation. Am J Transplant 2009;9(9):2197–202.
85. Maria VA, Victorino RM. Diagnostic value of specific T cell reactivity to drugs in 95 cases of drug induced liver injury. Gut 1997;41(4):534–40.

Hypersensitivity from Intravenous Iron Products

Andreas J. Bircher, MD[a],*, Michael Auerbach, MD[b,c]

KEYWORDS

- Intravenous iron • Adverse drug reaction • Hypersensitivity • Toxicity

KEY POINTS

- Parenteral iron substitution is increasingly used.
- Immune complex anaphylaxis has rarely occurred to high-molecular-weight iron dextrans.
- Severe adverse drug reactions to newer carbohydrate iron formulations are very rare.
- So far, mechanisms have not been elucidated.

INTRODUCTION

Among many physicians, it is generally thought that intravenous (IV) iron has an inherent risk of serious adverse events (SAE). Earlier preparations of high-molecular-weight iron dextrans (HMW ID) were associated with rare SAE consistent with anaphylaxis. Newer formulations, which are discussed in this review, are safe, albeit rarely adverse drug reactions (ADR) may occur. Some ADR are fueled by the misinterpretation of clinical signs and mismanagement of minor infusion reactions.[1] When the literature is reviewed, it becomes obvious that clinically significant toxicity or hypersensitivity is extremely rare. Here the authors review the available IV iron formulations, the clinical manifestations of adverse reactions, their epidemiology and perceived pathophysiologic mechanisms, and management of adverse events.

TERMINOLOGY

ADR are not infrequent and may result in severe symptoms. A variety of terms have been used for different ADR patterns.[2] The most common ADR are correlated to known pharmacologic or toxic drug properties, are predictable, and may occur in any exposed individual (type A). Hypersensitivity reactions are less common,

Disclosures: Dr A.J. Bircher has no relevant financial disclosures; Dr M. Auerbach has no relevant financial disclosures.
[a] Allergy Unit, Dermatology Clinic, University Hospital Basel, Petersgraben 4, Basel 4031, Switzerland; [b] Georgetown University School of Medicine, 3900 Reservoir road northwest, Washington, DC 20007, USA; [c] Hematology and Oncology, Private Practice, King Avenue #308, Baltimore, MD 21237, USA
* Corresponding author.
E-mail address: andreas.bircher@unibas.ch

Immunol Allergy Clin N Am 34 (2014) 707–723
http://dx.doi.org/10.1016/j.iac.2014.04.013
0889-8561/14/$ – see front matter © 2014 Elsevier Inc. All rights reserved.

unpredictable, do not depend on pharmacologic properties, and usually occur in susceptible individuals (type B).[3] These latter ones are classified into immunologically mediated reactions, such as allergy and nonallergic hypersensitivity (intolerance or pseudoallergic reactions, also referred to as anaphylactoid), and idiosyncratic reactions. These latter terms are not generally accepted and are used inconsistently. In a consensus statement, the World Allergy Organization proposed that reactions without a proven specific immunologic mechanism be referred to as *nonallergic hypersensitivity reactions* and *pseudoallergy* and *anaphylactoid* should no longer be used.[4] The term *hypersensitivity* should be used to describe objectively reproducible symptoms or signs resembling allergy and initiated by exposure to a defined drug at a dose tolerated by normal subjects. Allergy is a hypersensitivity reaction initiated by specific immunologic mechanisms, either antibody mediated or cell mediated. In non–immunoglobulin E (IgE)–mediated allergy, inflammation involves IgG antibodies or allergen-specific lymphocytes. The adjectives *immediate* or *delayed* refer to the delay of onset of symptoms after the last drug administration[2] and may indicate the probable underlying immunologic mechanism (antibodies [IgE] in immediate or T cells in delayed reactions).

The term *anaphylaxis* is also used inconsistently. It has been proposed that *anaphylaxis* should be the general term for an acute reaction defined as a severe, life-threatening generalized or systemic hypersensitivity reaction. The term *allergic anaphylaxis* should be used when the reaction is mediated by an immunologic mechanism (IgE or immune complexes). Conversely, anaphylaxis caused by any nonimmunologic cause could be referred to as *nonallergic anaphylaxis*.[4] Anaphylaxis should affect at least 2 organ systems (eg, skin and respiratory tract or respiratory and gastrointestinal tract); however, if acute hypotension after a very probable elicitor occurs, *anaphylaxis* is an appropriate term.[5]

Here the authors use the term *immediate-type hypersensitivity* for clinical manifestations e. presenting with urticaria or, bronchospasm, likely involving mast cells and basophils, and *delayed-type hypersensitivity* for manifestations likely including T-cell mechanisms, such as exanthemas. The adjective *allergic* should be used only for immunologically mediated reactions. The authors prefer the term *nonimmunologic* to *nonallergic anaphylaxis* if no specific immune mechanism is proven as in most cases of immediate iron hypersensitivity reactions.

IRON COMPOUNDS AS POTENTIAL ALLERGENS

Iron, an essential trace element, is one of the most common elements on earth. It is estimated that a healthy adult contains 35 to 50 mg of iron per kilogram of body weight or a total of 2 to 6 g. At least 70% is used in hemoglobin, myoglobin, and enzymes involved in intracellular oxidation-reduction processes, oxygen transport, and cellular respiration. As 99% of red cell iron is recycled, the daily need is between 1 and 2 mg/d for an adult because of physiologic loss in sweat and stool.

Metals are haptens; in order to form a complete allergen, a carrier protein, which is typically an endogenous protein, is needed. For nickel and some other metals, particularly in the setting of contact allergy, direct binding to the HLA molecule has been demonstrated.[6] Additionally, it has been shown that nickel and cobalt may initiate an innate immune response in the sense of a danger signal[7] that is needed to induce an immunologic response. For any other metal, including iron, such a mechanism has not been studied. In humans, iron has been rarely demonstrated to have antigenic or allergenic properties.[8] Some metals, such as cobalt, which are also part of essential molecules, such as the vitamin B12 complex, are well-known contact allergens on topical cutaneous exposure.[9]

To ensure better tolerance, iron products are administered in complexes as various salts or with carbohydrate carriers. A variety of different formulations are commercially available (**Table 1**). For HMW dextrans, also used as volume expanders[10] and still used in some iron preparations, IgG-mediated anaphylaxis has been documented.[11] Immune complexes formed by specific IgG binding to HMW dextrans, as with iron dextran hypersensitivity, have been shown to elicit a so-called immune complex anaphylaxis (Coombs and Gell type III).[12] Preexisting high levels of IgG and IgM antibodies, so-called dextran-reactive antibodies, have been identified. Some other carbohydrates, such as carboxymethylcellulose (E466), are held responsible for rare cases of anaphylaxis on the intramuscular (IM) administration of corticosteroid preparations containing this emulsifying agent.[13,14] Type I hypersensitivity is demonstrated here based on the presence of specific IgE. For other carbohydrates, such a mechanism has rarely been demonstrated. Recently, the disaccharide galactose-alpha-1,3-galactose has been shown to be an antigen in mammalian meat. The same antigen has been identified on the chimeric mouse/human antibody cetuximab, which has caused severe anaphylaxis on the first exposure in apparently previously sensitized patients.[15]

IRON PREPARATIONS

The liberation of catalytically active free iron is proportional to the instability of the carbohydrate complex and may lead to oxidative stress and hypotension.[16] IV iron formulations are colloids that consist of spheroidal iron-carbohydrate nanoparticles.[17] An iron-oxyhydroxide gel lies at the core of each particle. A shell of carbohydrate that stabilizes the iron-oxyhydroxide, slows down the release of bioactive iron, and maintains the resulting particles in colloidal suspension surrounds the core. IV iron agents share the same core chemistry but differ from each other by the size of the core and the type and density of the surrounding carbohydrate (see **Table 1**). Initially, only HMW ID were available and were associated with a high rate of anaphylactic reactions. The newer compounds have a considerably lower rate of ADR.

PATHOPHYSIOLOGY

Drug hypersensitivity reactions include all 4 Coombs and Gell types (types I–IV) as well as nonimmunologically mediated hypersensitivity reactions in which no specific initiating element, such as a drug-specific IgE-, IgG antibody, or T cell, can be demonstrated.[18]

In immediate IV iron hypersensitivity, several pathogenic models have been implicated. An IgE-mediated mechanism has not been convincingly shown.[19,20] However, with HMW ID, immune complex anaphylaxis (Coombs and Gell type III)[21] caused by preexisting dextran-reactive antibodies has been repeatedly demonstrated.[22]

Hypersensitivity reactions to IV irons have similarities to the so-called red man syndrome related to IV vancomycin administration (by direct stimulation of mast cells). It is a nonimmunologic reaction and is thought to involve direct stimulation of mast cells or basophils. An increase in serum histamine levels,[3] related to the rate of vancomycin infusion, has been shown. Therefore, it is recommended that vancomycin be administered over at least 1 hour.[23] The concomitant use of medications that cause nonspecific histamine release from mast cells may precipitate red man syndrome. Also, some infusion reactions from biologic drugs[24] show similarities (eg, toxicity caused by high doses or acute cytokine release [cytokine storm] caused by cell activation or cell death) that are also usually not immunologically mediated.[25] Other drugs include opioids, IV contrast agents, and muscle relaxants.[26]

Table 1
Iron products and their properties

Trade name	Currently Available Intravenous Iron Preparations					Investigational Agents (Not FDA Approved)	
	DexFerrum	InFeD, Cosmofer	Ferrlecit	Venofer	Ferumoxytol, Feraheme	Monofer Approved Europe	Injectafer Ferinject (Europe)
Carbohydrate	HMW ID (branched polysaccharide)	LMW ID (branched polysaccharide)	Gluconate (monosaccharide)	Sucrose (disaccharide)	Polyglucose sorbitol carboxy-methylether	Isomaltoside (linear oligosaccharide)	Carboxymaltose (branched polysaccharide)
Complex type	Type I; robust and strong	Type I; robust and strong	Type III; labile and weak	Type II; semirobust and moderately strong	Type I; robust and strong	Type I; robust and strong	Type I; robust and strong
Molecular weight measured by manufacturer (Da)	265,000	165,000	289,000–440,000	34,000–60,000	750,000	165,000	150,000
Labile iron release	–	–	+++	+/–	–	–	–
Total dose or >500-mg infusion	Yes	Yes	No	No	Yes	Yes	Yes

	DexFerrum	InFeD	Ferrlecit	Venofer	Feraheme	MonoFer	Injectafer
Premedication	TDI only	TDI only	No	No	No	No	No
Test dose required	Yes	Yes	No	No, yes[a]	No	No	No
Iron concentration (mg/mL)	50	50	12.5	20	30	100	30 / 50 (Europe)
Vial volume (mL)	1–2	2	5	5	17	1, 2, 5, 10	2, 10 / 1, 2, 10 (Europe)
Black box warning	Yes	Yes	No	No	No	No	No
Preservative	None	None	Benzyl alcohol	None	None	None	None

DexFerrum. Available at: http://www.americanregent.com/documents/Product16PrescribingInformation.pdf. Accessed September 4, 2013.

InFeD. Available at: http://pi.actavis.com/data_stream.asp?product_group=1251&p=pi&language=E. Accessed September 4, 2013.

Ferrlecit. Available at: http://www.products.sanofi-aventis.us/ferrlecit/ferrlecit.pdf. Accessed September 4, 2013.

Venofer. Available at: http://www.venofer.com/PDF/Venofer_IN2340_Rev_9_2012.pdf. Accessed September 4, 2013.

Feraheme. Available at: http://www.feraheme.com/downloads/feraheme-pi.pdf. Accessed September 4, 2013.

MonoFer. Available at: http://www.nataonline.com/sites/default/files/imagesC/Monofer_core_SPC.pdf. Accessed September 4, 2013.

Injectafer. Available at: http://www.injectafer.com/files/Prescribing_Information.pdf. Accessed September 4, 2013.

Abbreviations: FDA, Food and Drug Administration; LMW, low molecular weight; TDI, total dose infusion.

[a] A test dose is only required in Europe.

Data from Macdougall I, Geisser P. Use of intravenous iron supplementation in chronic kidney disease: an update. Iran J Kidney Dis 2013;7(1):9–22; and Muñoz M, García-Erce JA, Remacha ÁF. Disorders of iron metabolism. Part II: iron deficiency and iron overload. J Clin Pathol 2011;64(4):287–96.

CLINICAL MANIFESTATIONS

Generally, hypersensitivity reactions from drugs may include a large variety of different clinical manifestations on different organs. The clinical manifestation is an expression of the involved mechanism. After the introduction of iron dextran products, anaphylactic reactions, including urticaria, angioedema, bronchospasm, and anaphylactic shock, have been reported.[11] Typical hypersensitivity symptoms are listed in **Box 1**.

HISTORY

To better understand the origin of negative perception with IV irons' use, a brief review of the history is necessary. In the early twentieth century, parenteral iron usage, often via the IM route, was limited because of prohibitive toxic reactions.[27] In 1947, Nissim[28] demonstrated that IV iron as saccharide could be administered with relative safety, although infusion reactions were common. Given the safety and efficacy of oral iron, it is not surprising that a paper by Marchasin and Wallerstein[29] received little attention, reporting 37 patients treated with a total dose infusion of iron dextran and none with SAEs.

In 1954, the first iron dextran, IMFeron, an HMW ID, (no longer available) was introduced by Baird and Padmore[30] for the treatment of iron deficiency by the IM route. It was used in divided doses with infrequent adverse events, such as pain and pigmentation at the injection site. Rare episodes of anaphylaxis were reported. In 1980, the first large prospective study of IV iron in the United States[31] in 478 patients with iron deficiency who received full-dose replacement with HMW ID was published. Nearly all patients responded completely, but 3 had SAE; delayed reactions occurred in 8 patients, none of which were fatal. The researchers concluded that IV iron should only be used when iron deficiency cannot be treated adequately with oral iron. A black box warning was placed on the package insert that persists on all iron dextran products in the United States but not in Europe.

Box 1
Typical hypersensitivity symptoms to IV iron likely caused by an immune reaction

Immediate Symptoms

  Skin: pruritus, extended flush, urticaria, angioedema

  Respiratory: dyspnea, tachypnea, cough, bronchospasm, stridor

  Gastrointestinal: nausea, emesis, colic, diarrhea

  Cardiovascular: hypotension, hypertension, tachycardia, bradycardia, palpitations, chest pain, shock

  Central nervous system: dizziness, syncope, unconsciousness

Delayed Symptoms

  Fever

  Arthralgia, arthritis

  Lymphadenopathy

  Exanthems

Data from Farnam K, Chang C, Teuber S, et al. Nonallergic drug hypersensitivity reactions. Int Arch Allergy Immunol 2012;159(4):327–45; and Hoigné R, Breymann C, Künzi UP, et al. Parenteral iron therapy: problems and possible solutions. Schweiz Med Wochenschr 1998;128(14):528–35 [in German].

In 1989, erythropoiesis-stimulating agents (ESA) became available for use in dialysis. This class of drugs promised to eliminate the symptoms of anemia. However, enthusiasm for the use of erythropoietin (EPO), the first ESA to be approved in the United States, was limited. At the same time, seminal work by Eschbach and colleagues[32] and later Fishbane and colleagues[33] showed that when IV iron (but not oral) was given to hyporesponsive patients with iron-restricted erythropoiesis, marked synergy occurred. Iron dextran rapidly became standard in dialysis.

In 1991, IMFeron was removed from the market; but at the same time, a low-molecular-weight iron dextran (LMW ID), InFeD, became available. Between 1992 and 1996, virtually all patients undergoing dialysis received LMW ID. In 1996, another HMW ID (DexFerrum) was approved as an alternative. In 1999 and 2000, 2 iron salts, ferric gluconate (Ferrlecit) and iron sucrose (Venofer), were approved. Three retrospective studies on large dialysis populations,[34–36] using spontaneous adverse event reporting systems, reported a much lower incidence of SAE; these 2 iron products rapidly replaced iron dextrans. In 2004, Chertow and colleagues[37] reported that most SAE were caused by the HMW ID formulation, which has been corroborated by the preponderance of published evidence.[38]

Most of these concerns could have been precluded had the published evidence of Fishbane and colleagues[39] been more widely disseminated. They described an acute arthralgia and myalgia syndrome associated with the test dose. In 0.3% of patients, the acute onset of isolated chest oppression and back pain with or without facial flushing occurred (**Box 2**) but without further symptoms of anaphylaxis. After a short delay, symptoms resolved without treatment and rechallenges were tolerated. Unfortunately, these signs were considered as a prodrome to anaphylaxis; inappropriate intervention with drugs, such as diphenhydramine and epinephrine, converted a self-limited minor infusion reaction to a serious cardiovascular adverse event attributed to the IV iron. Similar misconceptions may arise when diphenhydramine is used as premedication for which there is no evidence to suggest a benefit. In a study of 135 patients receiving LMW ID preceded by premedication with cimetidine, dexamethasone, and diphenhydramine, most of the adverse events were considered secondary to premedication.[40]

Recently, 3 new IV iron formulations that promise to allow complete replacement dosing in 15 minutes have been approved. These formulations are ferumoxytol (Feraheme), ferric carboxymaltose (Injectafer, Ferinject in Europe), and iron isomaltoside 1000 (Monofer, Europe only). Using head-to-head comparisons of LMW ID versus iron sucrose, ferumoxytol versus iron sucrose, and ferric carboxymaltose versus iron sucrose, no differences in efficacy or safety could be identified.[41–45]

Box 2
Symptoms to IV iron likely caused by toxicity from free iron
Transient facial flushing
Chest oppression
Headache
Nausea, diarrhea
Back pain
Low-grade fever
Myalgia, arthralgia
If metallic taste, lower lumbar pain

ADR FROM IRON PRODUCTS

Reactions after the administration of IV iron can be divided into acute (immediately after the start of the infusion), delayed (hours to a day after the infusion), or long-term (mainly oxidative stress or infection). Although the literature is abundant with published evidence to theoretically support long-term reactions,[46] clinically relevant evidence is lacking. Following administration, iron is principally taken into the reticuloendothelial system where the carbohydrate shell is slowly degraded. Thus, elemental iron can be slowly released for erythropoiesis without causing toxicity. The metabolism of iron products is not similar to the physiologic iron process because IV administration bypasses the hepcidin-ferroportin pathway in the intestine, which protects against iron overload and regulates transferrin iron saturation.[47–50]

Iron Products and Immediate Toxicity

Toxicity related to IV iron administration is attributed to the effects of bioactive labile iron (see **Box 2**, **Fig. 1**). Yet, when appropriate dosing and proper administration protocols are followed, the symptoms are clinically insignificant, self-limited, and usually resolve without treatment. Furthermore, without any evidence, diphenhydramine is often used as premedication. This antihistamine is known to cause somnolence, diaphoresis, hypotension, and tachycardia; Barton and colleagues[40] reported that most adverse events were caused by the premedication with diphenhydramine.

To reduce the large amounts of labile iron causing toxicity, formulations were developed that shielded iron (see **Table 1**). Nonetheless, small amounts of labile iron are measurable following the administration of each formulation.[51] The currently approved IV iron formulations all share the iron-carbohydrate structure but differ from each other by the size of the core and the density of the surrounding carbohydrate determining the amount of labile iron that is released (see **Table 1**).

Following the release of LMW ID for use as an adjunct to ESA in dialysis-associated anemia, marked improvements in hemoglobin responses, energy, activity, cardiovascular function, cognition, sexual function, and survival were observed; SAEs were extremely rare. However, after the release of HMW ID in 1996, a small but clinically significant increase in SAEs was observed. Faich and Strobos[34] compared the spontaneous reports to the US and European drug agencies of SAEs to iron dextrans and noniron dextrans and noted a significantly higher rate of reactions and 31 deaths attributed to the iron dextrans. No deaths caused by the nondextran irons were reported. In 2 retrospective analyses,[35,36] a very low SAE rate with ferric gluconate as well as a negligible acute ADR rate even after previous iron dextran hypersensitivity were observed. It was subsequently concluded that ferric gluconate and iron sucrose were much safer than iron dextran, and more than 400,000 patients undergoing dialysis were switched from iron dextran to either ferric gluconate or iron sucrose.

Then in 2004, Chertow and colleagues[37] observed that most of the SAEs reported with iron dextran were caused by the HMW formulation and concluded that when HMW ID was avoided, SAEs were extremely rare, with an estimated incidence of less than 1:200,000 doses. Although using spontaneously reported ADR as an indicator of relative safety has been proscribed,[52] every prospective study and intrainstitutional retrospective study comparing the safety of the iron salts with LMW ID has shown no difference.[46] Ferumoxytol and ferric carboxymaltose have been prospectively compared with iron sucrose for efficacy and safety. As with LMW ID, no significant differences have been noted.[53]

An acute onset of arthralgia or myalgia and/or flushing may occur with any iron formulations. In extremely rare circumstances, these symptoms may be followed by

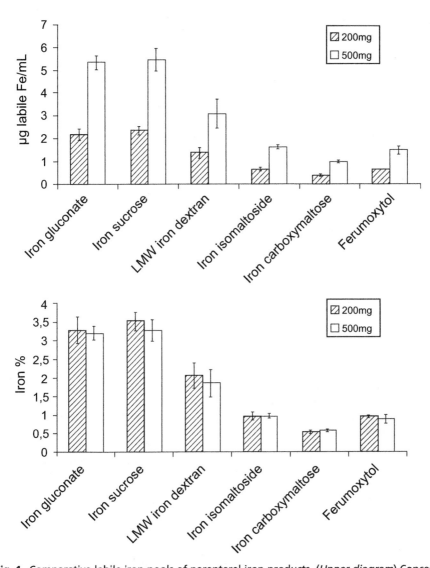

Fig. 1. Comparative labile iron pools of parenteral iron products. (*Upper diagram*) Concentration of the Ferrozine-detectable labile iron pool in μg/mL. The bars represent the average of at least 4 measurements. (*Lower diagram*) Ferrozine-detectable labile iron in percentage of the total used dose. For each measurement, the iron complex was incubated in human serum for 10 and 45 minutes, respectively. Thereafter, the Ferrozine reaction was performed; in each case, an intercept of a second-degree polynomial regression function of the absorption versus rime curve with the ordinate was calculated. These intercepts were extrapolated to an incubation time of t = 0 (where *t* is time) by linear regression, yielding the labile iron pool in serum for each intravenous iron product. Fe, iron. (*From* Jahna MR, Andreasen HB, Fütterer S, et al. A comparative study of the physicochemical properties of iron isomaltoside 1000 (Monofer), a new intravenous iron preparation and its clinical implications. Eur J Pharm Biopharm 2011;78:486; with permission.)

anaphylaxis. It is of note, however, that no increase of serum tryptase levels, a serologic marker for anaphylaxis, was documented during these reactions.[54] Based on a validated tool, the Ferrozine-detectable iron, the amount of labile iron after administration of either 200 mg (ferric gluconate and iron sucrose) or 500 mg (LMW ID, ferumoxytol, ferric carboxymaltose, iron isomaltoside), is highest with the 2 salts, much lower with LMW ID, and lowest with ferumoxytol, ferric carboxymaltose, and iron isomaltoside (see **Fig. 1**).[51] Therefore, the overwhelming likelihood is that they are minor systemic reactions to labile iron. These reactions resolve spontaneously and rarely recur with rechallenge. Pretreatment with methylprednisolone may decrease recurrence; in less than 1:1000 administrations, ranitidine and acetaminophen may be necessary.

Iron Products and Delayed Toxicity

Delayed arthralgias and myalgias infrequently occur after a total dose infusion or cumulative lower doses.[55] Premedication with corticosteroids abates or eliminates these reactions; but because they are mild and self-limited, the symptoms are also easily relieved with nonsteroidal antiinflammatory drugs. Other delayed reactions, with similar schedules, are low-grade fevers and headache.

Long-term toxicity remains a concern, but there are no prospective data on long-term outcomes with the use of IV iron. The most comprehensive work on this subject was done by Kalantar-Zadeh and colleagues[56] who examined time-dependent associations between IV iron administered and both all-cause and cardiovascular morbidity and mortality in patients undergoing maintenance hemodialysis. After extensive time-dependent and multivariate adjustment for case mix, administered IV iron and EPO doses, and surrogates of nutritional status and inflammation, the lowest all-cause and cardiovascular risk was associated with ferritin levels between 200 and 1200 ng/mL and transferrin saturations between 30% and 50%. Compared with those who did not receive IV iron, maintenance dosages of up to 400 mg per month were associated with improved survival. Supporting these conclusions, Feldman and colleagues[57] reported a slightly increased mortality in patients receiving more than 1 g of IV iron over a 6-month period; but after controlling for confounding variables, no morbidity with IV iron was present, thus, providing cautious support for the administration of greater than 1 g over a 6-month period if needed to maintain target hemoglobin.

Iron Products and Immediate Hypersensitivity

Despite the very rare occurrence of SAE,[19] there are some case reports of severe anaphylaxis. In a 38-year-old woman, IV ferric gluconate 125 mg was given over 10 minutes. The first dose was initially well tolerated; however, nausea, dizziness, and minor tongue swelling occurred several minutes later.[58] On her second course of therapy, premedication with dexamethasone, diphenhydramine, and prochlorperazine was given. Subsequently, epigastric pain, nausea, swelling of her lips and tongue, and hypotension occurred. The symptoms resolved after the administration of diphenhydramine, dexamethasone, morphine, cimetidine, IV fluids, and oxygen. The Naranjo probability scale indicated a probable relationship between the hypersensitivity reaction and ferric gluconate, but no investigation was done.[58] A 24-year-old primigravida received ferric gluconate and developed tongue swelling. Diphenhydramine was given and the infusion was continued. Suddenly hypotension (70/30 mm Hg, pulse 110 beats per minute) and severe angioedema of the face and tongue developed. Resuscitation was successful, and she delivered a healthy child 1 week later.[59] No allergy investigation was performed. A 42-year-old woman received 100 mg of IV iron sucrose (Venofer); after 15 minutes, generalized pruritus, burning of the tongue, and peribuccal hyperesthesia occurred.[60] Identical reactions occurred after premedication and iron sucrose and ferric carboxymaltose. Subsequent infusions were well tolerated. A patch test was negative, which is not surprising because it was likely the side effect of IV iron and not a T cell–mediated process. A particular case with a true allergic reaction to the casein component of oral iron proteinsuccinylate (Ferplex 40) was observed in a 4.5-year-old atopic child with a milk and fish allergy.[61] A skin test and IgE were positive to milk proteins. An immunoblot revealed binding to the proteinsuccinylate, indicating its allergenic property.

Iron and Delayed-Type Hypersensitivity

Drug-induced exanthemas have been described with IV iron products, suggesting a T cell–mediated reaction; however, it is unlikely that iron is the elicitor. Unlike with nickel and palladium, contact allergy to iron seems to be extremely rare. Some researchers question the existence of true positive patch tests to iron because of the potential contamination of tested iron agents with other metal contact allergens, such as nickel or cobalt. There are very few cases with positive patch tests with iron.[62,63] However, so far the optimal iron salt to be used in patch tests has not been established.

Iron and Long-term Toxicity and Infection

Human studies have shown transient increases in markers of oxidative stress with all forms of IV iron; however, no clinically negative outcomes associated with the increase in these markers has ever been reported.[54,64]

IV iron has also been theoretically implicated as a possible cause of increased infection rates.[65,66] However, no prospective study with defined infectious outcomes has ever shown an increase with millions of doses in dialysis-associated anemia, nondialysis chronic kidney disease, or chemotherapy-induced anemia, and several prospective and observational studies have shown the opposite.[57,67,68] Eleven studies examining IV iron in chemotherapy-induced anemia have shown synergy with ESA when IV iron was added to the treatment paradigm. One additional study[69] observed a hemoglobin increment with IV iron alone. In 6 of the 12, whereby a defined infection rate was evaluated, no increment in infections was observed.[69–74] This contention was corroborated in an extensive meta-analysis of IV iron in chemotherapy-induced anemia whereby no increment in infection was seen.[75] Finally, in a recent observational trial of 2547 perioperative patients who underwent elective lower limb arthroplasty or hip fracture repair, with or without ESA, observed not only reduced transfusion rates and length of hospital stay ($P = .0001$) but also no difference in infection rates.[76]

In summary, the current state of the literature regarding the risk of IV and infection is inconclusive; but based on the preponderance of published evidence, the risk of IV iron, if any, in causing increased morbidity because of infections is vanishingly small.

DIAGNOSIS AND MANAGEMENT

An allergological work-up of a drug hypersensitivity reaction is based on the assumption of an antibody- or T cell–mediated process. Subsequent prick and intradermal tests are typically used for the identification of an IgE antibody–mediated reaction, whereas intradermal tests with late readings and patch tests are typically used for the diagnosis of T cell–mediated reactions with readings after 24 or 48 and 72 or 96 hours.[77] For metal antigens, neither specific IgE antibodies nor a cellular in vitro assay have so far been commercially established. Typically in occupational situations, such as inhalatory exposure to platinum salts[78] or in anaphylaxis to platinum salts used in oncology,[79] an IgE antibody–mediated mechanism has been implicated. For other metals, this seems to be exceedingly rare. For immediate reactions basophil activation tests, that are used in drug hypersensitivity,[80,81] and for T cell–mediated processes lymphocyte activation tests are feasible. The determination of specific IgG and IgM antibodies has been established for dextrans to detect immune complex reactions from dextrans used as plasma expanders or anticoagulants.[82] However, for all in vitro tests, a standardized commercially available test is not on the market.

The only feasible test to identify a hypersensitivity reaction to a drug irrespective of the mechanism is a controlled reexposure or provocation test.[83] However, this carries the intrinsic danger of eliciting a life-threatening reaction. In some situations whereby a particular drug is indispensable, the procedure may help exclude a suspected hypersensitivity reaction.

If a patient has a probable hypersensitivity reaction after the administration of an iron product, the following information should be carefully obtained:

1. Brand and generic name of the product, including administered dose
2. Route of administration (perioral, IM, or IV [and velocity of infusion in the case of IV])
3. Morphology: exact description of clinical manifestations including all symptoms and signs (see "Clinical Manifestations"); nonspecific symptoms, such as metallic taste and lower lumbar pain, and so forth
4. Chronology: first onset of symptoms, their evolution, and disappearance
5. Response to treatment

From this description, a hypothesis on the potential mechanism can be made and the appropriate tests selected.

If suspected, a cutaneous or systemic mastocytosis should be excluded. The determination of baseline mast cell tryptase may be helpful in this situation. In the acute phase, mast cell tryptase can also be measured between 0.5 and 3.0 hours after the incident in order to demonstrate activation and mediator release from cutaneous mast cells.

For iron products, it is strongly discouraged to perform any prick or intradermal tests with undiluted or diluted solutions. First, an IgE-mediated mechanism, which could be identified by this technique, has not been demonstrated. Second, iron pigment may remain for prolonged periods. Skin tests for IgG-mediated reactions are not standardized and discouraged for the same aforementioned reasons. Finally, patch tests are only useful for T cell–mediated processes, such as eczema or exanthemas. These manifestations are exceedingly rare with iron, and the optimal patch test concentrations are not known. In vitro tests (such as the determination of specific IgG to potential antigens or allergens in iron formulations, basophil activation tests, and lymphocyte activation tests) are used in specialized laboratories for research purposes only.

Finally, provocation tests can be indicated in selected patients after a careful risk/benefit analysis.[83,84] For some iron products, test doses are recommended without evidence to support the recommendation.[1] There are many reports of an initial mild reaction (eg, urticaria) not recurring with rechallenge with the same iron preparation. In some patients, the selection of another formulation may be advisable. In the authors' hands, this approach without premedication was successful in most patients with a putative hypersensitivity reaction to iron products.

The systematic premedication including antihistamines, corticosteroids, and leukotriene antagonists, as often done before IV radiocontrast media, is not recommended.[85] It has not been shown that premedication is of benefit[58]; the premedication itself may lead to an ADR, including hypotension. In one patient, a so-called desensitization procedure with oral iron has been reported.[86]

SUMMARY

Although adverse events occur with all the formulations of IV iron, the frequency of SAE in prospective studies is extremely low; but the current reporting systems provide scarce or no data at all about the relative frequency among the available formulations. IV iron is generally safe and probably much safer than most physicians realize. It is effective in treating iron deficiency across a broad spectrum of anemias. Unlike oral iron, which is rife with gastrointestinal perturbation, which is reported in up to 70% of those to whom it is prescribed, adherence is 100%. Published evidence supports a larger and earlier role for IV iron and raises the question of whether it should be the frontline therapy.

REFERENCES

1. Auerbach M, Ballard H, Glaspy J. Clinical update: intravenous iron for anaemia. Lancet 2007;369(9572):1502–4.
2. Palmiere C, Comment L, Mangin P. Allergic reactions following contrast material administration: nomenclature, classification, and mechanisms. Int J Legal Med 2014;128(1):95–103.
3. Farnam K, Chang C, Teuber S, et al. Nonallergic drug hypersensitivity reactions. Int Arch Allergy Immunol 2012;159(4):327–45.
4. Johansson SGO, Bieber T, Dahl R, et al. Revised nomenclature for allergy for global use: report of the Nomenclature Review Committee of the World Allergy Organization, October 2003. J Allergy Clin Immunol 2004;113(5):832–6.
5. Sampson H, Muñoz Furlong A, Campbell R, et al. Second symposium on the definition and management of anaphylaxis: summary report–Second National Institute of Allergy and Infectious Disease/Food Allergy and Anaphylaxis Network symposium. J Allergy Clin Immunol 2006;117(2):391–7.
6. Gamerdinger K, Moulon C, Karp DR, et al. A new type of metal recognition by human T cells: contact residues for peptide-independent bridging of T cell receptor and major histocompatibility complex by nickel. J Exp Med 2003; 197(10):1345–53.
7. Schmidt M, Raghavan B, Müller V, et al. Crucial role for human Toll-like receptor 4 in the development of contact allergy to nickel. Nat Immunol 2010;11(9): 814–9.
8. Lansdown AB. Physiological and toxicological changes in the skin resulting from the action and interaction of metal ions. Crit Rev Toxicol 1995;25(5): 397–462.
9. Raghavan B, Martin S, Esser P, et al. Metal allergens nickel and cobalt facilitate TLR4 homodimerization independently of MD2. EMBO Rep 2012;13(12): 1109–15.
10. Bircher AJ, Hédin H, Berglund A. Probable grade IV dextran-induced anaphylactic reaction despite hapten inhibition. J Allergy Clin Immunol 1995;95(2): 633–4.
11. Bailie G, Clark J, Lane C, et al. Hypersensitivity reactions and deaths associated with intravenous iron preparations. Nephrol Dial Transplant 2005;20(7):1443–9.
12. Ring J, Behrendt H, de Weck A. History and classification of anaphylaxis. In: Ring J, editor. Anaphylaxis chem immunol allergy, vol. 95. Basel (Switzerland): Karger; 2010. p. 1–11.
13. Bircher AJ, Izakovic J, Bigliardi PL. Oral tolerance of carboxymethylcellulose in patients with anaphylaxis to parenteral carboxymethylcellulose. Ann Allergy Asthma Immunol 2004;92(5):580–1.

14. Bigliardi PL, Izakovic J, Weber JM, et al. Anaphylaxis to the carbohydrate carboxymethylcellulose in parenteral corticosteroid preparations. Dermatology 2003;207(1):100–3.

15. Wolver S, Sun D, Commins S, et al. A peculiar cause of anaphylaxis: no more steak? The journey to discovery of a newly recognized allergy to galactose-alpha-1,3-galactose found in mammalian meat. J Gen Intern Med 2013;28(2):322–5.

16. Potthoff SA, Münch HG. Safety aspects of parenteral iron supplementation therapies in patients with chronic kidney disease. Dtsch Med Wochenschr 2013;138(24):1312–7 [in German].

17. Danielson BG. Structure, chemistry, and pharmacokinetics of intravenous iron agents. J Am Soc Nephrol 2004;15(Suppl 2):S93–8.

18. Pichler WJ. Immune mechanism of drug hypersensitivity. Immunol Allergy Clin North Am 2004;24(3):373–97.

19. Novey HS, Pahl M, Haydik I, et al. Immunologic studies of anaphylaxis to iron dextran in patients on renal dialysis. Ann Allergy 1994;72(3):224–8.

20. Hoigné R, Breymann C, Künzi UP, et al. Parenteral iron therapy: problems and possible solutions. Schweiz Med Wochenschr 1998;128(14):528–35 [in German].

21. Zinderman C, Landow L, Wise R. Anaphylactoid reactions to dextran 40 and 70: reports to the United States Food and Drug Administration, 1969 to 2004. J Vasc Surg 2006;43(5):1004–9.

22. Kraft D, Hedin H, Richter W, et al. Immunoglobulin class and subclass distribution of dextran-reactive antibodies in human reactors and non reactors to clinical dextran. Allergy 1982;37(7):481–9.

23. Healy DP, Sahai JV, Fuller SH, et al. Vancomycin-induced histamine release and "red man syndrome": comparison of 1- and 2-hour infusions. Antimicrob Agents Chemother 1990;34(4):550–4.

24. Scherer K, Spoerl D, Bircher AJ. Adverse drug reactions to biologics. J Dtsch Dermatol Ges 2010;8(6):411–26.

25. Vogel W. Infusion reactions: diagnosis, assessment, and management. Clin J Oncol Nurs 2010;14(2):E10–21.

26. Levy JH, Marty AT. Vancomycin and adverse drug reactions. Crit Care Med 1993;21(8):1107–8.

27. Auerbach M, Coyne D, Ballard H. Intravenous iron: from anathema to standard of care. Am J Hematol 2008;83(7):580–8.

28. Nissim JA. Intravenous administration of iron. Lancet 1947;2(6463):49–51.

29. Marchasin S, Wallerstein RO. The treatment of iron-deficiency anemia with intravenous iron dextran. Blood 1964;23(3):354–8.

30. Baird IM, Podmore DA. Intramuscular iron therapy in iron-deficiency anaemia. Lancet 1954;267(6845):942–6.

31. Hamstra RD, Block MH, Schocket AL. Intravenous iron dextran in clinical medicine. JAMA 1980;243(17):1726–31.

32. Eschbach JW, Kelly MR, Haley NR, et al. Treatment of the anemia of progressive renal failure with recombinant human erythropoietin. N Engl J Med 1989;321(3):158–63.

33. Fishbane S, Frei GL, Maesaka J. Reduction in recombinant human erythropoietin doses by the use of chronic intravenous iron supplementation. Am J Kidney Dis 1995;26(1):41–6.

34. Faich G, Strobos J. Sodium ferric gluconate complex in sucrose: safer intravenous iron therapy than iron dextrans. Am J Kidney Dis 1999;33(3):464–70.

35. Coyne D, Adkinson NF, Nissenson A, et al. Sodium ferric gluconate complex in hemodialysis patients. II. Adverse reactions in iron dextran-sensitive and dextran-tolerant patients. Kidney Int 2003;63(1):217–24.

36. Michael B, Coyne D, Fishbane S, et al. Sodium ferric gluconate complex in hemodialysis patients: adverse reactions compared to placebo and iron dextran. Kidney Int 2002;61(5):1830–9.

37. Chertow G, Mason P, Vaage Nilsen O, et al. On the relative safety of parenteral iron formulations. Nephrol Dial Transplant 2004;19(6):1571–5.

38. Rodgers G, Auerbach M, Cella D, et al. High-molecular weight iron dextran: a wolf in sheep's clothing? J Am Soc Nephrol 2008;19(5):833–4.

39. Fishbane S, Ungureanu VD, Maesaka JK, et al. The safety of intravenous iron dextran in hemodialysis patients. Am J Kidney Dis 1996;28(4):529–34.

40. Barton JC, Barton EH, Bertoli LF, et al. Intravenous iron dextran therapy in patients with iron deficiency and normal renal function who failed to respond to or did not tolerate oral iron supplementation. Am J Med 2000;109(1):27–32.

41. Okam M, Mandell E, Hevelone N, et al. Comparative rates of adverse events with different formulations of intravenous iron. Am J Hematol 2012;87(11):E123–4.

42. Sav T, Tokgoz B, Sipahioglu M, et al. Is there a difference between the allergic potencies of the iron sucrose and low molecular weight iron dextran? Ren Fail 2007;29(4):423–6.

43. Moniem KA, Bhandari S. Tolerability and efficacy of parenteral iron therapy in hemodialysis patients, a comparison of preparations. Transfus Altern Transfus Med 2007;9(1):37–42.

44. Critchley J, Dundar Y. Adverse events associated with intravenous iron infusion (low-molecular-weight iron dextran and iron sucrose): a systematic review. Transfus Alternat Transfus Med 2007;9(1):8–36.

45. Macdougll IC (1), Strauss WE, McLaughlin J, et al. A randomized comparison of ferumoxytol and iron sucrose for treating iron deficiency anemia in patients with CKD. Clin J Am Soc Nephrol 2014;9(4):705–12.

46. Auerbach M, Al Talib K. Low-molecular weight iron dextran and iron sucrose have similar comparative safety profiles in chronic kidney disease. Kidney Int 2008;73(5):528–30.

47. Coyne D. Hepcidin: clinical utility as a diagnostic tool and therapeutic target. Kidney Int 2011;80(3):240–4.

48. Rosner M, Auerbach M. Ferumoxytol for the treatment of iron deficiency. Expert Rev Hematol 2011;4(4):399–406.

49. Nemeth E, Tuttle M, Powelson J, et al. Hepcidin regulates cellular iron efflux by binding to ferroportin and inducing its internalization. Science 2004;306(5704):2090–3.

50. Nemeth E, Ganz T. The role of hepcidin in iron metabolism. Acta Haematol 2009;122(2–3):78–86.

51. Jahn M, Andreasen H, Fütterer S, et al. A comparative study of the physicochemical properties of iron isomaltoside 1000 (Monofer), a new intravenous iron preparation and its clinical implications. Eur J Pharm Biopharm 2011;78(3):480–91.

52. Wysowski D, Swartz L, Borders Hemphill BV, et al. Use of parenteral iron products and serious anaphylactic-type reactions. Am J Hematol 2010;85(9):650–4.

53. Onken JE, Bregman DB, Harrington RA, et al. Ferric carboxymaltose in patients with iron-deficiency anemia and impaired renal function: the REPAIR-IDA trial. Nephrol Dial Transplant 2014;29(4):833–42.

54. Auerbach M, Ballard H. Clinical use of intravenous iron: administration, efficacy, and safety. Hematology Am Soc Hematol Educ Program 2010;2010(1):338–47.

55. Auerbach M, Chaudhry M, Goldman H, et al. Value of methylprednisolone in prevention of the arthralgia-myalgia syndrome associated with the total dose infusion of iron dextran: a double blind randomized trial. J Lab Clin Med 1998;131(3):257–60.

56. Kalantar-Zadeh K, Regidor DL, McAllister CJ, et al. Time-dependent associations between iron and mortality in hemodialysis patients. J Am Soc Nephrol 2005;16(10):3070–80.

57. Feldman H, Joffe M, Robinson B, et al. Administration of parenteral iron and mortality among hemodialysis patients. J Am Soc Nephrol 2004;15(6):1623–32.

58. Saadeh C, Srkalovic G. Acute hypersensitivity reaction to ferric gluconate in a premedicated patient. Ann Pharmacother 2005;39(12):2124–7.

59. Cuciti C, Mayer DC, Arnette R, et al. Anaphylactoid reaction to intravenous sodium ferric gluconate complex during pregnancy. Int J Obstet Anesth 2005; 14(4):362–4.

60. Sirvent-Pedreño A, Enríquez-Ascarza R, Redondo-Pachón MD, et al. Adverse reaction to intravenous iron: hypersensitivity or secondary side effect? Nefrología 2013;33(1):148–9.

61. Larramendi C, Marco F, García-Abujeta J, et al. Acute allergic reaction to an iron compound in a milk-allergic patient. Pediatr Allergy Immunol 2006;17(3):230–3.

62. Nater JP. Epidermale Überempfindlichkeit gegen Eisen. Hautarzt 1960;11: 223–4.

63. Baer RL. Allergic contact sensitization to iron. J Allergy Clin Immunol 1973;51(7): 35–8.

64. Scheiber Mojdehkar B, Lutzky B, Schaufler R, et al. Non-transferrin-bound iron in the serum of hemodialysis patients who receive ferric saccharate: no correlation to peroxide generation. J Am Soc Nephrol 2004;15(6):1648–55.

65. Brewster U, Perazella M. Intravenous iron and the risk of infection in end-stage renal disease patients. Semin Dial 2004;17(1):57–60.

66. Bullen J, Rogers H, Spalding P, et al. Iron and infection: the heart of the matter. FEMS Immunol Med Microbiol 2005;43(3):325–30.

67. Hoen B, Paul Dauphin A, Kessler M. Intravenous iron administration does not significantly increase the risk of bacteremia in chronic hemodialysis patients. Clin Nephrol 2002;57(6):457–61.

68. Brookhart MA, Freburger J, Ellis A, et al. Infection risk with bolus versus maintenance iron supplementation in hemodialysis patients. J Am Soc Nephrol 2013; 24(7):1151–8.

69. Steinmetz T, Tschechne B, Harlin O, et al. Clinical experience with ferric carboxymaltose in the treatment of cancer- and chemotherapy-associated anaemia. Ann Oncol 2013;24(2):475–82.

70. Beguin Y, Maertens J, De Prijck B, et al. Darbepoetin-alfa and intravenous iron administration after autologous hematopoietic stem cell transplantation: a prospective multicenter randomized trial. Am J Hematol 2013;88(12):990–6.

71. Pedrazzoli P, Farris A, Del Prete S, et al. Randomized trial of intravenous iron supplementation in patients with chemotherapy-related anemia without iron deficiency treated with darbepoetin alpha. J Clin Oncol 2008;26(10): 1619–25.

72. Henry D, Dahl N, Auerbach M, et al. Intravenous ferric gluconate significantly improves response to epoetin alfa versus oral iron or no iron in anemic patients with cancer receiving chemotherapy. Oncologist 2007;12(2):231–42.

73. Hedenus M, Birgegård G, Näsman P, et al. Addition of intravenous iron to epoetin beta increases hemoglobin response and decreases epoetin dose requirement in anemic patients with lymphoproliferative malignancies: a randomized multicenter study. Leukemia 2007;21(4):627–32.
74. Steensma D, Sloan J, Dakhil S, et al. Phase III, randomized study of the effects of parenteral iron, oral iron, or no iron supplementation on the erythropoietic response to darbepoetin alfa for patients with chemotherapy-associated anemia. J Clin Oncol 2011;29(1):97–105.
75. Gafter Gvili A, Rozen Zvi B, Vidal L, et al. Intravenous iron supplementation for the treatment of chemotherapy-induced anaemia - systematic review and meta-analysis of randomised controlled trials. Acta Oncol 2013;52(1):18–29.
76. Muñoz M, Gómez-Ramírez S, Cuenca J, et al. Very-short-term perioperative intravenous iron administration and postoperative outcome in major orthopedic surgery: a pooled analysis of observational data from 2547 patients. Transfusion 2014;54(2):289–99.
77. Brockow K, Garvey LH, Aberer W, et al. Skin test concentrations for systemically administered drugs – an ENDA/EAACI Drug Allergy Interest Group position paper. Allergy 2013;68(6):702–12.
78. Baur X, Bakehe P. Allergens causing occupational asthma: an evidence-based evaluation of the literature. Int Arch Occup Environ Health 2014;87(4):339–63.
79. Makrilia N, Syrigou E, Kaklamanos I, et al. Hypersensitivity reactions associated with platinum antineoplastic agents: a systematic review. Met Based Drugs 2010;2010. pii:207084.
80. Ebo DG, Leysen J, Mayorga C, et al. The in vitro diagnosis of drug allergy: status and perspectives. Allergy 2011;66(10):1275–86.
81. Leysen J, Sabato V, Verweij M, et al. The basophil activation test in the diagnosis of immediate drug hypersensitivity. Expert Rev Clin Immunol 2011;7(3):349–55.
82. Ljungström KG. Safety of dextran in relation to other colloids–ten years experience with hapten inhibition. Infusionsther Transfusionsmed 1993;20(5):206–10.
83. Aberer W, Bircher A, Romano A, et al. Drug provocation testing in the diagnosis of drug hypersensitivity reactions: general considerations. Allergy 2003;58(9):854–63.
84. Cernadas JR, Brockow K, Romano A, et al. General considerations on rapid desensitization for drug hypersensitivity – a consensus statement. Allergy 2010;65(11):1357–66.
85. Brockow K, Romano A, Aberer W, et al. Skin testing in patients with hypersensitivity reactions to iodinated contrast media – a European multicenter study. Allergy 2009;64(2):234–41.
86. de Barrio M, Fuentes V, Tornero P, et al. Anaphylaxis to oral iron salts. Desensitization protocol for tolerance induction. J Investig Allergol Clin Immunol 2008;18(4):305–8.

Index

Note: Page numbers of article titles are in **boldface** type.

Immunol Allergy Clin N Am 34 (2014) 725–737
http://dx.doi.org/10.1016/S0889-8561(14)00070-8
0889-8561/14/$ – see front matter © 2014 Elsevier Inc. All rights reserved.

immunology.theclinics.com

Moving?

Make sure your subscription moves with you!

To notify us of your new address, find your **Clinics Account Number** (located on your mailing label above your name), and contact customer service at:

Email: journalscustomerservice-usa@elsevier.com

800-654-2452 (subscribers in the U.S. & Canada)
314-447-8871 (subscribers outside of the U.S. & Canada)

Fax number: 314-447-8029

Elsevier Health Sciences Division
Subscription Customer Service
3251 Riverport Lane
Maryland Heights, MO 63043

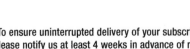

*To ensure uninterrupted delivery of your subscription, please notify us at least 4 weeks in advance of move.

Printed and bound by CPI Group (UK) Ltd, Croydon, CR0 4YY

03/10/2024

01040486-0011